# Medical Technology

## Series

# INSTRUMENT CHECK SYSTEMS

*Author:*

**Martha Winstead, M.S., M.T. (ASCP)**

*Chief of Quality Control*
*South Bend Medical Foundation, Inc.*
*South Bend, Indiana*

**Lea & Febiger**      **1971**      **Philadelphia**

Illustrations by Harry Lindstrand, Bluffton, Indiana

ISBN 0-8121-0260-6
Published in Great Britain by
Henry Kimpton Publishers, London
Library of Congress Catalog Card Number 68-18862
*Printed in the United States of America*

Other titles available

# Preface

The material in this monograph has been compiled over the last ten years from our experience in trying to check instruments, locate trouble, and eliminate it. It is interesting that at the beginning of this period, questions put to several company representatives were turned away with the comment that the instruments were better than any available means the user had for checking them; therefore, checking was not really necessary. Now the pendulum has swung—a full 180°. Some governmental regulations require that every function of each instrument be checked daily before using the instrument. There are, however, no directions yet available for checking every instrument. The check procedures now being worked out by users and manufacturers together will hopefully produce this information soon. Only with experience can checking procedures be evaluated and those eventually chosen that can reasonably be done at specific time intervals to safeguard the validity of the answers produced on the instruments.

General information about how a class of instruments works is not specific enough to check the function of individual instruments. We have therefore discussed specific instruments as examples of their class. The instruments chosen should not be considered as the best suited, or the least suited, for their purposes. They are the instruments with which we have had enough experience to work out the necessary checking procedures. While test directions are not exactly referable to other instruments, the points discussed for the examples can serve as leads to determine the precise information needed for other instruments.

The information in this monograph could not have been collected without the help of many people. Personnel in the service departments of the manufacturing and distributing companies have been helpful. Our own electronics men at the South Bend Medical Foundation, Don Dalke and Marlin Fuller, have had the patience of Job in working out the causes and corrections of the instrument problems. Special appreciation is due Dr. Jene R. Bennett, Director, and Ray Markey, Administrative Assistant. They have understood the problems enough to allow the necessary time for trial-and-error approaches to troubleshooting. The technical personnel throughout the Foundation have done much of the work to provide comparisons between one instrument and another, especially when trouble existed. To all of them, I would like to express my deep appreciation.

MARTHA WINSTEAD
*South Bend, Indiana*

# Contents

# Instrument Check Systems

# 1

# General Principles for Instrument Check Systems

The overall objective of check systems for our instruments in the clinical laboratory is to restrict the variation of the instrument's function to such an extent that the general level of precision chosen for the laboratory tests can be maintained. Without digressing to a discussion of the philosophy of quality control, it is necessary to state the following concepts as the limiting factors for establishing the general level of precision chosen for tests in any one laboratory:

1. The normal range for the test must have been established for the particular procedure using the particular instrument in the particular laboratory.
2. The allowable error for the test must have been calculated. Tonks' formula is the most commonly used generalization:[9]

$$\text{Allowable limit of error in \%} = \frac{(\frac{1}{4} \text{ of normal range})}{(\text{Mean of normal range})} \times 100.$$

Originally Tonks recommended that the allowable limit of error be $\pm 10\%$. Recently he modified this overall limit and suggested that $\pm 20\%$ may be the best attainable limit for enzyme methods such as amylase, LDH, acid, and alkaline phosphatase.[10] Usually the allowable limit of error in percent is equated to $\pm 2$ coefficient of variation (CV).

$$\text{Coefficient of variation} = \frac{1 \text{ Standard deviation}}{\text{Mean value}} \times 100.$$

Where standard of deviation (SD) is calculated by the replicate equation:

$$1 \text{ SD} = \pm \sqrt{\frac{\Sigma (\bar{x} - x)^2}{n}}.$$

3. The actual day-to-day error, or $\pm 2$ SD control values, must have been plotted and monitored. Not all tests will fit into Tonks' allowable error, but we must strive to limit the error to this value whenever possible and practical.

4. The value chosen for the control must, if possible, be that which most quickly detects problems within each test procedure for the particular constituent being determined.

When the general level of precision for laboratory tests is held within the limits thus described, the amount of error allowed for instruments must be held to a minimum. This is not easy to do, and if the instrument is not constantly monitored, the instrument alone can cause more error than is allowed for the whole procedure. On the other hand, out-of-control values are sometimes wrongly blamed on an instrument.

Failure to recognize two rather elementary contributions to laboratory performance of instruments can nullify the effectiveness of the most carefully constructed check systems for specific instruments. These include proper respect for the electrical circuits, especially grounding, and careful attention to basic equipment.

Stacy has estimated that 90 percent of the difficulties involved in instrumentation result from overloaded power lines or 60 cycle interference.[7] Many of these problems have been minimized by the manufacturers of our current instruments by such means as:

1. Including stable transformers within the instrument itself.

2. Shielding sensitive parts of the circuits, especially input leads.

3. Building containers for low-level impedance stages of the circuit.

4. Providing adequate grounding between the components of the instrument.

However, as Stacy points out: "None of these shielding measures can be effective unless the ground to which one attaches the shielding and the ground side of the circuit actually make good electrical contact with the ground of the power lines supplying the building." The radiators and water pipes frequently used as grounds in the laboratory are unsatisfactory for current sophisticated instruments. Many newer laboratories have "three prong" outlets and use only "three wire" plugs from instruments. However, to be an effective ground, the outlet must be connected to an earth electrode of low resistance. The entire system of the institution should be periodically reviewed and checked for the *actual* earth resistance of the system.[5] Factors that may change the grounding system include the following:

1. A plastic pipe or conduit coupling can completely nullify the low-resistance path to earth.

2. If the water table is gradually lowering, what was formerly an effective ground may result in simply an electrode in dry earth of high resistance.

3. Resistance of the soil increases with decreasing temperature so that during below-freezing periods the grounding system is much less effective.

4. Expansion of facilities, especially computer and communication systems, quickly overloads the grounding system.

Inadequate grounding is more dangerous than no grounding because it promotes a sense of false security.

As long as the grounding system is basically sound, a grounding plug may be used in one outlet of a double receptacle and a sensitive instrument in the other to reduce small interferences. Figure 1-1 illustrates the plug we find useful for the Coulter Counters and pH meters. The common side of the line is connected by a ½ amp fuse to the ground. One certainly cannot use such a plug until an electrician has actually verified that the wiring is standard and that the feedback on the

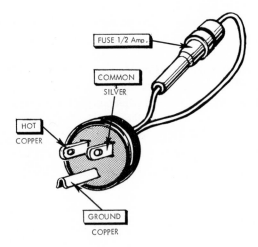

**Figure 1-1.** *Grounding plug for reducing line interference.*

common line is minimal. The user must also be careful to avoid ground loops when plugging several pieces of equipment together; only one ground is allowed for such combinations.

All laboratory personnel should be instructed concerning electrical hazards commonly present in the laboratory. The slightest shock felt while using equipment should be reported immediately, and the equipment should not be used again until it has been repaired. Low current of only 20 milliamperes through the body can cause fibrillation, and 100 milliamperes is almost certain to be fatal.[8] A résumé of safety precautions can be aptly quoted as a list of "Don'ts," author unknown.

## DON'TS

1. Don't by-pass fuses with jumpers, coins, etc.
2. Don't increase capacity of fuse before ascertaining circuit conditions.
3. Don't replace a fuse more than once unless you know why it has blown and have remedied the fault.
4. Don't work on equipment when hands or clothing are wet.
5. Don't risk contact between live circuits and rings, wristwatches, bracelets, zippers, etc.
6. Don't ever take shock intentionally. Testing outlets with the two-finger method is a way of demonstrating stupidity.
7. Don't use solvents containing alcohol for cleaning electrical equipment. Alcohol damages most types of insulation varnishes.
8. Don't use spring clips for grounding portable equipment.
9. Don't use water, soda and acid, foam, loaded stream or anti-freeze types of fire extinguishers on electrical fires. They may cause fatal shock. Use dry chemical, carbon dioxide, or vaporizing liquid.

The function of such basic equipment as water baths, centrifuges, and timers must be monitored consistently. Medicare regulations require that records show this information.[3, 4] However, each institution must establish practical time sequences and details for complying with the statement: "all equipment is in good working order, routinely checked and precise in terms of calibration."

A general classification of these items includes:

1. Temperature controlled spaces—Check temperature measuring devices against a National Bureau of Standards (NBS) certified thermometer. Some refrigerators and incubators must be equipped with a recording temperature device.
2. Autoclaves—Kilit Ampules* are convenient to check for adequate sterilization.
3. Balances—Evaluation includes condition of knife edge and pans. When one stamps on the floor, does the free-swinging pan vibrate? Are NBS weights used

*Available from BioQuest, Division of Becton, Dickinson & Co., Cockeysville, Md.

5

to check calibration? It is simpler to subscribe to a service contract from a reputable company than to attempt to check or service sensitive balances.

4. Centrifuges—Check various speeds with a photo-tachometer. Check the time and speed required to produce a constant volume for packed blood cells.

5. Timers—Check with reliable stopwatch.

6. Power supply, batteries and light sources—Check their output.

7. Volumetric measuring apparatus—Check calibration and delivery against certified equipment. From our experience it is impossible to check all items; spot checking appears the only practical approach.

8. Shakers and rotators—Check frequency of shakers and rotators for a given time period.

Ideally, the original evaluation of the instrument should also include a specific set of check procedures that can be recorded for later comparisons. In reality, laboratories presently fall short of the ideal situation for two reasons: (1) incomplete original evaluations are the usual circumstance for instruments that have been in use for some time, and (2) specific sets of check procedures for instruments have not been well identified. A suggested protocol for the original evaluation of automated instruments recently published could well be used also for other instruments.[2, 6] A generalized outline of this protocol is printed as the *Appendix*, page 307. Specific check procedures are also being developed slowly by individual users and manufacturers of instruments. There is, therefore, hope of approaching the ideal goal. Meanwhile, technologists can work with what information we do have to monitor instruments more effectively.

By judicious selection of the level of the control value to pinpoint the most vulnerable point on the calibration curve due to either the instrument or the procedure, the medical technologist can eliminate unnecessary control samples and also choose the most likely level at which a control value will detect a change in the instrument. For example, any colored solution read on a Coleman Junior spectrophotometer may be represented by Curve A of Figure 1-2. This example is the calibration of the Babson method for alkaline phosphatase.[1] Curve A is almost a straight line, and this is the response to be expected for a new photocell. Curves B and C, although they are the calibration curves for other Coleman Junior spectrophotometers, demonstrate the changes in slope for this calibration curve when the photocell ages. From A to B to C occurs with any colored solution when calibration curves are compared over a long period of time. If the chosen control value is at the high end of the calibration curve, this changing calibration curve will be readily detected. In Figure 1-2, a control value of 120 units would be ideal. When this principle is applied to the hemoglobin calibration curve, a value of 16 grams is the most efficient control range. With this range, the calibration change can be detected long before most of the patients' values are affected.

Still considering hemoglobin, two examples come to mind for out-of-control values that cannot be blamed on the spectrophotometer. The first instance involves shifts in the maximum absorbance wavelength for oxyhemoglobin when water used in the reagent (sodium carbonate) contained either ammonia-like contaminant

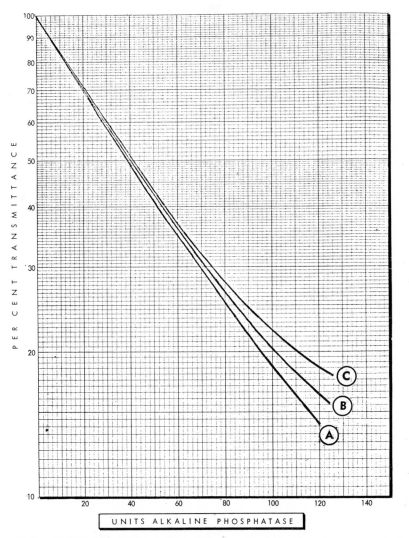

**Figure 1-2.** *Calibration curves for Babson alkaline phosphatase method using Coleman Junior spectrophotometers.*

or copper. The narrower the slit width, the more readily this shift will show up. Therefore, varying results will be obtained with routine colorimeters using 550 m$\mu$ filter, and/or the Coleman Jr. and Beckman DU spectrophotometers at 540 m$\mu$. The second instance involves the cyanmethemoglobin method when the diluent requires approximately 20 minutes to produce a solution with correct spectral characteristics. In this test the usual reading time of 2 to 5 minutes gave answers as much as one gram higher than the correct value.

One must, therefore, consider as many factors as possible in choosing the checking procedures for laboratory tests. To be considered are the peculiarities of

7

the instrument, the tests for which it is used, the reagents, and the people using the instrument. If the operator of the instrument can be persuaded to keep an accurate record of problems (symptoms, causes, and cures), this information can form the backbone of the check system for that instrument. There must be enough checkpoints to detect trouble with an instrument, but the system must remain practical. If a checkpoint doesn't really provide information after a reasonable trial period, it should be dropped. Laboratories have no time to play games; efforts put into all procedures must be well spent. Also there must be willingness to change even the best thought-out checking procedures. Instruments are continually being changed, and new instruments are being introduced. The process of building check systems must likewise change to keep the checking process valid.

Check systems for instruments mean different things to the three types of people involved with instruments: the manufacturer, the electronics technician, and the laboratorian. Their approaches will vary in relation to their own degree of expertise in electronics.

The manufacturer must ascertain that each component of his instrument meets his specifications. *Component* here relates to small single parts or to subunit modules. Often the equipment used to check the instrument is much more costly than the instrument itself. Therefore, the checking procedure used by the maker often cannot be directly followed either by the service department technician or the user. In the past, it has sometimes been hard to get from manufacturers specific information about how to check instruments. Even yet, schematics are sometimes withheld from the purchaser under the stated reason of protecting the privileged information of the manufacturer. More often the manufacturer has been reluctant to have repairs attempted by people less qualified than factory-trained representatives. As more instrumentation is used in medical laboratories, there is a growing need to include on the institution's staff electronics personnel who can service the instruments. Manufacturers are being requested to provide sufficient information about the instruments to allow as much repair work as possible in the field in order to decrease "downtime" of the instruments. The ideal working arrangement includes the cooperative efforts of the manufacturer, the electronics technician, and the operator; more and more such joint efforts are evolving.

The approach of the electronics technician is usually to get as much information as possible about malfunction from the operator of the instrument and then to attack the schematic. To him the output of the instrument is the final indication of malfunction. He will either work backward from the output or frontward from the input to isolate the defective electronic component. Stacy has broken down the lines of attack into five categories:[7]

1. Too little output per unit of input signal.

2. Zero level drift.

3. Varying gain or random instability.

4. Nonlinear output.

5. Oscillation.

He further develops each category into the systematic isolation of the cause of the problem. The user with enough time and electronic know-how may want to refer to Stacy's approach. Most electronic technicians have their own step-by-step isolation procedure. The most difficult problem to isolate is the one that appears intermittently. If the electronics technician does not happen to be able to catch this problem and isolate it (often by substitution of parts), he will usually react in one of two ways:

1. If he is located in the institution using the instrument, he will watch the instrument and wait for the malfunction to show up—hopefully with more definite and permanent symptoms. Once the problem has progressed this far, the defective part can be replaced. Meanwhile the observation of symptoms serves to provide experience for future similar episodes.

2. If the electronics technician is located in a service department some distance from the institution, his tendency is to replace any suspicious parts. Often the exact cause is never isolated.

The user's approach must be guided by what symptoms he can observe in the normal or correct operation of the instrument and the differences he sees when malfunction exists. By a deliberate process of learning what to look for in each instrument and observing the likely vulnerable portions of its function, the persistent operator can build his own check system. Once he has convinced the manufacturer and the electronics technician that he does share the responsibility of a properly functioning instrument, a joint effort can produce both check systems and maintenance programs.

At the South Bend Medical Foundation, Inc., our first efforts toward building a check system were centered around spectrophotometers. The final "system" includes ten functional characteristics: zero and 100%T, reproducibility, noise and/or drift, resolution, linearity, detector response, source of energy, stray energy, signal control (slit width, amplifier, or gain), and energy selector (wavelength calibration). Once these characteristics were determined to be essentially those necessary to check spectrophotometers, we began looking at other instruments.

The same parameters can be generalized, and similar functions can be identified in other instruments. All instruments have functions which must be checked for zero and maximum response, reproducibility, noise and/or drift, and linearity. Detector response represents the final signal that is translated into a measurable reaction; the count registered on the Coulter Counter, or the titration time of the Cotlove can be envisioned as a similar function for these instruments. Stray energy can be used to designate background counts for the Coulter, overshoot for the end point in the Cotlove, or even emission from contaminating substance used with a flame photometer or fluorometer.

## REFERENCES

1. Babson, A. L., Greeley, S. J., Coleman, C. M., and Phillips, G. E.: Phenolphthalein monophosphate as a substrate for serum alkaline phosphatase. Clin. Chem., *12:*482, 1966.

2. Broughton, P. M. G., Buttolph, M. A., Gowenlock, A. H., Neill, D. W., and Skentelbery, R. G.: Recommended scheme for the evaluation of instruments for automatic analysis in the clinical biochemistry laboratory. J. Clin. Path., *22:*278, 1969.

3. Department of Health, Education, and Welfare, Social Security Administration: Evaluation of quality control programs in laboratories. Form SSA-1557B, May, 1969.

4. ———: Independent laboratory survey report. Form SSA-1557, February, 1969.

5. Lange, A. Q.: Proper electrical grounding safeguards laboratory. Lab. Management, *5:*28, 1967.

6. Sharp, A. A., and Ballard, B. C. D.: An evaluation of the Coulter S Counter. J. Clin. Path., *23:*327, 1970.

7. Stacy, R. W.: *Biological and Medical Electronics*. New York, McGraw-Hill Book Co., Inc., 1960.

8. Stanley, P. E.: Hospital electrical safety and shielding. J.A.A.M.I., *2:*8, 1967.

9. Tonks, D. B.: A study of the accuracy and precision of clinical chemistry determinations in 170 Canadian laboratories. Clin. Chem., *9:*217, 1963.

10. ———: A quality control program for quantitative clinical chemistry estimations. Canad. J. Med. Techn., *30:*38, 1968.

# 2

# Spectrophotometers

The three most commonly used types of photometers have different levels of performance and degrees of instrumental sophistication. These photometers may be characterized as:

1. Simple instruments using filters and relatively insensitive components and limited to a few tests.
2. Wide bandpass spectrophotometers of intermediate complexity capable of reading most color-reaction tests.
3. More complex (narrow bandpass) spectrophotometers that permit assigning absorbance (OD) change to extinction values or kinetic studies.

The latter type has sufficient capacity for resolution to identify absorption peaks and to scan.

The performance of each instrument must be monitored, but the manner of monitoring increases in complexity in relation to the sophistication of the instrument. Most of the studies of performance have used data obtained with instruments in the third category. Wernimont used matrix algebra operations to examine the behavior of complete absorbance curves obtained with both simple instruments and group three types of instruments.[62] These conclusions were drawn from this study:

1. The instruments used in many laboratories are not well controlled.
2. Performance will not be improved merely by conducting more comparison studies.

Wernimont concludes: "It is economically wasteful to conduct comparison studies unless the performance of each individual instrument has been shown to be satisfactory."[62] Rand has even more specifically challenged all users of spectrophotometers with his assertion that "no spectrophotometric measurement can be considered reliable unless the instrument involved has been checked with suitable standards and found to meet specifications."[44] Obviously, then, the responsibility rests with each user to keep his own instruments in satisfactory working order and to use them properly.

Caster's evaluation in 1951 of errors applicable to the Beckman DU spectrophotometer[14] is still valid[18] and is just as appropriate for other instruments. Caster identified the errors as those affecting relative values and those affecting absolute values, adding an observation concerning corrective factors. These errors may be summarized as follows:

1. If the unit is used only to yield relative values (*i.e.*, to compare unknowns to standards in the same batch), very good and consistent results can be expected. A variation of ± 0.5% is reasonable and may be lower.
2. If calculations in "absolute values" are to be used (*i.e.*, extinction coefficients and kinetic reactions of A/time), considerable caution must be used because reproducibility and accuracy are far from identical. One should hesitate to attribute significance to discrepancies of 5% or less.
3. The proposal that a corrective factor be applied to an instrument whose value deviates from the mean value of a group of instruments is dangerous.[19] In view

13

of the complex and changing nature of these errors, such a practice may lead to a false sense of accuracy rather than any real improvement in the results obtained.

Any systematic scheme to check an instrument for proper function must include, as far as possible, the contribution each component makes toward the overall error of readings. It is difficult to separate the errors into individual causes. Almost all the parameters are present and function together even in testing for any given one.[14, 21]

Zero, 100%T, wavelength, and sampling errors can be easily isolated. Reproducibility, noise and drift, resolution, stray light, light leaks, and slit-width operation can be checked in a straightforward manner, but they contribute to other errors from which they cannot be completely isolated. In routine laboratories, it is almost impossible to separate errors due to the photometric scale (also called "linearity" or "photometric accuracy") from the aforementioned errors or from phototube response. This last, phototube response,[14] includes the phototubes themselves plus the energy source (including power supply), mirrors, and amplifiers. Miscellaneous errors include temperature, solvent transparency, sample cell, and the sample carrier.

## TESTS FOR FUNCTION

The individual function parameters will be discussed in general terms that are applicable to all instruments. A simple instrument will require a less comprehensive check system than a more sophisticated instrument, and one manually operated will differ somewhat from its recording counterpart. When indicated, available schemes given in the literature will be noted, followed by a detailed description of the system used for each instrument at the South Bend Medical Foundation. Each user may thus have several alternatives among functional tests and be able to choose those that seem most practical in his own laboratory.

### Zero and 100% Transmittance

The most important characteristics of any instrument are the stability of both the zero and 100%T.[11] The zero is more influential than the 100%T when working at high absorbance values, but the 100%T affects low absorbance values more. An error of 1 scale division at zero results in errors of about 8% at 5%T. Similarly, an error of 1 scale division at 100%T produces about 8% error at 90%T.[63]

While zero and 100%T are reset for readings taken in routine use of the spectrophotometer, they should periodically be thoroughly checked for stability. This check is particularly important for scanning instruments in which the 100%T is usually allowed a little wider range of deviation in the ultraviolet (UV) range.[11] For instruments with a shutter, a solid block should be used as an additional means of occluding light from the detector while checking the zero. Spiking or irregularity in a zero base line scan usually indicates that an amplifier tube has become weak or defective and should be replaced.

## Noise or Drift and Electronic Disturbances

The zero setting must be constant before useful readings can be obtained; [11, 14] by watching the needle for one minute, noise (fluctuation) or drift (constant change in one direction) may be detected. Should either be present in excess of the tolerance, it must be corrected before proceeding. Some of the more simple spectrophotometers (Coleman Jr., for example) tend to have a more stable zero than 100%T settings; for these it is worthwhile to check also the 100%T for noise and/or drift. Scanning instruments automatically include noise and/or drift consideration in their zero and 100%T checks. Some instruments are allowed to run for 8 to 15 hours in these checks.[11]

Noise and/or drift can usually be traced to one of four possible causes: moisture, some defective electrical connection, a fatigued or saturated photodetector surface, or an aging or unstable lamp. The moisture problem can usually be eliminated by regular replacement of the desiccant in some instruments or by leaving the exciter lamp turned on in other instruments.

Defective electrical connections are hard to trace but can sometimes be identified by slightly moving the cords or connections. If a solder joint gives way with a hard tug, it is a defective or "dry joint." Any proper solder joint normally has a tensile strength of a couple of tons per square inch.[18]

Sharp taps on the phototube housing will produce slight shifts in zero in almost any instrument. If shifts are large (or caused by gentle blows), the electrical circuitry must be checked, especially the amplifier.[24]

Shorts due to improper grounding may be detected by using a draftsman's electric "eraser" as a test for electronics disturbance.[11] In place of the "eraser," any similar vibratory device that creates a large amount of static will be satisfactory.

In ordinary use the photodetector's surface should not become fatigued or saturated, provided one follows the accepted routine to expose the detector to light only momentarily while readings are being made. Chances are that if the surface or the lamp is the problem, this component will cause failure of one of the specifically related check procedures and require replacement.

## Slit Width

The terminology for slit width,[31] spectral slit width, and bandpass, used in this discussion is consistent with that shown in Figure 2-1. The important consideration in spectrophotometry is not so much the actual slit opening in mm as it is the bandpass in $m\mu$ (*i.e.,* the average spectral range or range of $\lambda$ measured at half the peak transmittance for the slit). Instruments vary considerably in their bandpass, and the amount of control the operator has over this parameter is also variable. Whether the instrument has a fixed slit (and therefore a relatively fixed bandpass), a manual slit width to be set, or a programmed slit position to be chosen, the operator must be thoroughly familiar with the bandpass he is using.

Instruments using a grating as the monochromator make the choice of proper slit width simpler because their dispersion is almost identical for the entire wavelength range. For any given slit width, therefore, the bandpass is very nearly the

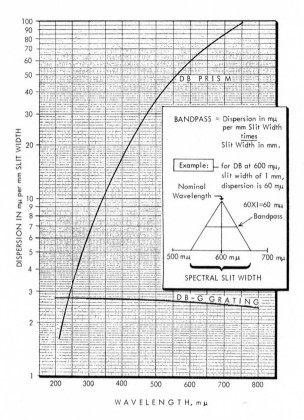

**Figure 2-1.** *Bandpass as produced by prism or grating. (Modified from Beckman Instruction Manual, 556-E, June, 1966.)*

same throughout the whole spectral range. The prism monochromator increases markedly in dispersion as the wavelength changes from the blue to the red spectral region, and the exact dispersion differs primarily with the manufacturer's choice of prism for the instrument. A 1 mm slit width at 250 m$\mu$ usually allows the spread of wavelengths passed to be only 4 m$\mu$ wide; at 700 m$\mu$ it allows a 85 m$\mu$ spread. The grating counterpart easily maintains a bandpass of about 2.7 to 2.5 m$\mu$ for the respective wavelength settings.

The general concept is that the narrower the slit widths the more accurate is the reading. The point has been made, however, that while slit widths should be reasonably small in analytical work it is more important that results be obtained at known widths (in m$\mu$).[9, 18, 22] A recent report from collaborative readings for the same absorbing solution stated that one of the main causes for divergent readings appeared to be variations in the slit width, *i.e.*, the bandpass used.[62] One cannot simply set the slit micrometer to a particular reading and be sure the bandpass for that setting has not changed unless the function has been checked. The same is true for a programmed slit position or even a fixed slit.

The bandpass may increase from a physical malfunction of the slit jaws or some change in the optical system which increases the dispersion. The easiest way to detect increase in bandpass is to note a decrease in resolution from time to time

16

using the same substance (*e.g.,* the holmium oxide filter or benzene vapor). This method does not, however, indicate the cause of the problem. (See this discussion under resolution, page 19).

The actual slit opening for programmed slits at a specific wavelength can be easily determined by finding the slit "pickup." The scan is stopped at the desired wavelength and then the slit micrometer is manually opened until the manual setting takes over. The reading on the micrometer is the actual slit width. A list of actual slit widths for selected wavelengths for each slit program is a necessity when a question arises as to whether the slit width has changed or not. The operator must have some base line for comparison.

The actual test for slit-function of the manual slit setting is the determination of minimum slit operation.[18] On the Beckman DU spectrophotometer this is done by noting either the minimum slit required to balance the meter at a given wavelength or the minimum slit at which energy is registered at a given wavelength. Both these tests relate more directly to source and detector efficiency. The changes noted with time are toward decreasing sensitivity. If, on the other hand, without replacement of components or repairs or adjustments on the instrument, the slit opening required becomes less, one should look for a slit "hang-up." Slits that "hang-up" or do not close properly produce a wider bandpass and cause loss in resolution. A relatively small increase in actual slit opening causes a much greater increase in energy passed by the slit because of the squared relationship. Twice the opening passes a $2^2$ energy increase for a continuous source lamp. An increased bandpass in any spectrophotometer must be detected quickly and once detected must be corrected immediately to prevent changes in calibrations made at even the maximum absorption wavelengths for particular tests.[65] Serious errors produced by large differences in bandpass have been reported many times.[9, 14, 17, 18, 44]

### Wavelength Calibration

Although repeated trials may give the same value over and over again, indicating high sensitivity and precision, and although the instrument may otherwise appear to be functioning properly, gross errors in wavelength may nevertheless render the values obtained highly unreliable.[21]

With rare exceptions,[10, 28] there is agreement that the mercury arc is the best single source of wavelength calibration for 205 to 1014 m$\mu$[21, 22, 44, 45 ,61] with 546.1 m$\mu$ as the reference line. "Current wavelength calibration at one point in the spectrum in no way assures calibration elsewhere."[44] Therefore, several lines must be checked, and these should span the entire spectral region used for any specific spectrophotometer The final wavelength adjustment is, then, that which gives the least minimum error for the several lines checked.

When the wavelength is put in the best average adjustment with the mercury lamp over the entire spectral range, current direct reading scales of wavelength are usually correct $\pm$ 1.0 m$\mu$.[21] Tolerances are closer for good grating instruments than for their prism counterparts. For example, the specifications of the Beckman DB spectrophotometer (prism model) for 220 to 334 m$\mu$ are less than 0.7 m$\mu$;

17

for 335 to 575 m$\mu$ less than 1.5 m$\mu$; and for 575 to 700 m$\mu$ they are less than 4.0 m$\mu$.[4] The specifications of the Beckman DB-G spectrophotometer (grating model) are less than 0.5 m$\mu$ throughout the scale.

Using the mercury lamp for calibration of the wavelength scale (or checking it) is not difficult but is time consuming. Peaks are best located when a relatively high sensitivity setting is used so that it is possible to use small slit widths. The wavelength should always be set from the same direction—against the spring-loading, which usually means from longer to shorter wavelengths.[18]

The published list of minimum slit widths for the lines is very helpful because it serves as an indication of the relative strength of the lines.[61] For our Beckman DU spectrophotometer, we attempted to locate all the lines and then chose seven (ranging from 253 to 1014 m$\mu$) sufficient for this purpose (See page 57).

In addition to the mercury lamps, the National Bureau of Standards (NBS)[21] lists other acceptable sources for wavelength calibration of non-recording spectrophotometers: helium lamp (8 lines between 388.86 and 1083 m$\mu$), hydrogen lamps, sodium arc, and cesium arc. Particular note is made of the 852.1 and 894.3 m$\mu$ lines for cesium because few lines are available in this area. The neon discharge tube is listed as not satisfactory for calibration between 750 and 1000 m$\mu$. Didymium and holmium glasses are also listed as unsatisfactory for calibrating non-recording spectrophotometers. Even for checking the wavelength calibration, the National Bureau of Standards prefers the emission lines of the lamps and arcs listed above. Use of these two glasses to check wavelengths of recording spectrophotometers is acceptable to the Bureau, provided the slit widths used are sufficiently narrow.

Holmium oxide has been proposed for wavelength calibration in the UV range,[40, 59] and the National Bureau of Standards (NBS)[21] lists 11 bands that have been checked on a Cary model 14 spectrophotometer (previously calibrated by other sources). This material is Corning 3130 glass, and for some melts, the 241 m$\mu$ band has been found unsatisfactory.[21, 40] NBS will supply this glass certified in the 241 area upon request in accordance with the NBS test for schedule 202.105.

Figure 2-2 shows the spectrum of holmium oxide glass using a Perkin-Elmer Model 350 spectrophotometer.[40] Such information is valuable for comparison with the data obtained on one's own instruments.

McNeirney and Slavin,[40] though stating that usual programmed slits make no change in the shape or position of the bands, do list the minimum bandpass that will cause the shapes to change. (See Table 2-1, page 22.) On conventional quartz or silica prism instruments using photomultiplier detectors, the first band to be altered as the slit width increases is the band at 536 m$\mu$. We have found this information valuable in alerting us to possible problems when our Beckman DB spectrophotometer scan showed changes in shape but prefer the 637.5 m$\mu$ peak, as discussed later.

Note should be taken that holmium oxide glass is not suitable for photometric standards for two reasons: (1) although no change in wavelengths is shown when

18

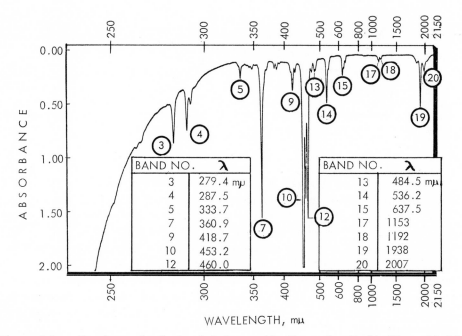

**Figure 2-2.** *Absorbance bands for holmium oxide filter using Perkin-Elmer Model 350 spectrophotometer. (From McNierney, J., and Slavin, W.: A wavelength standard for ultraviolet-visible-near infrared spectrophotometry. Appl. Optics, 1:365, 1962.)*

temperature is changed, transmittance values varied slightly[40] and (2) the transmittance values are too dependent on slit widths used.[21]

Edisbury points out that the quickest checks of wavelength calibration are the 656.3, 486.1, and 379.9 m$\mu$ hydrogen lines from the hydrogen or deuterium lamp already present in the instrument.[18] He cautions, however, that the first two cannot be picked out of the many fine lines present unless the instrument is already in fair calibration. He also states that the three lines are a satisfactory number to check on prism instruments and that two are enough for grating instruments. In the absence of anything better, Edisbury observes that a match or a taper dipped in table salt is sufficient to locate the major sodium lines.

## Resolution

The resolution of an instrument is the degree to which it can separate peaks (absorbance or transmittance) that occur at wavelengths close to each other. The customary test uses the doublets of 577 and 579 m$\mu$ of the mercury lamp spectrum.[7, 11] Resolution is expressed as the ratio of the depth of the valley (between the doublets) to the height of the doublets. The depth of the valley between 577 and 579 m$\mu$ should be at least one-fourth the height of the peaks. For example, if the peak height of 577 m$\mu$ is four divisions on the scale, the valley between the doublets should be one division on the scale.[7]

19

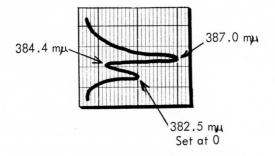

**Figure 2-3.** *Scan with holmium filter on Beckman DU spectrophotometer.*

After determining that our Beckman DU instrument meets this specification for resolution, doublets in the holmium filter spectrum (Fig. 2-3) are measured. These peaks are at 382.5 and 387 m$\mu$, with the valley at 384.4 m$\mu$. Valley depth is expressed as a proportion to the height of the 387 m$\mu$ peak (see p. 60).

Since this check involves only the use of the holmium filter, it can be used as a simple means of detecting any change in the resolution of the instrument. The same test can also be used for the Beckman DB and DB-G instruments. The observation of the shape of the 536 m$\mu$ band of this filter has also been suggested as a routine check for resolution,[40] but we prefer the 637.5 m$\mu$ band for a rough check on resolution.

The degree of separation of the peaks of benzene vapor between 240 and 260 m$\mu$ is a popular resolution check for recording instruments.[11, 18, 47, 48] Mercury vapor at 254 m$\mu$ and 185 m$\mu$ has also been proposed.[53] Water vapor is used for infrared (IR) range.[11, 47] The American Society for Testing Materials (ASTM) Committee E-13 Report includes four spectra listed as A, B, C, and D for increasingly better resolution of the benzene and water vapor spectra. Figure 2-4 shows the benzene spectra. The $\Delta\lambda$ expression on these spectra is the separation of two absorption bands that can just be distinguished. Condition A ($\Delta\lambda = 1.5$ m$\mu$) is stated as the lowest resolution that would probably be satisfactory for an instrument used in analytical procedure.

When the E-13 committee report was published in 1966,[42] the recommendation concerning resolution was changed somewhat. Recognizing that different analytical procedures can tolerate different requirements for resolution, the proposal now presented is that specific ASTM test procedures include the spectrum obtained at the resolution necessary. Identification of degrees of resolution is still labeled A, B, C, or D.

A decrease in resolution is caused by an increase in bandpass. While the bandpass can be the result of slit hang-up, the usual cause is some change in the quality of the components of the optical system—for example, a fogged source lamp or a cloudy mirror. Dust collected on the slit edges may produce the same effect. The Coleman Jr. spectrophotometer uses the filament of the exciter lamp, rather than an exit slit, to focus the beam. A dirty or fogged lamp quickly changes the bandpass in this instrument but can be easily detected. (See page 45.)

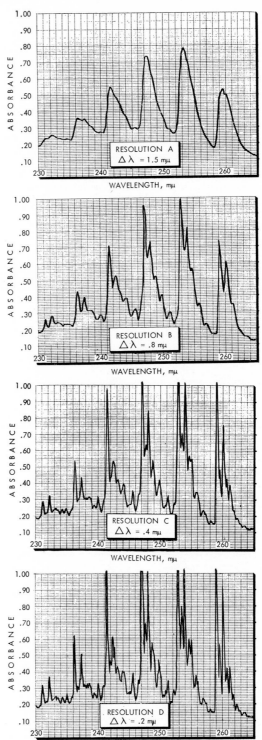

**Figure 2-4.** *Absorption spectra of benzene vapor showing four different conditions of resolution. (By permission from Proposed Methods for Evaluation of Spectrophotometers, Report of ASTM Comm. E-13. Proceedings, Amer. Soc. for Testing & Materials, June, 1958.)*

21

Prism instruments show increased bandpass (decreased resolution) first in the high dispersion red region. A fogged source lamp is enough to remove completely the two shoulders on the 637.5 m$\mu$ peak of the holmium oxide scan. If programmed slit operation is used and a change is noted in the shape of one of the peaks of this scan, the bandpass has increased to the minimum listed for that peak in Table 2-1.[40] The grating instrument, on the other hand, shows increased dispersion first toward the blue end of the spectrum. A change in the valley-to-peak height at the 385 m$\mu$ region is the best indication for loss of resolution caused by a fogged lamp in this instrument. Often a badly fogged lamp will not increase dispersion enough to be detected unless the operator is using very small slit settings.

### Reproducibility or Precision

Reproducibility or precision is probably the most popular of instrument checks. Each instrument has its own specifications for this test, and for manual instruments the range is from $\pm 2\%$ to about $\pm 10\%$ for the same "good precision" instrument.[18] More than $\pm 10\%$ may be observed between readings from different instruments of the same type. Recording instruments are usually allowed to deviate by the width of the pen.[11, 53] For this test any convenient sample can be used to take replicate readings, and it is often quicker to use the same sample as that used to check the photometric scale (*i.e.,* linearity). Thus, only one additional set of readings is required instead of two. Potassium diphthalate,[24] potassium chromate,[36, 38] screens,[47] and glass filters[11, 18] have been used.

For manual instruments it is convenient to use the neutral density filters that are also used to check linearity; for recording instruments, the holmium oxide filter.

### Stray Light and Light Leaks

The photo detector measures any radiation falling on it, whatever the wavelength of this energy might be. If wavelengths are present other than that set on the instrument dial, this extraneous energy is called "stray light."

**Table 2-1. Minimum Bandpass Showing Change in Holmium Oxide Peaks***

| Band† | m$\mu$ | Bandpass (m$\mu$) |
|-------|--------|-------------------|
| 9 | 418.7 | 4 |
| 10 | 453.2 | 7.5 |
| 12 | 460.0 | 5 |
| 13 | 484.5 | 4.5 |
| 14 | 536.2 | 6 |
| 15 | 637.5 | 12 |

* From McNeirney, J., and Slavin, W.: A wavelength standard for ultraviolet-visible-near infrared spectrophotometry. Appl. Optics, *1:*365, 1962.

† See Figure 2-2.

The wonder of stray light is not that it exists but that it can be reduced to levels such as the specifications of 0.2% in the ultraviolet (UV) and 0.1% in the visible range for the Beckman DU spectrophotometer. The source light, magnified five times by the mirror in the lamp house, is passed full strength (and consisting of all wavelengths) into the monochromator.[13] Through directional focus and refraction, the light must be purified $10^6$ times to reduce "stray" radiation enough for a true absorbancy of 1.0 to record accurately $\pm 1\%$.[32] The stray light, in this case, must be less than 1/3 of 1%. The shorter the wavelength, the greater the purification must be. At a wavelength of approximately 203 m$\mu$ the purification factor would have to be between 5 and 10 million to keep the stray light 1/3 of 1%.

The most frequent problem caused by stray light effect is decreasing the absorbancy of samples that do not themselves absorb light.[32, 55] Samples that significantly absorb stray energy give apparent absorption that will be too high.[55] Many apparent deviations from Beer's law can be directly attributed to these situations,[30, 43] but corrections of sample absorbance based on formulas for stray effect[30, 50] must be used with caution. Such calculations are based on the assumption that the sample is transparent at all wavelengths except that being currently measured. Most samples absorb enough in other parts of the spectrum to filter out appreciable amounts of stray energy. Potassium chromate and dichromate are examples of such samples.[18]

The aberration caused by stray light is a decrease in the maximum and minimum absorption peaks.[43] The effect is to increase the bandpass beyond the resolution of the instrument, and consequently the deviations are more serious when measurements are made on narrow absorption bands. Some absorbance bands reported in the 200 to 230 m$\mu$ range were spurious and actually were stray light

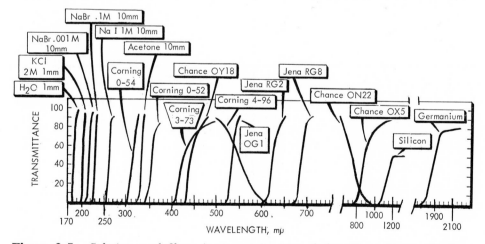

**Figure 2-5.** *Solutions and filters for measuring stray light. (From Slavin, W: Stray light in ultraviolet, visible, and near infrared spectrophotometry. Anal. Chem., 35:561, 1963. Reprinted by permission of the American Chemical Society.)*

23

measurements.[32, 50, 55] Checks for stray light are usually made in the UV portion but really should be made at both ends of the spectral range.[55] Stray light in a spectrophotometer is related to the amount of useful light present. In the midportion of the spectral range, where the energy level is high, instrument stray light will be much less. When the brightness of a source lamp decreases, the measured stray light will increase proportionally. A sharp-cut filter or solution easily checks the stray light in any region. Figure 2-5 shows some available materials and their ranges. Corning 4-96 is recommended for checking at 650 m$\mu$ upwards.[18] Many of these filters can also be used to reduce stray energy at specific areas when the instrument is being employed for readings in the common areas.

The Vycor* filter (Corning silica) has often been chosen for the routine stray light check. This filter cuts off at 220 m$\mu$, as shown in Figure 2-6. The recommended wavelength at which to read it is 205 m$\mu$ for manual instruments[18] and a 225 to 200 m$\mu$ scan for recording instruments.[11] Edisbury warns that readings taken at more than about 5 to 10 m$\mu$ beyond the cutoff edge will tend to underestimate the stray light if present, and readings at 20 m$\mu$ below the cutoff may underestimate by 50%. He also reminds us that, from a practical standpoint, stray light has such a catastrophic effect on results that it does not matter whether the amount is 1% or 5%. It must be eliminated or reduced as far as possible and as fast as possible.

Lithium carbonate read at 210 m$\mu$ has been reported as especially easy to use because a pinch of it may be added to distilled water and allowed to settle.[18]

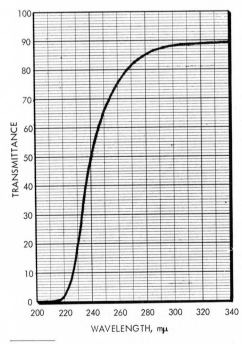

**Figure 2-6.** *Vycor filter transmittance on Beckman DB used to measure stray light.*

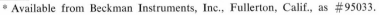

* Available from Beckman Instruments, Inc., Fullerton, Calif., as #95033.

Potassium chloride (KCl) has been used in preference to either Vycor or lithium carbonate.[55] The 15% W/V KCl has a steeper cutoff edge and when read at 190 m$\mu$ is a more stringent test. However, water absorbs at 180 to 190 m$\mu$ and must be distinguished from the absorbance for the KCl solution. The absorbance of this salt increases about 2% per degree C, and the exact wavelength at which the edge of the absorbance occurs is a function of the salt concentration. Slavin pointed out that KCl at 190 m$\mu$ may correctly give 0.5% stray light but Vycor may show only about half of this amount because Vycor itself absorbs a significant fraction of the stray light. He notes that the Vycor does record the correct stray energy measurement at 205 m$\mu$ (near its cutoff edge). Because most glasses fluoresce, this possibility also must be kept in mind with filters or with solutions in cuvettes, especially around 240 m$\mu$ where most silica materials have an absorption band.

The extremely low levels of the stray light signal in spectrophotometers make the readings rather difficult. Any device to expand the scale near the zero transmittance is recommended.[55] Screens* listed as 20W and 10S provide expansion of 100 and 15 times respectively. The expansion provided can be determined by measuring their transmittance on the spectrophotometer.

Nearby "stray light" will not be detected by the usual methods for testing UV monochromators for stray radiation but can be checked with saturated mercury vapor at relatively high temperatures.[58] This test is said to be required only for instruments used to record sharp absorbance peaks.

The chief causes of increased amounts of stray light are (1) dust and scratches or other imperfections on prism, lenses, or mirrors; (2) reflections from inside the collimator tubes, edge of the diaphragms, etc.; (3) energy from the room if the instrument or detector is not properly shielded;[20] and (4) secondary emission from the optical system caused by heat radiation or fluorescence.

A source of problems with stray light that might not occur to the user is the less-than-ideal combination of source lamp and detector for the wavelength being used. The 350 to 400 m$\mu$ range is accessible for either a tungsten or hydrogen (or deuterium) source. The tungsten, having more energy in the visible region than the hydrogen, is much more likely to produce stray energy in this near-UV region.[55] The hydrogen lamp is therefore preferable. Proper alignment of the hydrogen lamp and choice of silica envelope instead of glass for this lamp also increase radiation and reduce stray light.[18]

The photomultiplier and the lead sulfide detector present a similar problem in the 600 to 750 m$\mu$ range.[18, 55] The common 1P28 photomultiplier was shown to produce about 1.3% stray light at 740 m$\mu$, whereas the lead sulfide tube usually provides a broader spectral band and lower stray light.[55] Referring to the 1P28 photomultiplier Edisbury states that "a simple absorptionmeter with a 650-750 m$\mu$ filter would be much less costly and give better results without this misleading pretense at absoluteness or loss of reproducibility."[18]

Even the proper source and photodetector tend to increase stray light as they become less effective with age and use. The increased bandpass present when a

---

* Available from Perforated Products, Inc., Brookline, Mass.

source lamp becomes "frosted" from laboratory fumes increases stray light and decreases the maximum and the minimum for absorbance peaks.[65]

The third cause of stray light—energy from the room—can more properly be called a "light leak," but effects of stray light will be experienced if the light reaches the detector without passing through the monochromator. Stray light and light leaks can be differentiated, however, by repeated readings after increasing the slit width.[55] Stray light due to leaks will decrease rapidly as the slit width is widened; instrumental stray light (free from light leaks) will not vary much with changes in slit widths. Light leaks in the sample compartment or phototube house cause serious trouble, and the flashlight test is highly recommended for any optical electronic instrument.[11, 18, 24]

## Sensitivity or Photodetector Response

Sensitivity of an instrument is an illusive term, but since we often speak in terms of instruments losing sensitivity, we must find some definition of the original quality. Gibson's definition of sensitivity, as related to detectors, is probably as good as we can find: "relative response to an equal-energy spectrum."[20] Photodetector response, or the ability to record energy consistently, depends upon (1) the sensitivity and linearity of the detector itself; (2) the strength and stability of the power supply, light source, and amplifier tubes; (3) the cleanliness and focus of the mirrors; and (4) the linearity of the resistors and other components in the circuit.

Some instruments (Beckman DU, for example) have a sensitivity control setting to increase the gain of the amplifier. The operator usually chooses the lowest gain consistent with adequate signal in order to keep the noise or instability low. Using a different instrument, but one of the same type, Edisbury[18] reports the coefficient of variation (CV) as $\pm 6.7\%$ for the instrument's highest gain setting compared to $\pm 0.2\%$ for the lowest. The value of $\pm 0.5\%$ CV, obtained at about the midpoint between these two, represents the best compromise between responsiveness, slit width, and precision. For instruments without such sensitivity controls, the response of the detector is governed by all the contributing factors listed above. For optimum instrument performance each contributing factor must be considered separately and in relation to its most effective function.

## Photodetectors

The manner in which the photodetector of the spectrophotometer is checked will necessarily depend upon the detector and the way in which it is used, *i.e.,* direct reading or null balance. Choices of the detector are among barrier layer cell, phototube, and photomultiplier.

BARRIER LAYER CELL. Simpler instruments, such as the Coleman Jr., use the barrier layer cell almost exclusively. While this is a rugged detector for hard constant use, it may be nonlinear in its behavior.[8] A given light flux may produce different amounts of current on different photocells or at different wavelengths on the same photocell. The possibility of nonlinearity should be checked with suitable filters or solutions over its entire range of use.[8, 12, 18, 20] Even new cells are not linear at an illumination of 100 foot candles when the resistance in the external circuit is over 100 ohms.[8] Instruments using this cell often have a resistance over 100 ohms but are compensated by using low levels of illumination. The Coleman Jr. instrument, for example, has a resistance of 500 ohms, but illumination is about 0.2 to 0.3 footcandles. Improper electrical contacts can greatly increase resistance in the external circuit. These cells are factory tested for linearity but are not individually tested for spectral sensitivity.

There is no information available from Coleman Instruments regarding loss of linearity with age or use. Loss of sensitivity starts immediately after production and ranges from 2 to 5% per 500,000 footcandle hours. At about 3,000,000 footcandle hours a more sudden, sharp drop occurs. Great variability also has been recorded for shelf life. For cells in use, the chief cause of nonlinearity is said to be saturation at high light intensities or for long periods of time. Occlusion of the cell, when readings are not being made, prolongs the effectiveness of the photocell.

Nonlinearity from causes other than saturation has been reported.[8, 12] Cannon and Butterworth described a photocell whose response gave a linear Beer's law plot but whose absolute absorbance was different by a factor of about 2.[12] The response of the photocell has since been explained as defective because of mercurial "poisoning."[18] This incident alerts the operator to what *can* happen. Mercury can modify the semiconductor properties of selenium.[8] Manufacturers warn that excessive heat, moisture, and active vapors (such as mercury and sulfur) affect the stability of photocells. Checking eleven Klett Summerson photometers, Beeler observed no direct correlation between nonlinearity of photocells and the ages of the instruments. Both linear and nonlinear photocells produced straight line plots of concentration versus absorbance. The difference between these lines was in their slopes. He stated that "no confidence can be placed on linearity of the photocell merely because one obtains straight line plots of concentration versus absorbance."[8]

A rough check of a barrier layer cell can be made by reversing the leads of the cell in connection with a 1.5 volt battery and measuring the current output on a microammeter.[18] The current through a cell 25 mm in diameter should not exceed 50 to 100 microamps.

In our experience with Coleman Jr. spectrophotometers the only criteria for judging the presence of defective photocells is the inability to set 100% T at 400 m$\mu$.

PHOTOTUBES.    Phototubes commonly used are not equally sensitive for both the blue and red ends of the spectrum. Usually, blue sensitive tubes (cesium antimony) are used for the 325 to 625 m$\mu$ range but can be extended downward to about 200 m$\mu$ by changing to a hydrogen source.[22] The red sensitive tube (cesium oxide) is used in the 600 to 1000 m$\mu$ range. Problems in nonlinearity have been reported only for the latter tube;[24] however, any phototube may exhibit a lack of uniform response or relative spectral sensitivity.[37] For these reasons the calibration settings must exactly duplicate the settings used in the test measurement (*i.e.,* slit widths and concentration ranges).

27

The most accurate estimate of photon flux is made when the phototube is used at about 10% of its maximum sensitivity.[37] Since this response can change with time and use, the sensitivity of the phototube should be monitored. Its sensitivity is measured in terms of its "minimum slits."[7] At a specified wavelength (instrument has been zeroed with dark current), with the shutter open, the slit width is increased enough to zero the meter needle. Such a slit width reading in millimeters is called the minimum slit width for that wavelength. Obviously the more sensitive the tube, the smaller will be the minimum slit width. Specifications for these minimum slit widths differ among instruments, depending upon the intensity of the source and the efficiency of the optical system. The outer surface of these tubes should be kept free of dust, moisture, or smudges. Besides decreasing the light allowed to pass, dust can provide a short circuit.[7] The outside surface should be cleaned with alcohol about every three months.

PHOTOMULTIPLIER. The photomultiplier (PM) is about 100 times more sensitive than the blue or red sensitive tubes and therefore has become the detector of choice in many instruments. The 1P28 (Cs-Sb photosurface) is used in the range from 200 to about 650 m$\mu$. For full-range work extending to 750 m$\mu$, the R-136 is recommended.[4]

Although manufacturers may check their photomultiplier tubes for linearity, circuitry in the instrument may produce a slightly nonlinear response.[57] Since ratio-recorders rely entirely on detector response, checking linearity is mandatory for these instruments.

Edisbury has listed three precautions for photomultiplier tubes:[18]

1. Photomultiplier tubes may be ruined if daylight overloads the surface. Even exposure to daylight with the voltage supply "off" raises the dark current enough to require a recovery rest period.[37]

2. These detectors are more sensitive to heat than phototubes are. Operating at 25°C (or lower where possible) will minimize dark current and noise.

3. Cleanliness of the outside of this tube is extremely important because of the high potential involved. Dust is attracted even around the socket and pins. Cleaning is accomplished best with a suction tube that has a small brush attached.

Sensitivity of the photomultiplier is so high that measurement of minimum slits is rather futile. The best indication we have seen for deterioration of this detector has been the loss of accuracy on neutral density filters or the requirement of increasing slit widths for reading the same filters over a period of time.

## Power Supply

The power supply should be serviced only by a qualified electronics technician; laboratory personnel should adopt a strict "hands-off" policy and should seek the expert assistance of such a person.

If minimum slit specifications for the phototubes can be met, it can also be concluded that the power supply is adequate in strength. One reference in the literature reports decreased strength of the power supply. A battery-operated unit is said to have shown a fivefold precision drop caused by failing "B" batteries.[45] Fluctuation or instability of the instrument is the most likely problem caused by the power supply. Instability can best be detected by a drift in the dark current. Fluctuations of minimum slits (*i.e.,* changing sensitivity) were observed in one Beckman DU spectrophotometer that started to blow fuses several times a day. The unit was old and insulation was cracked in many places. Replacement of the power supply corrected the problem.

Simpler instruments are now usually stable on line voltage because some type of voltage regulator is either included in the instrument or installed in the line ahead of the instrument. Current voltage regulators and/or transformers are much more efficient than those used several years ago. While fluctuations in the instrument from this cause are relatively uncommon, the user must still be alert for the possibility and should protect the instruments as much as possible from excess line fluctuation by providing several separate circuits into the laboratory.

## Source Lamp

The tungsten incandescent lamp is the most suitable source for the range from 350 to 1000 m$\mu$.[18, 20] It has adequate intensity, the intensity can be kept constant, and the spectrum is continuous. When first turned on, these lamps vary in the length of time required to stabilize. It saves time in the long run to note the time required for each lamp. Some are stable at once and others may take several minutes. With use, the inside of the lamp surface will build up a deposit of metallic tungsten. Edisbury states that the lamp has become inadequate for good spectrophotometry as soon as this film is detectable.[18]

The hydrogen or deuterium lamp, whose spectrum is nearly continuous from about 200 to 400 m$\mu$, changes in brightness with age.[18, 53] After a few hundred hours, the performance falls off so that larger slit widths are required. Such a lamp in instruments with programmed slits may seemingly function properly and be undetected until long past the time it should have been replaced. Weekly checks should be made to detect decreased energy from the lamp. Either the requirement of increasing slit widths or physical examination of the lamp should detect the problem.

With the lamp off, inspect it by looking straight into the aperture, using a dental mirror, if necessary.[18] If the lamp is approaching the need for replacement, the metal around the aperture will be discolored over about a millimeter in area and the aperture will be enlarged. Spattered metal may also form a film inside the envelope in front of the aperture, but the film may not be detectable when the lamp is turned on. Failure to fire is often a sign that the lamp will soon need replacing. When the lamp does not fire properly, a pinhole glow starts eroding the metal parts to produce the condition described above.

The deuterium lamp has about three times the output of the hydrogen lamp and also lasts longer in terms of hours of service. For these reasons, the deuterium lamp seems to be replacing the hydrogen lamp. The same general precautions are required, whichever lamp is used for the source energy of the spectrophotometer. The lamp must be properly aligned (*i.e.,* "peaked") for maximum intensity. Stepwise directions are given in the instrument manual for this operation. Misalignment is a common cause of loss of instrument sensitivity,[18, 24, 53] and erroneous extinction values have been traced to this cause.[24]

In addition to the necessity for maintaining a clean inside surface, the outside surface must also be kept clean. Chemical "frost" collects on this surface and should be wiped off as necessary.[65] Maximum absorbance peaks that have shifted to slightly higher wavelengths when the bulb is dirty have returned to their normal wavelengths when the bulb is wiped clean. Transmittance values for one Coleman Jr. instrument were also affected to the extent that a hemoglobin solution of 15.6 grams gave a 2.16 gram error (17%). The intensity of the lamp energy also is dependent upon proper cleanliness and alignment of the rest of the optical system, particularly the mirrors.

### Mirrors

Proper alignment of mirrors is usually the means by which the final peak intensity of the source is accomplished. This procedure is included in each instrument manual. "Fogging" of mirrors occurs with time, producing stray light in the spectrophotometer. The best way to delay the process is to protect the instrument from dust and fumes as much as possible. Even moisture from the breath should be excluded from the inside portions of the monochromator.[18] Edisbury suggests wearing a surgical mask when peering closely into the inner parts of the instrument.

The more accessible mirrors can be carefully wiped with alcohol or a mild detergent on a cotton applicator. In general, success in cleaning mirrors is minimal. They usually have to be replaced when the fogging of the surface is due to accumulations of more than a very thin coating. McDaniel uses collodion to paint the mirror and then peels it off like fingernail polish.[39] He reports success with this procedure three or four times without causing stray light, but we have not had this kind of success.

### Amplifier Tubes

Only the more sophisticated instruments include amplifier tubes in their structure. In general, the amplification can be checked from time to time by noting the amount of deflection of the meter needle caused by a slight turning of the transmittance control.

Shorts,[24] noise or drifts,[7] and photometric scale difficulties[20] have been traced to defective amplifier tubes. Many times these tubes are not of a type that can be removed and checked on a tube tester. If their function is suspected, they should be tested by substitution. If the difficulty does not disappear, the tubes are not at fault. An unusual example of tube problems is illustrated in Figure 2-7. During a test procedure with a biuret solution, a tube in the amplifier circuit (#5654, 6AK5) of our Beckman DB spectrophotometer caused the strange looking scan in part A. This solution ordinarily produces the scan shown in part B. Note that the left edge of the oscillating line follows the contour of the correct curve. The

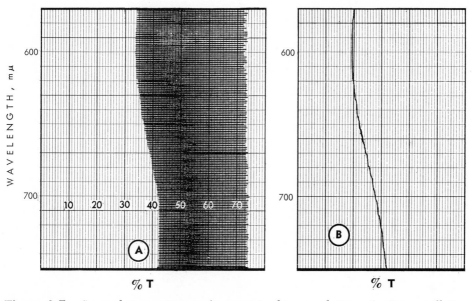

**Figure 2-7.** *Spectral transmittance for protein biuret solution. A. Pen oscillating (defective amplifier tube). B. Normal scan.*

defective tube checked "satisfactory" on a high grade tube checker and was isolated only by substitution. Edisbury points out that replacement of amplifier tubes, phototubes, and photomultiplier tubes according to the manufacturer's recommendations is probably cheaper in the end because nominally identical tubes may not be precise enough for delicately balanced amplifier circuits.[18]

### Load Resistors and Switches

Resistors in the detector circuit (either phototube or photomultiplier) must conform to Ohm's law for the instrument to function accurately.[20] Nonlinearity caused by these resistors has been reported,[24] but noise and drift are more frequent problems.[7] If the resistors are suspect, they can only be replaced. Resistor switches, when dusty, may produce the same symptoms as defective resistors. The switch can be cleaned with carbon tetrachloride or preferably with a commercial "switch cleaner" spray.

### Sample Cells

Sample cells (or absorption cells) must maintain a specified path length and must not contribute to the absorbance of the material. The cell window materials, their appropriate wavelength ranges, and the tolerances shown in Table 2-2 are representative of those generally used in clinical laboratories.

Regardless of the type of cell used, the following precautions are necessary to keep sampling errors at a minimum:

31

**Table 2-2.  Specifications for Beckman Absorption Cells***

| | Far-UV Silica | NIR Silica | Standard Silica | Pyrex† | Vycor† |
|---|---|---|---|---|---|
| Guaranteed transmittance (%T) | 60%T @ 170 mμ 70%T @ 180 mμ 75%T @ 220 mμ | 60%T @ 170 mμ 70%T @ 270 mμ 80%T @ 1000, 1500 & 2700 mμ | 65%T @ 220, 240 & 270 mμ (100 mm) 70%T @ 220, 240 & 270 mμ (10, 25 & 50 mm) | 65%T @ 320 mμ | 65%T @ 320 mμ |
| Light path | Within 0.5% of a specified length | Within 0.5 % of a specified length | Within 0.5% of a specified length | Within 0.5% of a specified length | Within 0.5% of a specified length |
| Spectral range | 170 to 2600 mμ | 220 to 3500 mμ | 220 to 2600 mμ | 320 to 2500 mμ | 320 to 2500 mμ |
| Matching tolerance (For cells in matched sets) | Within 3%T @ 1700 mμ, 2%T @ 220 & 2200 mμ | Within 3%T @ 220 2%T @ 240 & 270 3%T @ 1000, 1500 & 2700 mμ | Within 3%T @ 220 mμ 2% @ 240 & 270 mμ | Within 4%T @ 320 mμ | Within 4%T @ 320 mμ |

\* From Beckman Bulletin 85B. Courtesy Beckman Instruments, Inc.
† Pyrex and Vycor are registered trademarks of Corning Glass Works.

1. CLEAN CELLS. The transmittancy for cells of different materials (Table 2-2) may be regarded as a means of determining whether or not a cell is clean (tolerance ± 1%T). Edisbury measured the effect of an unremoved fingerprint on an empty cuvette at 360 and 240 m$\mu$ and found an average increase in absorbance of 0.006 and 0.072 respectively.[18] The absorbance for distilled water vs air when 10 mm pathlength cuvettes of quartz or silica are used is 0.083 to 0.093 at 240 m$\mu$ and that for glass is 0.025 to 0.035 at 650 m$\mu$.[47]

2. MATCHED CELLS. "Matched" pairs of cells (Corex or Silica) have in the past commonly been different by as much as 4% to 6%[45] and quartz cells by 0.5%.[14] The tolerance is better now, but individual cells must be checked among themselves at a specific wavelength. Rotating the cell 180 degrees should not give an absorbance difference greater than 0.005, and matched cells should not differ more than 0.003.[47]

3. TEMPERATURE EFFECTS. Ideally, solutions should be maintained at a constant temperature whenever absorbance readings are made. Variations due to temperature differ both in amount and direction of absorbance change.[22, 24, 45, 49] Absorbance peaks may even show their wavelengths shifted somewhat.[49]

4. TURBIDITY EFFECTS. Apparent variations in transmittancy may be due to a turbidity forming in the solution.[14] Solvents (including water) should be checked for transmittancy before being used, especially after storage.[24]

5. CELL POSITION. The cell must be in a mechanically stable, reproducible, and exact position.[20] Micro cells require extra care in centering.[1] Improper positioning and failure to fill the cells adequately can account for a 20% to 50% error.[14] Centering the cell in the light path may be checked by blowing tobacco smoke into the area[18] or by adding a drop of fluorescein to water in the cuvette. At about 490 m$\mu$ the fluorescent pathway is easily seen if the room is darkened somewhat. We prefer this method over blowing anything into a sample compartment.

## Linearity

In the following discussion the term *linearity* is used for the same instrument characteristic that other authors call overall performance, photometric scale, or photometric accuracy.

Only when all components of the instrument are functioning properly can the linearity be confirmed. Theoretical arguments about linearity of a transmittance scale versus absorbance scale in terms of instrument function are beyond the scope of this discussion. There are, however, three useful points that relate to instrument linearity resulting from transmittance versus absorbance readout construction. Tarrant states that instruments vary in different ways as they get older.[57] The potentiometer slide wire of a transmittance instrument continues to produce corresponding results, but an absorbance instrument will produce low absorbance results, the error being proportional to the absorbance. This idea emphasizes the operator's responsibility to check his instrument continually.

33

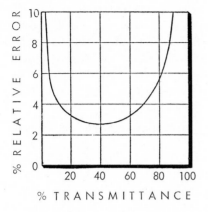

**Figure 2-8.** *Relative analysis error as a function of transmittance. (From Ayres, G. H.: Evaluation of accuracy in photometric analysis. Anal. Chem., 21:652, 1949. Reprinted by permission of the American Chemical Society.)*

Slavin points out that the most accurate portion of the photometric scale differs for absorbance and transmittance instruments.[52] Gridgeman showed that the optimum transmittance was 37%T with little difference in accuracy at 20%T to 60%T, assuming no error in setting zero or 100%T.[25] Slavin found Gridgeman's theory valid for transmittance instruments only. Instruments designed for readout in absorbance provide more precise data at the high end of the absorbance scale. One must note, however, that even though Slavin did his work on a Perkin-Elmer model 4000-A spectrophotometer, the paper includes no statement that his observations should not apply to instruments outside the UV range. Gridgeman's

Table 2-3.   Relative Analysis Error for Different Transmittance*

| Transmittancy % | % Relative Analysis Error per 1% Photometric Error |
|:---:|:---:|
| 95 | 20.8 |
| 90 | 10.7 |
| 80 | 5.6 |
| 70 | 4.0 |
| 60 | 3.3 |
| 50 | 2.9 |
| 40 | 2.7 |
| 30 | 2.8 |
| 20 | 3.2 |
| 10 | 4.3 |
| 5 | 6.5 |

* From Ayers, G. H.: Evaluation of accuracy in photometric analysis. Anal. Chem., 21:652, 1949. Reprinted by permission of the American Chemical Society.

34

paper specifically stated that infrared, visible, and ultraviolet spectrophotometers were alike in his theory.

Ayres has shown that Ringbom plots provide the simplest way to delineate the %T range over which a given method can retain best accuracy.[2] Recognizing the optimum %T reading as 36.8 and also the relatively good range as 20%T to 60%T, he gives the relative error at 95%T as 20.8% and at 5%T as 6.5%. (Fig. 2-8 and Table 2-3.)

The 90%T to 100%T range is often used for reading of clinical laboratory tests. Although the relative analysis error per unit photometric reading error is large, the results are a practical compromise because of the nature of the test (normal ranges are very low concentrations of the test constituent) and/or because they can be checked against calibration curves covering the same range. These calibrations should be checked by plotting Ringbom graphs to see exactly what the error is. From these graphs one may detect the concentration changes that would greatly improve accuracy (Fig. 2-9). In Figure 2-9 the hemoglobin calibration

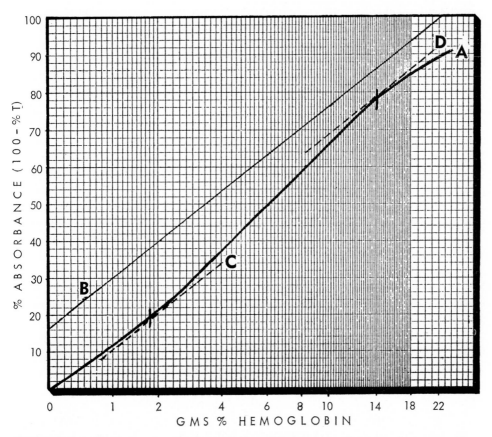

**Figure 2-9.** *Ringbom plot for hemoglobin calibration on Coleman Jr. spectrophotometer.*

curve was plotted from zero to 22 gms%. The most accurate portion is 2.3 to 14 gms. and has a relative error of 3.5% for every 1% photometric error. (The 10-fold concentration range representing this line spans 12 to 78 on the 100%T scale. The error is $\dfrac{230}{78-12} = 3.5$). If a 5% relative error per 1% photometric error is acceptable, more of the calibration curve can be used. The slope for 5% error must be $\dfrac{230}{5} = 46$ span on the 100%T scale. This slope is drawn so that any 10-fold concentration of hemoglobin spans 46: for example, 1 gm = 30 and 10 gm = 76. The lines parallel to this slope and also tangent to the inflection points of the calibration curve limit the concentration range which has 5% relative error per 1% photometric error. In the Figure 2-8 example this range would be 1.8 to 14 gms.

Any feeling of asssurance about tests that read in the 90%T to 100%T range when calibration curves are used obviously vanishes when tests are read in absolute absorbancies. These test procedures require checking of absorbance scale in this range with absolute standards. As with calibration curves, it would be much better to change concentrations so that the 90% to 100% is avoided. Test values whose transmittance readings are below 20% are easier to manipulate for better accuracy than those between 90%T and 100%T. One can always use less sample or make a greater dilution.

The ideal check for linearity "would be a series of samples whose respective transmittances do not vary with wavelengths, which do not displace the beam, which do not reflect strongly, and for which the transmittances are known. No such materials are available."[21] It has recently been reiterated that checking the fulfillment of Beer's law does not yield an adequate proof of linearity.[46] Reule uses a light addition method to calibrate one instrument and then uses this instrument to check others. His method, however, is outside the realm of clinical laboratories as is also the use of rotating sectors.[21] For simpler instruments used to compare unknowns with standards, proof of Beer's law is probably satisfactory.[14,18]

Spectrophotometers used to record absolute absorbance values can be checked by reading solutions whose extinction values have been proven, or more conveniently, by reading filters whose absorbances have been previously calibrated. Solutions cited by numerous authors include copper sulfate, potassium chromate, cobaltous ammonium sulfate, potassium dichromate, potassium nitrate and potassium acid phthalate. The same precautions are required in this test procedure as were listed for the routine use of sample cells, page 31. In addition, differences in the accuracy of the wavelength setting can have marked effects on this procedure.[26,28]

Table 2-4 gives the wavelengths usually listed for maximum absorbance peaks for these solutions. Precise concentrations and precautions are necessary for using each, and the technologist is urged to check the reference listed for the solution

**Table 2-4. Solutions for Measuring Photometric Accuracy and Their Maximum Absorbance Wavelengths**

| Solution | Wavelength $m\mu$ | Reference |
|---|---|---|
| Potassium dichromate (in 0.01N $H_2SO_4$) | 257, 350 | 18 |
| Potassium chromate (in 0.05 N KOH) | 275, 380 | 21 |
|  | 273, 373 | 18 |
| Potassium acid phthalate | 281 | 19 |
| Potassium nitrate | 302 | 18 |
| Copper sulfate | Gradual increase from 350 to 750 | 21 |
| Cobaltous ammonium sulfate | 510 | 21 |

of his choice. A few selected values for the NBS standard solutions of potassium chromate and copper sulfate are listed in Table 2-5. The choice between potassium chromate and potassium dichromate deserves a particular note of caution. Johnson warns that dichromate in 0.01 N $H_2SO_4$ appears to differ both in absorbance and in maximum absorbance wavelength when solutions are compared by concentration and pathlength combinations which should give identical results[34] (Fig. 2-10). He proposes using the chromate dissolved in M/20 disodium hydrogen phosphate buffer (pH 9.1). In his experience, this solution has conformed to Beer's law over a concentration range of 25 to 1 and is satisfactory in 1 cm cells from 500 $m\mu$ down to 205 $m\mu$.

The solution recommended by the NBS is potassium chromate (0.04 gm per liter in 0.05 N KOH).[21] For wavelengths lower than 260 $m\mu$ solutions less than 6 months old should be used;[27] above 260 $m\mu$, solutions 5 years old have remained satisfactory. On the other hand, Edisbury,[18] though not particularly enthusiastic about using any solutions for this purpose, chooses the dichromate over the chromate. He states that in acid solutions the former has had more consistent absorbancies reported for observed maximum absorbance peaks. The 273 $m\mu$ peak for chromate has been reported variously between 0.189 to 0.199 absorbance, and the 373 $m\mu$ peak for the same material has been from 0.247 to 0.249.

Rand's recent report of the work done with potassium dichromate by the Standards Committee of the American Association of Clinical Chemists concludes that if the pH is carefully controlled this solution is useful as a check of the entire spectrophotometric measurement system (*i.e.,* instruments, cuvettes, and operator

37

**Table 2-5.** Selected Values of Spectral Transmittance for Standard Potassium Chromate*
and Copper Sulfate† Solutions. 1 cm cell, 25° C.‡

| Wavelength, $m\mu$ | Potassium Chromate %T | Copper Sulfate %T |
|---|---|---|
| 220 | 35.8 | |
| 275 | 17.5 | |
| 300 | 70.9 | |
| 313.2 | 90.5 | |
| 350 | 27.6 | 97.9 |
| 375 | 10.2 | |
| 400 | 40.2 | 99.5 |
| 450 | 92.7 | 99.7 |
| 500 | 100.0 | 99.4 |
| 550 | | 96.5 |
| 600 | | 85.5 |
| 650 | | 59.7 |
| 700 | | 29.7 |
| 750 | | 15.2 |

* Potassium chromate: 0.0400 gm/liter in 0.05 N potassium hydroxide. Distilled water used as reference.

† Copper sulfate ($CuSO_4 \cdot 5\ H_2O$): 20.000 gm and 10.0 cc sulfuric acid (specific gravity 1.835) per liter.

‡ From Gibson, K. S.: Standards for checking the calibration of spectrophotometers (200 to 1000 $m\mu$). National Bureau of Standards Circular #LC-1017, Washington, D. C. Reissued January, 1967.

technique).[4] The material is minimally affected by temperature and is available in high purity from the National Bureau of Standards (SRM #136d). The 0.0500 gm/liter concentration is 0.01 N $H_2SO_4$ for an absorptivity of 10.70 with an uncertainty of less than 0.3%.

Henry, Cestaric, and Goodwin consider cyanmethemoglobin standard read at 540 $m\mu$ a convenient check for the photometric scale of their modified Beckman DU spectrophotometer.[29] Their day-to-day variation from 0.560 absorbance is given as less than 0.001. It is interesting that the hemoglobin standard is one of those certified by the College of American Pathologists and the sample to check the instruments used in the certification is an NBS carbon yellow filter.[16]

Filters, though much easier to use than solutions, are susceptible to temperature changes and except for "neutral density filters" are correlated to definite wavelengths and are subject to effects of slit widths. Even "neutral density filters" are somewhat different at wavelengths other than that specified.

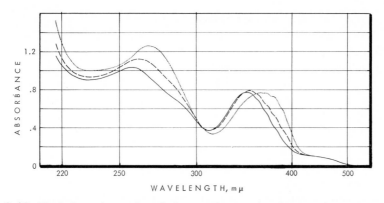

**Figure 2-10.** *Variation of wavelength for maximum absorbance of potassium dichromate solutions (all in 0.01 N H₂SO₄ and expected to have the same absorbance): _____0.00133% in 5 cm cells; _____ 0.0664% in 0.1 cm cells; .......... 2.5% in 0.025 mm cells. (From Johnson, E. A.: Potassium dichromate as an absorbance standard. Phot. Spect. Group Bull., 17:505, 1967.)*

The National Bureau of Standards certifies and sells four filters: selenium orange, carbon yellow, copper green, and cobalt blue.[21,41] The range covered by these filters is shown in Figure 2-11. The recent reevaluation of the absorbance values for these filters concluded that the filters could be considered "permanent" absorbance standards for about ten years.[35] The cobalt blue filter, however, has not changed at all in that period. These filters are available in 30 mm disks or 51 mm squares and cost approximately $175 each. The sizes are not convenient for many spectrophotometers, and it is unfortunate that different sizes cannot be specified. A user would be very reluctant to buy the filter at that cost and then try to cut it

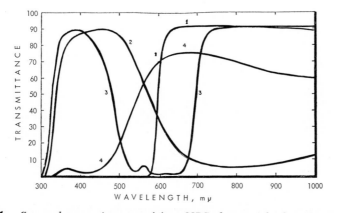

**Figure 2-11.** *Spectral transmittances of four NBS glass standards: 1. selenium orange; 2. copper green; 3. cobalt blue; 4. carbon yellow. (From Gibson, K. S., and Belknap, M. A.: Permanence of glass standards of spectral transmittance (R.P. #2093). J. Res. NBS., 44:463, 1950.)*

to size himself. The certified transmittance is from 390 to 750 m$\mu$ at 25°C; for an additional fee, other wavelengths may be calibrated as desired. The estimated uncertainty of each value and the effect of temperature change on transmittance at each wavelength is reported for each filter.

Chance ON-10 filter* has been highly recommended for checking the photometric scale between 390 and 750 m$\mu$. Slavin suggested three thicknesses: 1, 2, and 3 mm;[54] Edisbury considers the 1 and 3 mm sufficient and measures them at 402, 445 and 640 m$\mu$.[18] The spectral curves for the 1, 2, and 3 mm thickness of this filter are shown in Figure 2-12. This filter had proven stable for 5 years at the time it was reported in 1962. A slight oxidation film is said to form with age, but this can be removed with alcohol.

Hilger's rhodiumized silica filter has recently been recommended as suitable for the visible and the UV range.[18] This filter is manufactured in England and is apparently not yet available in the United States of America.

While considering filters for checking photometric accuracy, one might think of either the holmium oxide or didymium filter already being used for other testing. The NBS will not recognize either didymium or holmium oxide filters for this use.[21] Screens have been stated to be superior to solutions for checking linearity,[28] but screens are considered inferior to glass filters,[60] and have been judged inadequate for photometric standards.[54]

The inconvenience of solutions and the high cost of calibrated filters have led to the compromise of checking the photometric scale occasionally by one of these methods and then more frequently using a cheaper set of "neutral density filters"

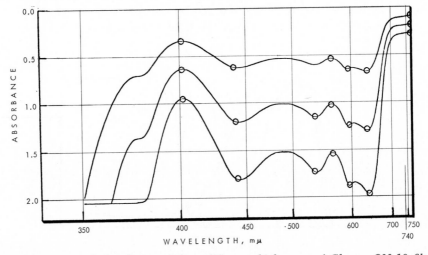

**Figure 2-12.** *Spectral absorbance of three different thicknesses of Chance ON-10 filter. (From Slavin, W.: Photometric standard for ultra-violet-visible spectrophotometers. J. Opt. Soc., Amer., 52:1399, 1962.)*

---

\* Available from Alpha American Corp., Rockford, Ill.

as a reproducibility check. These filters* have stated values of 0.3, 0.6, and 0.9 absorbance but are reproducible from time to time within ± 0.005 on the Beckman DB spectrophotometer with a 5-inch recorder. Readings for these filters have varied from this range only when a detector required replacement. Prior to the advent of these glass filters Gilford gelatin sandwich filters were used, but they separate with time.

Rand recommends that linearity of wide bandpass instruments be checked by comparing the absorbance of standards read on these instruments with those obtained on narrow pass instruments.[44] He also suggests a similar comparison be used to express the sensitivity of the wide bandpass instruments.

Edisbury recommends plotting a daily reading of the photometric standard on the usual ± 2 SD control chart, shown in A of Figure 2-13.[18] He used a manual instrument and observed the minimum slit at which this value was determined. A weekly average of these slit width values was plotted on another chart, shown as B of Figure 2-13. The trend for wider slits was corrected by replacing the hydrogen lamp and the mirror. These changes are indicated as 3a and 3b respectively. Incidents 1, 2, 4, and 5, noted in Figure 2-13B, were stated to be minor adjustments

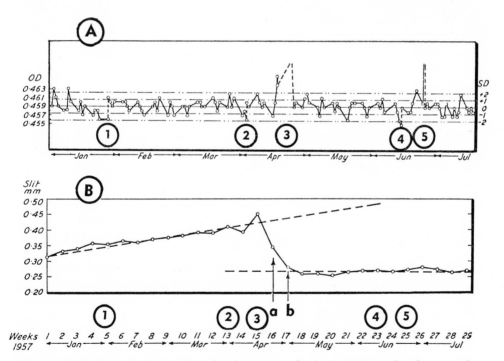

**Figure 2-13.** *Control charts for absorbance standard: A. Mean absorbance value ± 2 SD; B. Weekly average for slit widths used to obtain the values shown in A. (By permission from Edisbury, J. R.:* Practical Hints on Absorption Spectrophotometry. *New York, Plenum Press, 1967.)*

---

* Available from Arthur H. Thomas Co., Philadelphia, Pa., as #9104–N25.

on a slipping cam and a connector spring. Edisbury reminds us that if these minor adjustments had not been detected quickly and repaired, they would have become major problems later.

As Gibson and Belknap emphatically state, tests for linearity are to be used to *check* the instrument, and these values may not be used to *correct* the instrument.[23] If discrepancies occur, the causal factor or component must be found and corrected.

## CHECK SYSTEM FOR THE COLEMAN JR. SPECTROPHOTOMETER

While the Coleman Jr. spectrophotometer is a simple instrument, its satisfactory performance is directly proportional to the user's understanding and care of the optical system. The entire optical system of this instrument is based on the condition and position of its exciter lamp. The base of this lamp is said to be "pre-focused," meaning that the filament has been aligned and the lamp can only fit in the socket one way. This position of the lamp then determines that the filament will be precisely vertical so that it can focus the light through the sample as a relatively homogeneous band of wavelength covering 35 m$\mu$ (or 20 m$\mu$ for some models). The lamp is screened by the manufacturer, and the user should be careful to use the correct one for this instrument. A similar lamp used in the Coleman Universal Model spectrophotometer does not require the bandpass to be so carefully screened. Since the Coleman Jr. does not use an exit slit, the lamp focus determines the bandpass.

As the lamp condition changes with age or becomes coated with a film inside or outside, the bandpass changes and the wavelength calibration itself can change. For this reason, it is necessary to check the wavelength calibration daily before the instrument is put into use. The calibration filter supplied by the company has the transmittance expected at 610 m$\mu$ printed on it. The knurled wavelength adjustment screw can be regulated enough to set the proper %T at 610 m$\mu$, but it can also be set to read the proper % T at about 565 m$\mu$. The latter setting would then render the whole wavelength scale incorrect. (See Figure 2-14.) The user must familiarize himself with the color of the light passing through the sample compartment, especially at 610 and 565 m$\mu$. A small white card dropped into the sample compartment makes the color easier to see. The color from the blue end through the red end of the spectrum should gradually and smoothly fade from one color to the next. Any blotchy appearance or slanted bands of color indicate malfunctions and must be corrected immediately. Blotchiness can occur with damaged grating. Slanted bands of color usually are caused by lamp filaments improperly mounted on the lamp base. While looking at this color, glance at the photocell front and be sure it is clean. No readings can be correct if a smudge disperses the light hitting the photocell.

In order to eliminate effects caused by humidity, the instrument should be left on continuously. When the instrument is not in use, the cuvette holder is positioned

42

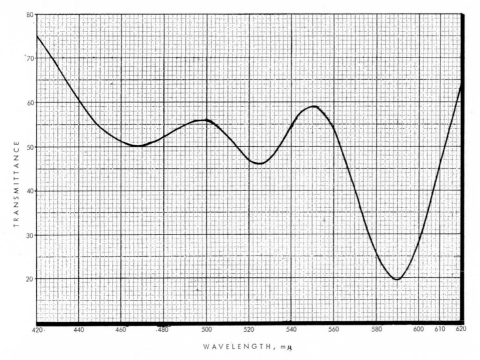

**Figure 2-14.** *Spectral transmittance for didymium filter, using Coleman Jr. spectrophotometer.*

so as to occlude the light from the photocell. A check sheet for this instrument is shown in Figure 2-15.

### Didymium for Wavelength Calibration

1. With the cuvette holder at a 90° angle to its usual position, occlude the light from the photocell and read zero. Adjust if necessary.
2. Set instrument at 610 m$\mu$.
3. With the cuvette well empty and the top covered, set 100%T against air.
4. Read the didymium filter. If it does not read within 1.5%T of its stated value, adjust as described in the manual.
5. Change the wavelength to 465 m$\mu$ and set 100%T against air.
6. Read the didymium filter and record the %T on the check sheet.

### Noise and Drift

The zero and 100%T are checked for each sample read on the Coleman Jr. instrument. As a check for noise and drift, zero and 100%T are set and each observed for one minute. The most common drift occurs at 100%T and often is caused by failure to fit the 6-pronged plug on the electric cord snugly into the instrument.

43

COLEMAN JR. DAILY CHECK

Hospital _____ Instrument # _____          Month _____ Year _____

| Date | Didymium 610 mμ ±1.5%T | Reaction Time 5-9 sec. | Nickel Sulfate | | | | | | Elec. Shorts | Tech. | Remarks |
|---|---|---|---|---|---|---|---|---|---|---|---|
| | | | 400 mμ %T < 4%T | 460 mμ %T 28±3 → OD .509-.602 | 510 mμ > 68%T | 550 mμ %T 54±2 → OD .252-.284 | OD 460/550 | 700 mμ < 2%T | | | |
| 1 | | | | | | | | | | | |
| 2 | | | | | | | | | | | |
| 3 | | | | | | | | | | | |
| 4 | | | | | | | | | | | |
| 5 | | | | | | | | | | | |

**Figure 2-15.** *Coleman Jr. daily check sheet.*

44

Flecks of dirt on the potentiometer windings for the coarse or fine galvanometer adjustment can cause drift. When dirt is the cause, the galvanometer index light "jumps" when the adjustment knob is touched. Several firm turns of the knob in each direction will usually correct the problem.

## Reaction Time

The current models seem much better in reaction time than were some of the older ones. If one has only newer models in use, this check need not be done daily.

---

### Reaction Time

1. With a stopwatch, check the reaction time required for the galvanometer needle to stop when a colored solution is read. Choose any solution which will read about midpoint, *i.e.* 40%T to 50%T.
2. Record this time on sheet provided. An instrument functioning well should have a reaction time of less than 9 seconds.

---

## Stray Light, Bandpass, and Linearity

Stray light, bandpass, and linearity are all checked by reading nickel sulfate at the appropriate wavelengths. A set of sealed 25 mm cuvettes containing nickel sulfate and a carbon tetrachloride blank are available commercially.* It is convenient when using several instruments to keep the AOCS standard set for reference and prepare a set for each instrument. The directions for preparation are:[15]

1. Carefully clean and dry a pair of Coleman Catalog No. 6-300B, 25 × 105 mm cuvettes.
2. Dissolve 20 gm of Special Reagent Grade (Cobalt free) $NiSO_4$ $6H_2O$ in distilled water. Add 1 ml of concentrated HCl and dilute to exactly 100 ml in a volumetric flask. Filter 15 ml of this solution into one of the cuvettes and stopper immediately with a paraffin-coated cork.
3. Reference solution. Into a 100 ml graduate, pour 1 ml of concentrated HCl and dilute to 100 ml with distilled water. Into the second selected cuvette pour 15 ml of this solution. Stopper immediately with a paraffined cork.
4. Indelibly mark each cuvette for permanent identification.

The solutions in these sealed cuvettes will remain clear and stable for long periods of time. Their continuing value as standards will depend largely upon the care with which their optical surfaces are maintained. Store them upright at a temperature no lower than 5°C and no higher than 30°C. Use them only at 25°C to 30°C.

We have used some of these sets for 5 years now, but some have developed leaks around the corks and have had to be replaced. The secret to successful corking

---

* Coleman Catalog #6-404/405 A.O.C.S. calibrating standard.

seems to be to immerse the cork in warm paraffin for about an hour before inserting it into the cuvette. The cuvette top should be completely dry. After pushing the cork into the cuvette, dip the whole top in warm paraffin several times.

## Nickel Sulfate

See spectral transmittance curve (Fig. 2-16)

1. Read the nickel sulfate against its blank at 400, 460, 510, 550 and 700 m$\mu$, referencing blank at 100%T for each wavelength.
2. Record each %T on the chart provided and compare each to the specifications shown in Table 2-6.

**Table 2-6.** Specifications for Nickel Sulfate Transmittance on Coleman Jr. and Coleman Jr. II Spectrophotometers

| Wavelength | Coleman Jr.* | Coleman Jr. II† | Significance of Reading‡ |
|---|---|---|---|
| 400 m$\mu$ | Less than 4%T | Less than 4%T | Stray light |
| 460 m$\mu$ | 28%T ± 3 | 17%T ± 3 | Wavelength dial calibration accuracy |
| 510 m$\mu$ | 68%T or higher | 77%T or higher | Peak transmittance |
| 550 m$\mu$ | 54%T ± 2 | 57%T ± 2 | Wavelength dial calibration accuracy |
| 700 m$\mu$ | Less than 2%T | Less than 2%T | Stray light |

* From Service Department, Scientific Products: Personal communication.

† From author's experience using two instruments.

‡ From Coleman Technical Report #T-198: A procedure for monitoring the performance parameters of Coleman Jr. spectrophotometers, 1965.

3. Convert %T to OD for the 460 and 550 m$\mu$ readings. If the OD values for 460 and 550 m$\mu$ shift in opposite directions, the cause could be inaccurate wavelength settings. Recheck or readjust (if necessary) the 610 m$\mu$ point with the didymium and repeat the 460 and 550 m$\mu$ readings for nickel sulfate. If the shift in OD is in excess of ± 0.020, is not in opposite direction for 460 and 550 m$\mu$, or is in opposite direction but not corrected by changing didymium adjustment, the possible causes for the problem must be investigated. Consultation with the manufacturer is often necessary, and usually professional repair service is required.

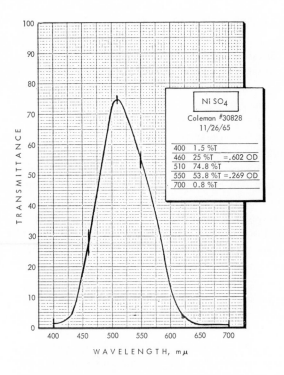

Figure 2-16. *Spectral transmittance for nickel sulfate solution, using Coleman Jr. spectrophotometer.*

The specifications for the readings at 400 and 700 m$\mu$ must be strictly held, but some latitude can be tolerated in the 460 and 550 m$\mu$ readings.[33] The main consideration in all the readings, except the 400 and 700 m$\mu$, is how much *change* there is in the readings from time to time.

The stray light detected by the readings at 400 and 700 m$\mu$ (usually 700 m$\mu$ does not increase nearly as much as the 400 m$\mu$) can be caused by an old or dirty exciter lamp. If the specifications are not met, the lamp should be cleaned and the readings repeated. Once in a while, a new exciter lamp is defective. The usual reason is that the base and filament do not appear to be perpendicular to each other. Lamps should be checked before sending the instrument to the manufacturer for repair. If the reading is still too high, the instrument should be sent in for repair. Under these circumstances, the instrument usually requires a new grating. Although replacement seems simple, the grating should not be replaced by the user. Rigid company specifications for alignment require equipment and techniques not ordinarily available in the laboratory.

The width and general character of the bandpass is interpreted in the consideration of the reading at 510 m$\mu$. If the filament of the exciter lamp is not focused properly, there will not be sufficient energy to produce a %T as high as 72 at 510 m$\mu$. This wavelength is the minimum absorption peak for nickel sulfate. Decreased readings for this minimum absorption (maximum transmittance) can be caused by the increased bandpass that occurs from film on the outside of the exciter lamp,[65] dirty or damaged slit opening in the cuvette housing, or deteriorating

47

diffraction grating.[15] If the 510 m$\mu$ reading is less than 72 or has decreased by 3%T from the exciter lamp change,[15] the slit should be examined visually by moving the cuvette holder. A cotton swab can be used to clean the slit edges. Incidentally, a dense smudge from something spilled over the front surface of the photocell can give this same dispersion of light. If cleaning the slit doesn't correct the problem, (and it usually doesn't, despite periodic cleaning of the slit surface), the next step is to clean or replace the exciter lamp. If the reading still is outside specifications, the manufacturer should be consulted. Usually the instrument has to be sent in for a grating replacement.

To replace a grating for a 3%T change in this reading will strike some users as absurd. It is true that the instrument can be recalibrated for whatever test procedures are read on it and it can continue to be used for a variable length of time. However, once a grating starts to change, it may produce inaccurate readings at some wavelengths and not at others. For example, when one grating was removed, there was a small bubble on its surface. We cannot swear the bubble hadn't been there originally, but we know that minimum absorption readings for the instrument changed. In the process of recalibrating the instrument the only curve that was different was the one for bilirubin read at 540 m$\mu$. When the 510 m$\mu$ reading was found to have reached the 3%T difference, the instrument was sent in for repair, and the grating was changed.

Bandpass that is monitored with a 590 m$\mu$ reading on the didymium filter may yield valid information,[65] but the didymium filter in this thickness provides no area in which stray light can be detected. Nickel sulfate does not have this limitation.

The readings at 460 and 550 m$\mu$ serve two purposes: a wavelength check and a linearity or proportionality check. An error in wavelength is said to cause the two readings to shift in opposite directions.[15] An easy independent wavelength check can be made by using a holmium oxide filter.* Although none has been permanently mounted in a size for the Coleman Jr., the 10 x 25 mm glass can be taped to a card and slipped into the cuvette holder or a cuvette.

Figure 2-17 shows the spectral transmittance curve for the holmium oxide filter. Since the maximum absorbance is widely separated from the 610 m$\mu$ spot for which the instrument is calibrated, this spread should provide a sensitive wavelength check. However, there are three bands in the region of 440 to 460 m$\mu$, and the 35 mm slit leaves some uncertainty as to the location of the unresolved peak to be expected for individual instruments.

Assignment of linearity interpretation to the interrelation of the 460 and 550 m$\mu$ readings of nickel sulfate appears a little nebulous.[15, 33] If a shift occurs in these two readings and if the shift is in the same direction for both, the instrument's linearity is said to have changed. A clearer evaluation of the change is evident if the %T readings are converted to absorbance. The relationship of the 460 m$\mu$ to the 550 m$\mu$ reading should be about 2 to 1; a change from the original relationship is said to be more important than the closeness of the 2 to 1 ratio. If this relationship has changed, the instrument should be sent to the manufacturer for repair.

---

* Available from the Arthur H. Thomas Co., Philadelphia, Pa., Catalog #9104 N25.

48

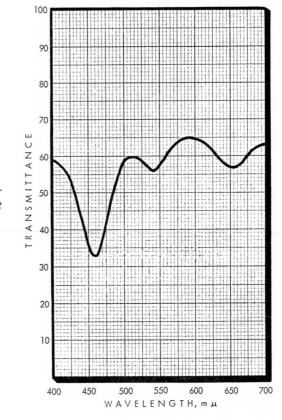

**Figure 2-17.** *Spectral transmittance for holmium oxide filter using Coleman Jr. spectrophotometer.*

## Electrical Shorts

When the side of the case is tapped, the galvanometer needle will bounce slightly but should go back to rest at its original setting. Meter needle drift (after it quits bouncing) has been found when the plug to the electric cord has not been snugly seated in the intrument. If this is not the cause, the instrument must be checked for shorts by an electronics technician.

## CHECK SYSTEM FOR BECKMAN DU SPECTROPHOTOMETER*

The entire check system for the Beckman DU spectrophotometer is to be run monthly, and indicated portions are to be done daily. Special attention must be paid to the desiccant; it often needs replacement more frequently than once a month during periods of high humidity. Perform all the tests on one phototube, switch to the other, and (after it has had sufficient time to warm up) repeat the tests using that tube. Directions for performing each function check are coded

---

*Parts of this discussion are from Winstead, M.: A check system for proper function of the Beckman DU spectrophotometer, Amer. J. Med. Techn., *28*:67, 1962, and are reprinted with permission of the publisher.

BECKMAN DU FUNCTION SHEET

Date *10/20/64*                                                    Instrument #  ___*73769*___

I.  Slits, 0%T, 100%T, Noise and Drift - Sensitivity Control CW

|  | Red Tube |  | Photomultiplier Tube |
|---|---|---|---|

700 mμ:                                              540 mμ:

  A. 0%T *OK*  ; with Block *OK* [N D] ✓✓✓        A. 0%T *OK*  ; with Block *OK* [N D] ✓✓✓

  B. Energy noted *3/4 → .01*  mm SW               B. Energy noted *½ → .01*  mm SW

  C. 100%T;CK selector *OK* [N D] ✓✓               C. 100%T; CK selector *OK* [N D] ✓✓

II.  Switch accuracy - Sensitivity Control CW

  700 mμ:  A.  CK→1 reads *100.0*%T              540 mμ: A.  CK→1 reads *100.0* %T
         B.  1→0.1 reads *101.0*%T                     B.  1→0.1 reads *101.0* %T
         C. 0.1→1 reads *100.0*%T                      C. 0.1→1 reads *10.0* %T
         D. 1→CK needle is *100.0* 100               D. 1→CK, needle is *100.0* 100

III.  Reproducibility with      Gilford filter - Sensitivity Control Center  *#506 filter: A .109 valids; B1.1, C2.07*

  700 mμ SW .05                                   550 mμ SW .03

  A. *.104*  ;B *1.13* ;C *2.10*                   A. *.110*   ;B. *1.12* ;C. *2.05*

IV   Sensitivity of Phototubes (minimum slit widths) - Sensitivity Control CW

  700 mμ *.088* 850 mμ *.054* 1000mμ *.051*        540 mμ *.0175*

V.  Tungsten energy measurement:  (2.0 mm slit width)              *290* mμ

VI.  Sensitivity of Amplifiers.

  700 mμ-sensitivity control CCW                   540 mμ-sensitivity control CW *(@ 2 off scale)*

X 99.0%T drives needle left *1* div.             99.0%T drives needle left *@ 12 (@ 2 off scale)* div.

  101.0%T drives needle right *2* div.             101.0%T drives needle right *5* div. X

VII.  *Wavelength calibrated with holmium filter - sensitivity Center

  638 mμ,SW 0.05, *638.0* mμ= *68.0* %T          361 mμ,SW 0.08, *360.8* mμ= *9.6* %T
                                                  536 mμ,SW 0.01, *536.4* mμ= *44.0* %T

* 700/mμ A.108, B2.15, C 2.14                    * 559mμ A.109, B 1.10, C 2.06

VIII.  Resolution with holmium filter (locate peak with sensitivity control CCW)

                                                  382.5 peak set at zero
                                                  387.1 peak position right *10* div.
                                                  384.4 valley position left *8* div.

IX.  Stray light with 7 mm (thickness) didymium - sensitivity control Center

  580 mμ, SW 0.1 = *.38* %T                       340 mμ (with filter),SW 0.15 = *.20* %T
                                                  580 mμ, SW 0.01 = *.20* %T

X.  Linearity with Gilford filters - sensitivity control Center

  600 mμ, SW .08:A *.113* , B. *1.09* C. *2.10*    340 mμ, SW .15: A *.256* ,B *1.92* ,C *2.50*
  700 mμ, *,SW .05:A. *.114* , B *1.18* C. *2.15*   550 mμ*,SW .03: A *.111* ;B *1.08* ,C *2.05*
  800 mμ,SW .03: A *.089* B. *1.72* C. *2.35*      600 mμ,SW .02: A *.112*,B. *1.06* ,C *2.00*

XI.  Electrical Disturbance: A. Taps *OK*  B. Vibro-Graver *OK*  -

XII.  Light Leaks  *none*

XIII.  Desiccant  ✓ OK;        changed

  *  Repeat test for reproducibility and record in III.

**Figure  2-18.**  *Sample of monthly check of Beckman DU spectrophotometer. The Gilford filter set has since been replaced with glass filters.*

BECKMAN DU SPECTROPHOTOMETER DAILY CHECK

| | Red Phototube | | | | | | | Photomultiplier Tube | | | | | | |
|---|---|---|---|---|---|---|---|---|---|---|---|---|---|---|
| Date | 0%T 700 mμ | N* or D | 100%T 700 mμ | N* or D | Sens. Min. SW 700 mμ | Holmium filter 637.5 mμ peak | Holmium filter %T (SW .05) | 0%T 540 mμ | N* or D | 100%T 540 mμ | N* or D | Sens. Min. SW 540 mμ | Holmium filter 536.2 mμ peak | Holmium filter %T (SW .01) |
| | | | | | | | | | | | | | | |
| | | | | | | | | | | | | | | |
| | | | | | | | | | | | | | | |
| | | | | | | | | | | | | | | |
| | | | | | | | | | | | | | | |
| | | | | | | | | | | | | | | |
| | | | | | | | | | | | | | | |
| | | | | | | | | | | | | | | |

* √ to denote noise or drift *absent;* X to denote noise or drift *present.*

**Figure 2-19.** *Daily check sheet for Beckman DU spectrophotometer.*

to the monthly check sheet, and an example of typical results is shown as Figure 2-18. The daily check sheet is illustrated in Figure 2-19.

Routine details of technique include the following:

1.  Focus and check the energy whenever a lamp is replaced.
2.  Allow the following warm-up times: 1 hour for power supply; 15 minutes for lamp and either phototube.
3.  Correct cause of noise or drift if it is present. The instrument will be more easily and accurately operated.
4.  For the photomultiplier tube, use the lowest possible switch sensitivity (power supply) consistent with that required to set the %T range for given slit widths.
5.  *Always* use the Corex filter for wavelengths between 325 to 400 m$\mu$ with the tungsten lamp source.
6.  Adjust final wavelength settings from longer to shorter m$\mu$.
7.  Adjust final slit width settings from narrower to wider openings.
8.  For routine readings attempt to keep the sensitivity control between midrange and two and a half (2½) turns from CW (clockwise).
9.  Locate peaks at CCW (counterclockwise) sensitivity control position and then change the sensitivity control midrange for reading the %T values.

### Noise or Drift, Slit Operation, and Zero

The zero setting must be constant; by watching the needle for one minute, noise (fluctuation) or drift (constant change in one direction) may be detected. Should either be present in excess of the tolerance, it must be corrected before proceeding. Provision has been made in the slit operation test and on the check sheet to detect noise and drift.

The zero setting is an adjustment for the dark current and also a function of slit operation. The proper physical closing of the slit (and also the shutter) can be separately determined by the use of a metal block inserted in the sample holder.

---

### I: A, B.  *Slit Operation*

A.  Zero opening
    1.  Set slit width at 0, %T dial at 0, sensitivity control at CW (clockwise) limit, and selector switch at 0.1. Sample is air.
    2.  Adjust wavelength to 700 m$\mu$ for the red tube.
    3.  Adjust the dark current to zero the needle. Leave in this position for one minute and watch for noise or drift. If present, check the sheet in the box provided. Tolerance: ½ division per minute.
    4.  Open shutter; the needle should remain at zero.

B.  Block test.   Pull sample carrier into position for the block and open the shutter. The needle should remain at zero.

C. Slit opening
1. Remove the block and open the shutter. The needle should still be at zero.
2. Open slit slowly and note when energy begins to move the needle. Tolerance should show about three fourths of the way toward 0.01 from 0 slit.

D. Repeat A through C using photomultiplier tube at 540 m$\mu$.

## 100% Transmittance

Maintenance of a steady 100% T setting is also necessary for any readings to be reliable. On the Beckman DU spectrophotometer the selector switch on CK with the shutter open completes a circuit in which a fixed resistor replaces the slide wire potentiometer. This circuit also must be equivalent to a selector switch position 1 with % T dial at 100 when the shutter is open.

### I:C.    100% T Noise and Drift

Adjust the instrument for 700 m$\mu$, using the red tube. Sensitivity control is fully CW; sample is air.

1. With selector switch on CK and % T at 100 and shutter "off", adjust the needle to zero with dark current.
2. Open shutter and adjust slit width to zero the needle. Leave in this position and note noise or drift. Tolerance: ½ division per minute.
3. Change selector switch to 1. The needle must remain zeroed.
4. Repeat all tests at 540 m$\mu$ with photomultiplier tube, power supply sensitivity at 4. Tolerance: 0.1 division on meter scale.

If noise and/or drift occurs with the shutter open in this test, the difficulty is probably in the phototube house. The desiccant is a likely possibility, or the cause could be electronic. If this reading is not stable, the problem must be corrected before proceeding.

## Switch Accuracy

On the Beckman DU spectrophotometer the selector switch at CK is equivalent to the selector switch at 1 with % T dial at 100. Changing the switch to 0.1 expands the % T to 10% T scale tenfold. The absorbance scale likewise is expanded, and readings are made by adding 1.0 to the observed absorbance.

The switch positions that expand the scale and change the selector from CK to 1 are each governed by a separate resistor. Failure of switch and % T to function interchangeably denotes that one or both resistors are defective and should be replaced. Occasionally the % T cam can be manually advanced only as far toward

0 as 0.25%, and a "backward" check is necessary. If the usual check meets the tolerance, then this "backward" check need not be done.

---

## II. *Switch Accuracy*

Adjust instrument for 700 m$\mu$, using the red tube. Sensitivity control is fully CW; sample is air.

1. With selector switch at CK and shutter closed, zero the needle with the dark current.
2. Open the shutter and adjust slit width control to zero the needle.
3. Change selector switch to 1 and adjust needle with %T dial. Record the %T which should be 100. Tolerance: 100.0 ± 0.1%T.
4. With selector switch at 1 and %T dial at 10, zero the needle with the slit width control.
5. Change the selector switch to 0.1 and zero the needle with the %T dial. Read the %T; it should be 100. Tolerance: 100.0 ± 1.0%T.
6. Repeat all steps at 540 m$\mu$ with the photomultiplier tube, power supply sensitivity at 4.

If tolerance of #3 or #5 is not met, reverse the order of switching (*i.e.,* from 0.1 to 1, etc.) before declaring the resistor defective.

NOTE: For 1 → CK, leave %T dial at 100 with selector switch on 1. It should also be 100 on CK.

---

## Reproducibility or Precision

Reproducibility is proved by reading the same sample several times. Neutral filters (described under linearity, page 62) are chosen for several reasons: they are convenient to position; the usual sampling errors are avoided; and wavelength settings are not critical.

The positioning of the cell (*i.e.,* sample carrier) must be mechanically stable, reproducible, and exact. Micro cells require extra care in centering.

The pull knob of the sample positioner is fastened to a shaft that screws into the block end of the carrier base. This positioning shaft can become loosened and throw cells far from center. Centering should be visually checked with fluorescein from time to time, but this knob should not be continually adjusted. The sample compartment should be replaced in such instances.

---

## III. *Reproducibility*

Adjust the instrument for 700 m$\mu$, using the red tube, slit width of 0.5 mm, and sensitivity control "Center."

1. Set selector switch on CK and adjust dark current.

2. Open shutter (air as sample) and zero the needle with the sensitivity control.

3. Read the neutral density filters and record the OD.

4. Repeat twice at spaced intervals as shown on check sheet.

5. Repeat for photomultiplier tube at 550 m$\mu$ (power supply sensitivity 4) and slit width of 0.03 mm.

   Tolerance: ± .005 from established values on this instrument.

## Phototube Response

The ability of the phototube to record energy consistently depends upon (1) the sensitivity and linearity of the tube itself; (2) the strength and stability of the power supply, light source, and amplifier tubes; (3) the cleanliness and focus of the mirrors; and (4) the linearity of the resistors in the phototube circuit. Each of these components must be checked.

PHOTOTUBES. The Beckman DU spectrophotometer includes a red-sensitive phototube and either a blue-sensitive or a photomultiplier tube. The cutoff points for these tubes are given as 600 to 1000 m$\mu$, 325 to 625 m$\mu$, and 325 to 600 m$\mu$, respectively, when used with the tungsten lamp. The photomultiplier can be used down to 200 m$\mu$ if the hydrogen lamp is used.

The sensitivity switch on the power supply enables the user to decrease the sensitivity of the photomultiplier tube to any one of the 10 levels desired. The usual sensitivity switch setting for routine work is "4" or "5." At this level, readings are completely stable when the instrument has been put in "good trim."

Sensitivity of the phototube is measured in terms of its "minimum slits." At a specified wavelength (the instrument having been zeroed with dark current and the shutter being open), the slit width is increased enough to zero the meter needle. Such a slit width reading in millimeters is called the *minimum slit width* for that wavelength. The more sensitive the tube, the smaller will be the minimum slit width.

---

IV. *Phototube Sensitivity*

Sensitivity control should be fully CW.

Minimum slits allowable for wavelength

| | | |
|---|---|---|
| A. Red tube: | 700 m$\mu$ | 0.1 mm |
| | 850 m$\mu$ | 0.079 mm |
| | 1000 m$\mu$ | 0.13 mm |
| B. Blue tube: | 300 m$\mu$ | 2.0 mm |
| | 500 m$\mu$ | 0.079 mm |
| | 600 m$\mu$ | 0.15 mm |

*Continued on page 56*

C. Photomultiplier tube: Use either (1) or (2) below
 (1) Sensitivity switch on 5    540 m$\mu$                0.03    mm
 (2) Select sensitivity switch setting to approximate 300 m$\mu$ = 2.0 mm;
     check 500 m$\mu$ and 600 m$\mu$ as for blue tube above.

---

POWER SUPPLY.    If minimum slit specifications for the phototubes can be met, it can also be concluded that the power supply is adequate. Its lack of stability can best be detected if there is drift in the dark current.

SOURCE LIGHT.    The incandescent lamp for the range of 325 to 1000 m$\mu$ is satisfactory. The intensity of this light, however, must be absolutely constant. The lamp used in the Beckman DU spectrophotometer is a standard 32 candlepower automobile headlight bulb (G.E., Mazda #2331). Being unscreened for stability, it should be the first cause suspected for noise or drift in the dark current.

If the energy of the light is satisfactory, a slit width of 0.2 mm will allow the meter needle to zero at a wavelength lower than 305 m$\mu$. If the energy does not meet this requirement, the next step is to clean and refocus the lamp; replace it if it cannot be proved satisfactory.

---

### V.    *Tungsten Lamp Energy*

1. With the photomultiplier tube in position (power supply sensitivity at 4), set the sensitivity control fully CW. Push the Corex filter in (*i.e.*, not in use).
2. With the selector switch on CK, zero the needle with dark current.
3. Adjust the slit width to 2.0 mm and open the shutter.
4. Rotate the wavelength knob until the meter needle reaches zero.
5. Record the wavelength indicated on the dial. Tolerance: must be below 305 m$\mu$.

---

AMPLIFIER TUBES.    In the Beckman DU spectrophotometer the two amplifier tubes, #2531 and #2532, are placed in the circuit so that both contribute at all times. The bias switch on the top of the power supply #73600 (or the screw in the back of older units) controls the voltage on the screen of the #2532 tube. This functions as a coarse adjustment in conjunction with the dark current control. The proper bias setting is one that will allow the meter needle to zero approximately when the dark current control is in a position within 1 revolution from its CW limit.

---

### VI.    *Amplification*

1. Set the sensitivity control fully CCW, using the red tube; set the wavelength at 700 m$\mu$.

2. With selector switch on CK, zero the needle with dark current.

3. Set selector switch on 1 and %T control at 100. Open shutter and adjust the needle to zero with the slit width control.

4. Move the %T to 99 and then 101. Note the needle deflection by the number of divisions on the meter scale.
Tolerance: The needle should move 3 divisions for 99 and for 101.

5. Repeat above for photomultiplier tube at wavelength of 540 m$\mu$ but set the sensitivity control on CW.
Tolerance: The needle should move off scale for 99 and for 101.

WAVELENGTH CALIBRATION.  The mercury arc is the best single source of wavelength calibration for 205 to 1014 m$\mu$ with 546.1 m$\mu$ as the reference line.

The published list of minimum slit widths for the mercury lines indicates the relative strength of the lines. Location of the seven lines shown in Table 2-7 is sufficient.

Table 2-7.  Selected Mercury Emission Lines for Wavelength Calibration or Check for the Beckman DU

| Wavelength* (m$\mu$) | Tolerance Allowed† (m$\mu$) | Minimum Slit‡ Width (mm) |
|---|---|---|
| 1014.0 | 6.0 | 0.02 |
| 577.0 | 1.0 | 0.07 |
| 546.1 | 0.6 | 0.015 |
| 435.8 | 0.4 | 0.01 |
| 334.1 | 0.15 | 0.04 |
| 280.4 | 0.15 | 0.36§ |
| 253.6 | 0.1 | 0.01 |

* South Bend Medical Foundation selection.
† Beckman Instruments, Inc. tolerance.
‡ Walker, I. K., and Todd, H. J.: Wavelength calibration of spectrophotometers. Anal. Chem., 31:1603, 1959.
§ A value was not listed by Walker and Todd; this is our value.

If tolerances are not met, the calibration must be adjusted as directed in the manual for the instrument. Day-to-day checking of the wavelength scale is done with a holmium oxide glass filter.*

The spectral transmittance curve for the holmium filter on our Beckman DU spectrophotometer is shown in Figure 2-20. The absorbance peaks chosen for wavelength checks were as widely separated as possible for each phototube.

* Corning CS 3–138 of glass #3130 available from Beckman Instruments, Inc. and Arthur H. Thomas Co.

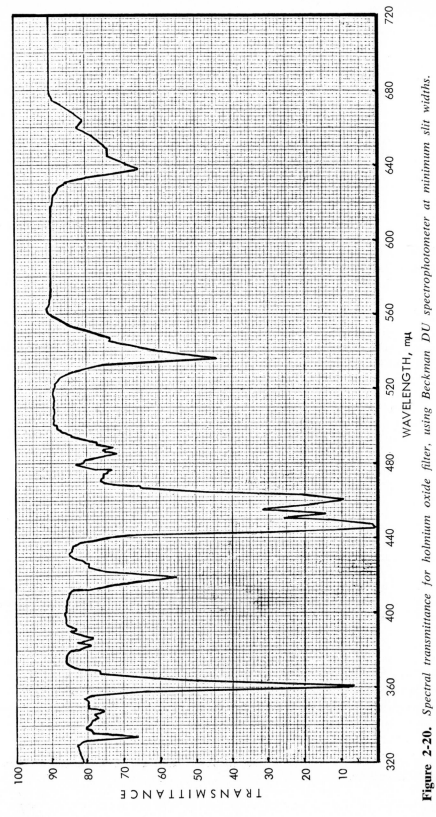

**Figure 2-20.** Spectral transmittance for holmium oxide filter, using Beckman DU spectrophotometer at minimum slit widths.

58

Peaks are best located with the sensitivity control at its CCW limit in order to use the smallest possible slit width; but once found, the peak's transmittancy values are measured with the sensitivity control approximately center and at the slit widths indicated.

Find the absorbance peaks as follows:

1. Zero the instrument with dark current in the usual manner against air as the sample.
2. Set the selector switch on 1, the %T dial at about 50, and pull the holmium filter into sample position.
3. Open the shutter and adjust the slit width so that the meter needle is on scale.
4. Slowly rotate the wavelength knob (from long toward short m$\mu$) and constantly adjust the slit width to keep the needle on scale.

When a maximum absorbancy peak is passed, the needle will swing *right* to a maximum and then go *left*. The exact peak is indicated by the maximum needle swing to the right. Read off the m$\mu$ as closely as possible, using a magnifying glass to estimate between marks on the scale. Leave the wavelength knob in its position and proceed to measure the %T of the peak as follows:

1. Again zero the instrument with dark current.
2. Adjust the slit width for the wavelength as given below and with the shutter open, zero the needle with the sensitivity control.
3. Read the %T of the peak using the 0.1 switch when the %T goes below 10.

---

## VII.  *Wavelength Calibration Check with Holmium Filter*

*absorbance→*                                    *transmittance←*

Find the absorbance peak with sensitivity control
CCW and read the %T using specifications below:

For the red tube:

637.5 m$\mu$ = _____ m$\mu$

SW of 0.05 mm gives %T

Tolerance $\pm$ 1.2 m$\mu$

For the photomultiplier tube,
power supply sensitivity = 4

360.9 m$\mu$ = _____ m$\mu$
(filter in use)

SW of 0.08 mm gives _____%T

Tolerance $\pm$ 0.2 m$\mu$
536.2 m$\mu$ = _____ m$\mu$
SW of 0.01 mm gives _____%T
Tolerance $\pm$ 0.6 m$\mu$

---

RESOLUTION.  Routine checking of resolution is done by measuring doublets in the holmium filter spectrum at 382.5 and 387 m$\mu$ and the valley at 384.4 m$\mu$

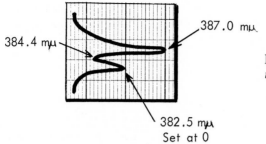

384.4 mμ

387.0 mμ

382.5 mμ
Set at 0

**Figure 2-21.** *Scan with holmium filter on Beckman DU spectrophotometer.*

(Fig. 2-21). The heights of the two peaks are not identical, but it is possible to keep both peaks and the valley on the meter scale while rotating the wavelength adjustment from one peak to the other. All other controls (*e.g.,* slit width and sensitivity control) are left in the same position throughout.

## VIII.   *Resolution Using Holmium Filter*

Sensitivity control is CCW. Start with sensitivity on power supply at 5.

1. Using minimum slit widths, locate the 382.5 mμ maximum absorbance peak.
2. Turn the %T knob until the meter needle is at 0.
3. Slowly rotate the wavelength knob to locate the 387 mμ maximum absorbance peak. The needle will move right. If it goes off the scale, lower the sensitivity on the power supply and start over. Note the final position of the needle, *e.g.,* right 10 divisions.
4. Slowly rotate wavelength knob to locate valley at 384.4 mμ. Note the final position of the meter needle, *e.g.,* left 8 divisions.
   Tolerance: Valley value should be three fourths the 387 mμ value ± 1 division.

Stray Light and Light Leaks.   Stray light is customarily measured in the UV range (below 230 mμ) with a Vycor filter. If one is not routinely using the instrument in this range, the 7 mm didymium can be used for measuring this error in the visible range. The spectral transmittance curve for the didymium filter (Fig. 2-22) indicates the wavelengths to be chosen for the test.

## IX.   *Stray Light*

1. Set the selector switch on CK and zero the needle with dark current.
2. Using the photomultiplier, set the wavelength dial at 210 mμ and the slit width at 0.1 mm.

*Continued on page* 62

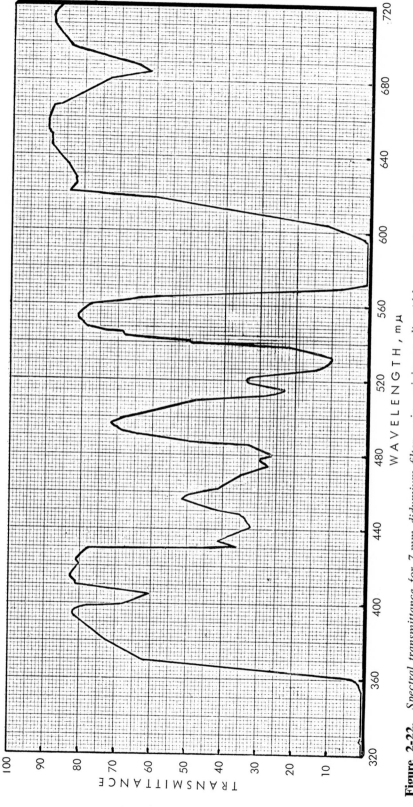

**Figure 2-22.** *Spectral transmittance for 7 mm didymium filter, using minimum slit widths on Beckman DU spectrophotometer.*

3. Open the shutter and zero the needle (air is sample) with the sensitivity control.
4. Pull the Vycor filter into sample positions and record the %T, using the 0.1 selector switch.
5. For *didymium* filter, use red tube at 580 and 340 m$\mu$ with 0.1 mm slit width.

Tolerance: less than 0.5%T.

---

Stray light and light leaks can be differentiated by repeating readings with a much wider slit width. Stray light due to leaks will decrease rapidly as the slit width is widened. Instrumental stray light (free from light leaks) will not vary much with changes in slit widths.

---

## XII.   *Light Leaks*

1. Use the photomultiplier tube with the sensitivity on the power supply at 6. The wavelength setting does not matter. Turn the lamp off.
2. With the shutter closed, zero the needle with dark current control.
3. Set the slit width at 0, the %T dial on 0, and the selector switch on 0.1.
4. Open the shutter.
5. Play the beam of a strong flashlight on the seams and sides of phototube house and cell compartment.
6. If the meter needle fluctuates, light is leaking through and must be corrected.

---

LINEARITY.   Tests for linearity are to be used to check the instrument. These values may not be used to *correct* the instrument. If discrepancies occur, their cause must be found and corrected.

A set of three approximately neutral density filters (sold commercially as Gilford filters*) come installed in a block similar to the Beckman sample carrier. They are individually calibrated by Eastman Kodak Co., Rochester, N. Y., and have approximately 0.1, 1.0, and 2.0 OD values at 550 m$\mu$. Included with each set are spectral transmittance curves for 400 to 700 m$\mu$ so that they may be checked at other wavelengths.

---

## X.   *Linearity Using the Gilford Filter**

Read each filter at the wavelengths and slit widths indicated.

1. Zero the dark current, and balance the needle with the sensitivity control while the shutter is open.

---

* Available from Gilford Instruments, Inc., Oberlin, Ohio.

2. For the red phototube use: 600 m$\mu$, SW 0.08 mm
   700 m$\mu$, SW 0.05 mm
   800 m$\mu$, SW 0.03 mm

3. For the photomultiplier tube use: 340 m$\mu$, SW 0.15 mm
   550 m$\mu$, SW 0.03 mm
   600 m$\mu$, SW 0.02 mm

Tolerance: For 400 to 700 m$\mu$ $\pm$ 0.020 from calibrated value accompanying the filters.

For other wavelengths: $\pm$ 0.020 from own established values.

---

* NOTE: Some difficulty has arisen from separation of the gelatin filters. Glass filters are available from Arthur H. Thomas Co., Catalog #9104, N25. These filters are not as precisely calibrated as the Gilford filters.

ELECTRONIC DISTURBANCES. If noise or drift occurs when both phototubes are used and the desiccant is known to be satisfactory, the problem is probably caused by the power supply or an unstable lamp. The difficulty may also be caused by either of the phototubes. In this case the defective tube must be replaced.

Sharp taps on the phototube housing will produce slight shifts in zero in almost any instrument. If shifts are large (or caused by gentle blows), the #2532 amplifier tube should be replaced.

Shorts due to improper grounding may be detected with any vibratory device that creates a large amount of static (*e.g.*, a Burgess vibro-graver*).[11]

---

## XI: A, B.  *Shorts*

Place photomultiplier tube in position with power supply sensitivity at 4 and sensitivity control CCW (fully counter clockwise).

A. Taps on phototube house
   1. Set selector switch on CK with shutter "off" and adjust needle with dark current.
   2. Gently tap top of phototube house and watch for needle shift.

B. Electronics disturbance
   1. Set selector switch on 0.1, %T at 0, and with shutter "off" zero needle with dark current.
   2. Open shutter and zero needle with slit width control.
   3. Move the electric vibratory device about one inch over cables and phototube house. Note any shift in needle.

Tolerance: one division on meter

---

* Fisher Scientific Company, Pittsburgh, Pa.

**Table 2-8, continued**

| Symptom | Cause | Correction |
|---|---|---|
| | 3. Mechanical stop of zero incorrect | Can be corrected by operator but contact manufacturer for specific instruction |
| IV. Phototube response—sensitivity specifications not met for single phototube | 1. Defective or improperly focused lamp | Refocus and replace if necessary |
| | 2. Defective amplifiers | Replace one at time #2531 & #2532 |
| | 3. Defective resistor | Replace |
| | 4. Dirty or defective resistor switch | Clean or replace |
| | 5. Defective phototube | Replace |
| V. Tungsten energy—too low; *i.e.*, m$\mu$ above 305 | 1. Defective or improperly focused lamp | Refocus and replace if necessary |
| | 2. Phototube improperly focused | Refocus |
| VI. Stray light reading too high | 1. Dirty or scratched mirrors | Replace |
| | 2. Light leak | Locate and correct |
| VII. Flashlight test denotes light leak or needle position changes when operator moves near instrument during measurements | Screw not tight in compartment or some other failure to be light tight | Tighten all plate screws and tape seams if necessary |
| VIII. Shorts<br>  A. Taps | 1. Defective #2532 amplifier tube | Replace |
| | 2. Any short in the circuits | Locate and repair |
|   B. Vibro-graver | 1. Loose connections at terminal parts | Tighten |
| | 2. Poor insulation on cable | Wrap with tape temporarily and have cable replaced |
| | 3. Short to ground (case probably) | Have electrician repair |

* From Winstead, M.: A check system for the proper function of the Beckman DU spectrophotometer. Amer. J. Med. Tech., *32:*35, 1966.

**Table 2-9. Checklist, Beckman DK2 Recording Spectrophotometer, Visible and Near Infrared (with Tungsten lamp)\***

| Check for: | Settings and Conditions | Requirements | Result |
|---|---|---|---|
| 100% $T$ from 700 to 350 m$\mu$ | PM: 1 ×<br>S: 10<br>TC: 0.2<br>R: 0–100 T<br>Sc-time: 20 | Deviation from 100%<br>$< 1\%$ | |
| Slit width | 400 m$\mu$ ⎫ PM: 1 ×<br>500 " ⎬ S: 10<br>600 " ⎭ TC: 0.2 | $< 0.10$ mm.<br>$< 0.05$<br>$< 0.05$ | |
| Noise level | 650–600 m$\mu$<br>S: 300<br>TC: 0.2<br>PbS<br>R: 0–100 T<br>Sc-time: 20<br>Set on approx. 95% T | Noise<br>$< 7\%$ | |
| 100% $T$ from 3000 to 700 m$\mu$ | PbS<br>S: 10<br>TC: 0.2<br>R: 0–100 T<br>Sc-time: 5 | Deviation from 100%<br>$< 1\%$ | |
| Slit width | 600 ⎫ PbS<br>800 ⎬ S: 50<br>1000 ⎬ TC: 0.2<br>2850 ⎭ | $< 0.10$ mm<br>$< 0.05$<br>$< 0.05$<br>$< 0.20$ | |
| Wavelength accuracy and resolving power | Slowly scan the atmospheric H$_2$O bands from 2.7–2.8 $\mu$<br>S: 300<br>Slit: 0.03 mm<br>TC: 0.6<br>Sc-time: 50<br>R: 0–100 T<br>"Energy" (single beam) | Transmission maximum at:<br>2722 m$\mu$ $\pm$ 2m$\mu$<br>minimum at:<br>2720 m$\mu$ $\pm$ 2 m$\mu$<br>$\dfrac{T\,(2722) - T\,(2720)}{T\,(2722)} > 0.25$ | |

\* Spruit, F. J., and Keuker, H.: A routine system of maintenance and performance tests for spectrophotometers (Beckman DK2 and DU). Phot. Spect. Group Bull., *16*:468, 1965.

Explanations of symbols used in Tables 2-9 and 2-10.

        S = sensitivity control (0—300 in arbitrary units).

        R = range selection (0—100% in transmission or 0—1 in absorbance).

      TC = time constant control (four positions available, 0.1, 0.2, 0.6, and 2.0).

Sc-time = scanning time (seven positions available, 1, 2, 5, 10, 20, 50, and 100 minutes).

    PbS = lead sulphide photocell.

    PM = photomultiplier (two sensitivity ranges available, marked ×1 and ×20).

      T = transmittance; A = absorbance.

  Note: 0—100% T implies setting *range switch* and *function switch*.

      PM×20 implies setting detector optics to PM and amplifier input to PM×20.

**Table 2-10.** **Checklist, Beckman DK2 Spectrophotometers, Ultraviolet (with Hydrogen Lamp)***

| Check for: | Settings and Conditions | Requirements | Result |
|---|---|---|---|
| 100% transmittance from 400 to 225 $m\mu$ | Record 100% T at<br>PM: $1 \times$<br>S: 50<br>R: 0–100 T<br>TC: 0.2<br>$H_2$-lamp<br>Sc-time: 5 | Deviation from 100%<br><br>$< 1\%$ T | |
| Slit width,<br>$H_2$ lamp | 220 $m\mu$   S = 50<br>240   ”<br>260   ”   PM = $1 \times$<br>300   ”<br>400   ”   TC = 0.2 | $< 0.7$ mm<br>$< 0.5$ mm<br>$< 0.4$ mm<br>$< 0.3$ mm<br>$< 0.3$ mm | |
| Limit of workable wavelength range | S: 300<br>PM: $20 \times$<br>$H_2$-lamp | slit width at 185 $m\mu$<br><br>$< 1.4$ mm | |
| Noise level | 350–300 $m\mu$<br>S: 300<br>PM: $20 \times$<br>TC: 0.2<br>R: 0–100 T<br>Sc-time: 10<br>$H_2$-lamp<br>Set on approx. 95% T | noise<br>$< 7\%$ | |
| Agreement between transmission and absorbance | R: 0–100 T and 0–1 A<br>S: 50; TC: 0.2 | Difference between T = 100% and A = O, $\triangle$ A $< 0.001$ | |
| Photometric accuracy | PM: $1 \times$<br>S: 50<br>R: 0–100 T and 0–1 A<br>$H_2$-lamp<br>ca 25 mg $K_2Cr_2O_7$/litre in 0.05 N KOH, 1 cm cell | E (1%, 1 cm) 275 $m\mu$: 190 $\pm 2$<br>373 $m\mu$: 249 $\pm 2$<br>at 20°C.<br><br>(calculated from both transmittance and absorbance) | |
| "Switch" point | as above<br>Set on wavelength at which T = 39.9% | 39.9% T = 0.399 A $\pm 0.001$ | |
| Wavelength accuracy | Record $H_2$ lines on "Energy" at slit width $\leqslant 0.02$ mm<br>379.9 $m\mu$, 399.1 $m\mu$<br>486.1 $m\mu$, 581.3 $m\mu$ | Tolerated deviation:<br>$< 0.3$ $m\mu$    $< 0.4$ $m\mu$<br>$< 0.5$ $m\mu$    $< 0.6$ $m\mu$ | |
| Resolving power in ultraviolet | One drop of benzene in 1 cm cell, slowly scan over 270 – 250 $m\mu$<br>PM: $1 \times$<br>S: 50<br>R: 0–100% T<br>TC: 0.2<br>Sc-time: 20 | $\dfrac{T\ (259.3) - T\ (259.5)}{T\ (258.4)} > 0.15$ | |

* Spruit, F. J., and Keuker, H.: A routine system of maintenance and performance tests for spectrophotometers (Beckman DK2 and DU). Phot. Spect. Group Bull., *16*:468, 1965.

DESICCANT. Failure to keep fresh desiccant in the instrument, particularly in the phototube house, may cause noise or drift. It is not sufficient to watch the indicating window for a color change and to assume, if none appears, that the desiccant is satisfactory. The container should be taken out, opened, and inspected. When fresh, the silica gel is dark blue; it changes to pink and then becomes colorless as it is spent.

The desiccant in the monochromator is not so critical as that in the phototube house. It should be changed every three months but does not need to be examined more frequently.

## XIII. *Desiccant*

1. Remove the plate on the phototube house and take out the desiccant container.
2. Look at the silica gel. If it is dark blue, mark "OK" on check sheet.
3. If it is not dark blue or if it has been in use 3 months, change it. If the latter is the case, also change the desiccant in the monochromator.

In testing specific functions of the Beckman DU spectrophotometer we have accumulated some information about symptoms, causes, and remedies. They are listed in Table 2-8. This list is far from complete, and is included to make it easier for other users to pinpoint difficulties they can easily correct.

## CHECK SYSTEMS FOR RECORDING SPECTROPHOTOMETERS

Cahn and Henderson published a check system for the Beckman DK spectrophotometer in 1958.[11] Their system was rather elaborate and appeared to be aimed more at proving the capabilities of the instrument than at checking the system daily or weekly. Twelve functional points were checked individually in the ultraviolet, visible, and infrared regions. The functions were 100% stability, 100% line; stray radiation; resolution; photometric accuracy; reproducibility; slit width, noise; zero stability; light leaks; electrical disturbance; and switching.

Spruit and Keuker worked Cahn and Henderson's criteria into a more practical weekly check system for the Beckman DK spectrophotometer.[56] Since the journal in which the system was printed is not readily accessible, Tables 2-9 and 2-10 are included to give a résumé of this check system. The authors note that the 100% T should be checked much more frequently than once a week; they also state that the complete instrument, including the monochromator, should be extensively inspected and cleaned once a year. Rectifier tubes should be checked every 3 months and other tubes every 6 months. Transmittance and absorbance slide wires should be cleaned every 6 months and replaced every 2 to 3 years.

Slavin recommends the following check system for the Perkin-Elmer Model 350 recording spectrophotometer:[53]

*Daily:*

REPRODUCIBILITY. Two scans of a material whose absorbance values cover a range of 1.5 A units.

WAVELENGTH. In UV, visible, and near IR using holmium filter (8 points noted).

PHOTOMETRIC SCALE. Visible with 3 thicknesses of Chance ON-10 filter; absorbance 0.2 to 2.0 with 9 bands noted. UV to NIR with metal screens, absorbance 1 and 2.

*Weekly:*

SOURCE ENERGY. Using the hydrogen lamp, record slit setting required.

STRAY ENERGY. With 2 M KCl.

RESOLUTION. Hg vapor using 3 slit widths.

This system is said to require about ½ hour for the daily and 1½ hours for the weekly procedures. Slavin considers the scheme detailed enough that it is highly unlikely that malfunctions will escape detection.

Edisbury has two additional points included in his weekly scheme for checking spectrophotometers.[18] He records the 100% T (or zero absorbance) and holds the tolerance to 1% T. If the reading exceeds tolerance, he checks mirrors on the beam chopper. His second check is valid only for instruments that have separate absorbance and transmittance presentations by either switch or cam arrangement). He scans the portion from 0.35 to 0.45 absorbance and then repeats as % T. A reading of 0.399 absorbance should equal 39.9% T and should not differ by more than 0.01 absorbance. He considers the check of photometric scale (reading a filter) necessary as a *daily* procedure.

Tarrant,[57] in his critique of results obtained on 94 recording spectrophotometers, concluded that thirteen possible causes can affect the absolute values: width of band (resolution); stray light; wedge effect in cells; cell cleanliness; sample purity; linearity of detector (in ratio-recording instruments); linearity of optical attenuator (in optical-null instruments); spillage of one beam into another (optically or electrically); faulty synchronization (optically or electrically); integrating time constant; lag, friction, and imbalance in the servomechanism; linearity of slide wires; and recording errors from such things as play in pen bearings.

## CHECK SYSTEM FOR THE BECKMAN DB SPECTROPHOTOMETERS

Since the Beckman DB spectrophotometer is a double beam instrument, errors caused by noise or drift and variations in source energy or detector sensitivity are greatly reduced. When the magnitude of such variables continues to increase, however, the instrument cannot compensate for them and they appear. The use of the instrument for scanning adds other variables such as programmed slits and automatically changing dynode voltages on the photomultiplier. Interrelationship between components makes it more difficult to pinpoint one specific cause for a change in a scan related to resolution, wavelength, etc. One must look at several check procedures together and compare them today with what they were previously.

The time table for frequency of specific check procedures will vary somewhat in institutions as the specific use of the instrument varies. Our spectrophotometer is used primarily for absolute absorbance changes in enzyme tests and scanning for substances such as amniotic bilirubin. After the operator has become thoroughly familiar with the spectra of holmium oxide and has seen changes as they parallel the more specific check procedures, he can, in our opinion, use this scan as a single *daily* procedure. Other weekly and monthly checks are indicated by the record sheets shown as Figures 2-23 and 2-24.

Our Beckman DB spectrophotometer is equipped with tungsten and deuterium lamps, and the 1P28 photomultiplier detector. The power supply is the Beckman #73600, and the recorder is the 5-inch Beckman linear log. There is always some lag in the recording of a reading seen on the spectrophotometer meter; we attempt to keep this at a minimum. We also keep the recorder synchronized with the meter needle rather than ignoring the meter and depending only upon the recording.

In preparation for the monthly check of the DB, we follow two procedures to assure that the recorder is operating properly:

1. Check the gain control of the recorder by measuring the dead band.[6]

   a. Press "Record" push button and set the recording at about 50%T with the spectrophotometer "Ref" control.

   b. With the pen recording, use a pencil to displace the pen holder about 2%T in one direction and then in the opposite direction. When released, the pen should return to its original line within 0.5%T.

2. Check the log vs. linear slide wire adjustment of the recorder:

   a. Set the recorder to "log" and at 500 m$\mu$, block the sample until the meter reads about 40%T (or 0.400 OD). Make the final adjustment with the 100%T adjustment knob.

   b. Switch the recorder to "linear." The line being drawn by the recorder pen should not move more than ± 0.5%T.

A few trouble-shooting ideas may be helpful. These are the most common problems we have seen:

1. Excessive noise (not seen on DB meter needle) is likely to come from defective settings of the gain and/or damper control.

2. "Stepping" is traceable to a weak amplifier or gain.

3. If the pen cannot be adjusted to the 0 and/or 100%T lines, the mercury battery is probably defective. This battery does not gradually weaken but suddenly ceases to function. It usually lasts about a year. The "spare" should be kept refrigerated.

The following check procedures for the Beckman DB spectrophotometer are separated into double beam (normal mode) and single beam operation for convenience in testing. Usually the technologist performs all the tests in double beam before switching to single mode.

71

WEEKLY CHECK

Instrument #_____

| Date | 0%T | Scan 700–205 mμ Set at 500 mμ | | | | | Single Wavelength | |
|---|---|---|---|---|---|---|---|---|
| | | 100%T | | | | | 0%T | 100%T |
| | | Max. Diff. | N* or D | 370 mμ | 220 mμ | | | |
| | 0.2%T | ±2.0%T | ±0.5%T | %T | %T | | | |
| | | | | | | | | |
| | | | | | | | | |
| | | | | | | | | |
| | | | | | | | | |
| | | | | | | | | |
| | | | | | | | | |
| | | | | | | | | |
| | | | | | | | | |
| | | | | | | | | |
| | | | | | | | | |
| | | | | | | | | |
| | | | | | | | | |
| | | | | | | | | |
| | | | | | | | | |
| | | | | | | | | |
| | | | | | | | | |

\* Noise and/or drift

**Figure 2-23.** *Weekly check sheet for Beckman DB spectrophotometer.*

FOR BECKMAN DB

Month_____     Year_____

| Holmium Filter | | | | | | Reed | Remarks |
|---|---|---|---|---|---|---|---|
| Wavelength | | | Reproducibility | Accuracy | Resolution | Vibrat | |
| 279.3 | 360,8 | 637.5 | %T diff. | %T, 637.5 m$\mu$ | Appearance 637.5 m$\mu$ | | |
| ± 0.7 | ± 1.5 | ± 4.0 | ± 0.5%T | ± 0.5%T | | | |
| | | | | | | | |
| | | | | | | | |
| | | | | | | | |
| | | | | | | | |
| | | | | | | | |
| | | | | | | | |
| | | | | | | | |
| | | | | | | | |
| | | | | | | | |
| | | | | | | | |
| | | | | | | | |
| | | | | | | | |
| | | | | | | | |
| | | | | | | | |
| | | | | | | | |
| | | | | | | | |

MONTHLY CHECK

Instrument # ____________________

| Date | Resolution | Linearity | | | Stray Light | | | Slit Operation | | |
|---|---|---|---|---|---|---|---|---|---|---|
| | B/A | 560 mμ | | | Vycor | Didymium | | Manual | Narrow | Zero |
| | | .3 ___ | .6 ___ | .9 ___ | 210 | 340 | 580 | 500 | 500 | 500 |
| | 0.6 ± 0.1 | < ± 0.005 | | | < 0.5%T | | | < .2 mm | .04 ± .02 | No diff. |
| | | | | | | | | | | |
| | | | | | | | | | | |
| | | | | | | | | | | |
| | | | | | | | | | | |
| | | | | | | | | | | |
| | | | | | | | | | | |
| | | | | | | | | | | |
| | | | | | | | | | | |
| | | | | | | | | | | |
| | | | | | | | | | | |
| | | | | | | | | | | |
| | | | | | | | | | | |
| | | | | | | | | | | |
| | | | | | | | | | | |
| | | | | | | | | | | |
| | | | | | | | | | | |

**Figure 2-24.** *Monthly check sheet for Beckman DB spectrophotometer.*

## FOR BECKMAN DB

Year _____

| Single Beam Operation | | | | | | Tech. | Remarks |
|---|---|---|---|---|---|---|---|
| D$_2$ lamp scan | | | Tungsten lamp scan | | | | |
| 656.3 | 720 | 595 | 700 | 595 | 350 | | |
| ± 4 m$\mu$ | %T | %T | %T | %T | %T | | |
| | | | | | | | |
| | | | | | | | |
| | | | | | | | |
| | | | | | | | |
| | | | | | | | |
| | | | | | | | |
| | | | | | | | |
| | | | | | | | |
| | | | | | | | |
| | | | | | | | |
| | | | | | | | |
| | | | | | | | |
| | | | | | | | |
| | | | | | | | |
| | | | | | | | |
| | | | | | | | |

## Double Beam Operation

### Reed Vibration Amplitude

Reeds must have enough amplitude to allow quick adjustment of the instrument from "Idle" to "On." When the amplitude is adjusted properly, a bright single line should be visible in the center of the swing.

---

### *Reed Vibration*

1. With the power switch in "On" position, shine a flashlight into sample compartment so that it lights the exit slits.
2. Peer down from above through the small hole in the center of the top of the sample compartment (over the exit slits).
3. If the center line is wide or appears double, consult the instrument manual for directions for adjusting the amplitude of vibration of the reeds.

---

The reed amplitude should not change from time to time, and for some instruments this check will need to be done infrequently. With other instruments it may need to be checked daily. Although the sample compartment (cuvette carrier portion) of the Beckman DB-G spectrophotometer can be lifted out, the user of the Beckman DB must *not* remove the sample compartment of that instrument. There is no separate cuvette carrier portion, and the whole compartment comes out in one piece. The alignment of the sample compartment is the means by which sample positioning is fixed. It is a critical adjustment, and once the permanent portion of the compartment has been removed, an experienced serviceman must use an oscilloscope to align the compartment.

If the reed adjustment is incorrect, it must be corrected at once. If it is allowed to continue to become further out of adjustment, the response of the instrument is decreased, instability of readings may occur, and then there may be no response at all.

### 0% T

The 0% T test is almost always satisfactory. In three years of checking, on only two occasions has the base line been known to drift on our Beckman DB. Vibrating mirrors that lost their synchronization caused the base line to drop below zero in the 700 to 600 m$\mu$ and in the 450 to 250 m$\mu$ regions. A weak or defective amplifier tube can cause spiking or irregularity of the zero base line.[7]

---

### *0% T*

1. With power control switch in "On" position, allow instrument to warm up 15 minutes.

2. Set wavelength at 500 m$\mu$; set programmed slit at "narrow."

3. With sample beam blocked, adjust meter to zero against air, using zero adjustment control.

4. Set wavelength at 700 m$\mu$ and scan to 205 m$\mu$. Switch to deuterium lamp at 350 m$\mu$.

5. Maximum difference allowable is $\pm 0.2\%$T (from value at 500 m$\mu$) and must be exactly the same at a single wavelength.

## 100% T

In our experience, the 100%T line has consistently dropped more than 2%T during the scan when the source lamp has needed replacing. If the tungsten lamp gets weak enough, the 637.5 m$\mu$ peak of the holmium oxide scan shows very poor resolution and even a shift in wavelength (discussed later under tungsten lamp scan). Changing the lamps when the 100%T line decreases more than 2%T

### *100% T, Noise, and Drift*

1. Set programmed slit at "narrow"; set 0%T with sample blocked.
2. Set 100%T against air at 500 m$\mu$.
3. Scan 700 to 220 m$\mu$. Switch to deuterium lamp at 350 m$\mu$.
4. Record readings at 370 and 220 m$\mu$.
5. The maximum difference allowable throughout scan is $\pm 2.0\%$T. It must remain exactly the same at any single wavelength. The noise allowed is $\pm 0.5\%$T.

avoids the wavelength shift for the 637.5 m$\mu$ holmium peak caused by the blackened lamp.

The 100%T line can also drop as the result of a dirty optical system, a weak detector, or a defective amplifier. Consult the manufacturer if changing the lamp or cleaning the optical system does not correct this problem.

## Wavelength with Holmium Filter

Major wavelength shifts have occured from vibration of the counter on which the instrument was sitting and from accidentally moving the adjustment of the

### *Wavelength with Holmium Filter*

1. Adjust 0%T and 100%T at 500 m$\mu$ against air, using the linear recording position.

*Continued on page* 78

2. Scan holmium glass filter from 700 to 250 mμ (cut in deuterium lamp at 350 mμ).

3. Locate and record mμ peaks for those listed as 279.3 mμ, 360.8 mμ, and 637.5 mμ.

4. Wavelength of peaks must be within the following specifications of those stated for the filter used with this instrument:[6]

| | |
|---|---|
| 279.3 mμ | ± 0.7 mμ |
| 287.6 mμ | ± 0.7 mμ |
| 333.8 mμ | ± 0.7 mμ |
| 360.8 mμ | ± 1.5 mμ |
| 418.5 mμ | ± 1.5 mμ |
| 536.4 mμ | ± 2.0 mμ |
| 637.5 mμ | ± 4.0 mμ |

On subsequent checks of the same filter, readings should be within the following range from those originally read on the same instrument:

220 to 234 mμ less than ± 0.35 mμ

335 to 574 mμ less than ± 1.0 mμ

---

collimating mirror. The shift for the 637.5 mμ holmium peak from the former cause was to 627 mμ and from the latter cause to 576 mμ. In both cases the resolution of this peak remained good. Notice in Figure 2-25 that this peak has two rather distinct notches on the long wavelength side. Loss of resolution sometimes is severe enough that this side of the peak is smooth. As was mentioned earlier, blackening of the tungsten lamp causes poor resolution and wavelength shift of this peak. It is extremely useful always to look at this peak and evaluate it qualitatively for loss of resolution and quantitatively for wavelength shifts. The 536.4 mμ peak has been reported as the first to reflect wavelength shifts in a prism instrument,[40] but we find the 637.5 mμ peak more useful.

On a few occasions we have had to use the holmium oxide filter to "correct" the wavelength adjustment. For this purpose the 536.4 mμ peak seems most useful. After such corrections we have had the manufacturer's serviceman check the wavelength at the earliest convenient time. Using a mercury pen light, he has always found our wavelength to be within specifications.

## Reproducibility with Holmium Filter

---

### *Reproducibility with Holmium Glass*

1. Back up the recorder and repeat scan of the holmium glass filter.

2. The two scan lines must be within 0.5%T of each other. Usually they will superimpose.

---

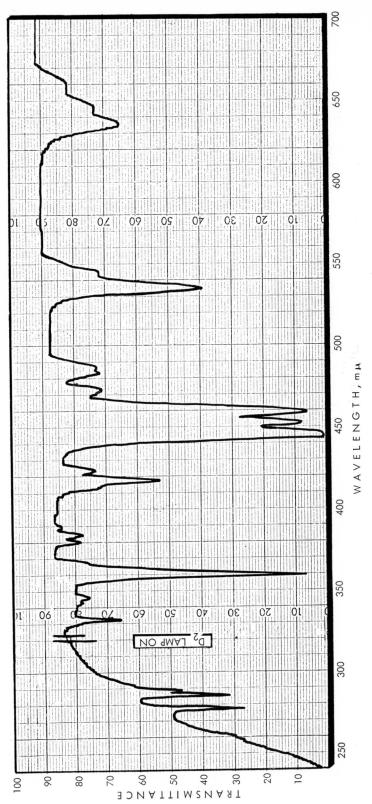

**Figure 2-25.** *Spectral transmittance for holmium oxide filter, using Beckman DB spectrophotometer.*

79

### Resolution with Holmium Filter

As has already been mentioned, a good idea of the resolution can be formed from glancing at the shape of the 637.5 mμ peak on this holmium scan. The peak obtained on the Beckman DB spectrophotometer will change its shape before a difference in the calculated ratio will appear. Recording the ratio of the B/A, however, provides a basis for comparison over a long period of time.

---

### Resolution with Holmium Filter

1. Using a scan already run with holmium glass filter, locate the doublet at 382 and at 387 mμ (Fig. 2-26).

**384 mu**

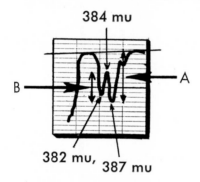

B ——→ ——→ A

382 mu, 387 mu

**Figure 2-26.** *Scan with holmium filter on Beckman DB spectrophotometer.*

2. Count the height (in spaces on graph) of A (the 387 mμ peak from its base).
3. Count the chart divisions representing the valley B (at 384 mμ).
4. Record the value for B/A.
   Tolerance: 0.6 ± 0.1.

---

### Accuracy with Holmium Filter

Testing accuracy would be more properly done with one of the National Bureau of Standards calibrated filters or a solution such as potassium chromate or copper sulfate. As has been pointed out earlier, this test and the linearity test check reproducibility more than accuracy. However, if the readings differ from those previously obtained, trouble exists, and one must stop to look for it. Slit hang-up was found after one such "trouble" alarm.

---

### Accuracy with Holmium Filter

1. Using the scan already run with holmium glass, locate the 637.5 mμ peak.
2. Read the %T of this peak and record it on the chart.
3. Look up the original value for this peak. The current value must be within ± 0.5%T of the original value or ± 1.0%T of the stated value of the filter.

---

## Linearity with Neutral Density Filters

Three filters with absorbance values of 0.3, 0.6, and 0.9 are available from Arthur H. Thomas Co. (#9104-N45). Since these filters are inexpensive, one may well doubt their reproducibility and/or their permanency. They have been demonstrated to be within the range of the reproducibility we get on our instrument. Figure 2-27 shows the scan of these filters from 760 to 360 m$\mu$. One could choose some other points to check the reproducibility of these filters, but we have used only the 560 m$\mu$ point. One surprising incident occurred in which we got 0.31, 0.62, and 0.93 in the morning; then on replacing the PM tube in the afternoon we got 0.301, 0.603, and 0.910.

---

### *Linearity with Neutral Density Filters*

1. Using the "log" recording position, adjust the zero absorbance against air at 500 m$\mu$.
2. Scan the 0.3 filter from 600 to 500 m$\mu$.
3. Back up the recorder to the starting point and repeat the scan with 0.6 and 0.9 filters on the same graph.
4. Record the absorbance of each at 560 m$\mu$ and note their proportionality.
5. Each filter's absorbance at 560 m$\mu$ must agree within $\pm$ 0.005 of its established value.

---

## Stray Light

Watching the holmium scan at 443 m$\mu$ has been suggested as a rough check for stray light if this peak pulls away from zero %T.[7] In our experience this is not a sufficient check. A Vycor reading of 2%T at 210 m$\mu$ has been registered while the holmium peak still hung at zero.

---

### *Stray Light*

*Ultraviolet*—using Vycor* filter.

1. Using the linear recording position, adjust the instrument against blocked sample cell for 0 and against air for 100%T, at 240 m$\mu$.
2. Scan the %T of the Vycor filter from 240 to 200 m$\mu$.
3. Record the %T at 210 m$\mu$ on the chart.
   Tolerance: must be less than 0.5%T.

*Visible*—using 7 mm didymium filter.

1. Adjust the instrument (linear recording) for 0 with sample blocked and for 100%T set against air at 360 m$\mu$.

*Continued on page* 83

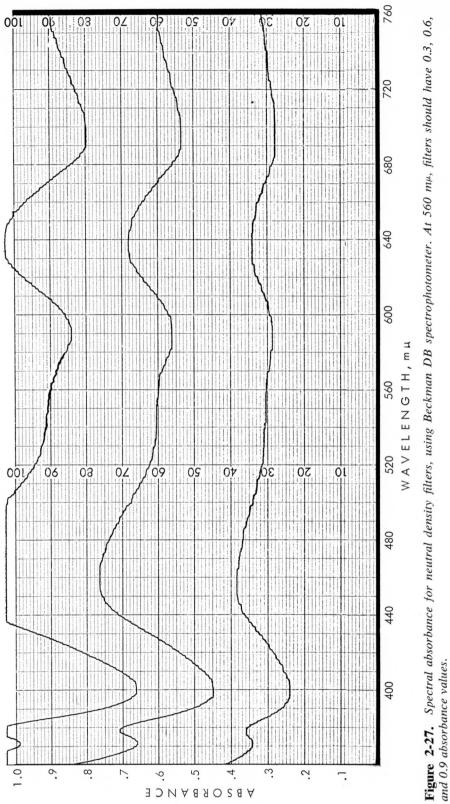

**Figure 2-27.** *Spectral absorbance for neutral density filters, using Beckman DB spectrophotometer. At 560 mμ, filters should have 0.3, 0.6, and 0.9 absorbance values.*

82

2. Scan the %T for the didymium filter from 360 mμ to 320 mμ.

3. Record the %T at 340 mμ on the chart.

4. Set 100%T vs. air at 500 mμ and scan the didymium filter from 600 mμ to 550 mμ.

5. Record the %T at 580 mμ on the chart.
   Tolerance: The value for 340 mμ and/or 580 mμ must be less than 0.5%T.

---

* Available from Beckman Instruments, Inc., Fullerton, Calif. as #95033.

The lack of sensitivity at the red end of the spectrum in the 1P28 photo-multiplier makes one very nervous about the stray light in this range. It would be desirable to use some filter to check stray light in the 650 to 700 mμ range, but we have not yet found a satisfactory one. A saturated solution of copper sulfate remains the only recommended check for this range.[7] Tolerance: less than 0.4%T.

The filters used automatically in the Beckman DB-G at specified wavelengths offer some protection against energy of extraneous wavelengths. These filters do not completely rule out the possibility of stray light for this instrument. We have not yet detected stray light, however, in our instrument for the 210 or 580 mμ checks.

## Slit Width of Programmed Slit

The actual slit width of the programmed slit is measured at a given wavelength. Any wavelength that is practical for the user may be chosen. The slit opening may be measured by two methods: (1) slit pickup and (2) equal %T. The slit pickup method is quicker but will give slightly less accurate results for the "narrow" program. The differences reflected in this method are those that result from the positioning of the cam follower and the slit-adjustment arm when the program slit selector lever is placed into the respective slot. When the selector is placed in the "medium" program, the angle of the slit-adjustment arm and the follower cam is changed. Unsatisfactory values for the slit settings are obtained when determined by slit pickup. The equal %T method is preferable for both program settings but must be used for the "medium" setting.

---

### Slit Width by Slit Pickup

1. Set the slit lever in "Narrow" position.

2. Set the wavelength at 500 mμ.

3. With the instrument ON, rotate the micrometer slit control CCW until you can feel a drag on the micrometer. This is the manual slit adjustment overriding the programmed slit and indicates the width in the operation.

4. Note the width indicated in millimeters on the micrometer. At 500 mμ the slit width should be 0.04 mm.

---

### Slit Width by Equal % T

1. Set the slit selector lever in the proper position.
2. Set the wavelength at any desired position.
3. Adjust the meter to read 50% T using the reference control.
4. Change the slit selector level to manual.
5. Open the slit micrometer until meter again reads 50% T. Read the setting in millimeters of the micrometer. This is the actual slit width of the programmed slit at the respective wavelength.

Obviously the range of settings for the various wavelengths is dependent upon the adjustment of the slit cam follower of a particular instrument at a particular time. The 500 m$\mu$ value for the "narrow" program given in the instruction manual is the only one specified by the manufacturer. The value of this check procedure is to know what slit widths are in use. If the slit program malfunctions, a difference in slit pickup will be detected.

## Manual Slit Opening (when manual slits are used)

The check procedure for manual slit opening is intended to detect a change in the sensitivity of the detector or a decrease in the efficiency of the optical system and source. The instruction manual for this instrument contains specific instructions for adjusting the manual slit zero.[4] The readings obtained for the slit opening will depend upon the zero setting of the manual slit for each instrument, and values obtained on other instruments may well vary from those given as our setting. The variation should be relatively small, however, if the instruments meet the specifications for slit zero (*i.e.,* ± 2 divisions from the zero mark on the micrometer).

### Manual Slit Opening

#### (*with manual slits*)

1. Set slit selector to manual slit opening position.
2. Set the micrometer slit adjustment on the zero stop position and note the background level of the meter.
3. Turn the micrometer adjustment in a CCW direction until the meter reading begins to increase.
4. The point at which this increase begins is the *manual slit zero position*. (Be sure to return the micrometer adjustment to zero stop before using the instrument in the programmed slit position).
   Tolerance: 0.02 mm or less.

## Function Tests Using Single Beam Operation

### *Slit Zero for Programmed Slit Operation*

1. Start with the instrument in double beam mode. Set 0%T with block in sample position, adjust 100%T against air at 500 m$\mu$.
2. Occlude the reference with block and set programmed slit. Switch to single beam.
3. Adjust to 100%T by use of dynode voltage control.
4. Switch to manual slit position with micrometer completely clockwise.
5. Needle should return to 0%T. If it does not, slits are hanging and should be serviced.

Another check for slit operation before calling for professional assistance is to switch the instrument into single beam mode, any wavelength, and set the slit adjustment micrometer on zero.[7] Open the slits 4 divisions on the micrometer and set the %T to read 20. Open the slits 4 more divisions and the %T should read 80 $\pm$ 10. Since the detector sees the square of the increase in slit opening, the increase in energy above should be $2^2$. If the detector is adequate, failure of the square law indicates inaccurate slit opening.

## Wavelength with Hydrogen or Deuterium Lamp

Beckman Instruments considers the check for wavelength with the hydrogen or deuterium lamp more accurate than the check with the holmium oxide filter. Figure 2-28 shows the spectral energy response of our deuterium lamp as currently adjusted. The sharp, strong peak at 656 m$\mu$ indicates a good check for wavelength adjustment. Much more information can be observed from this scan; in fact, the additional observations are more important than the wavelength parameter.

### *Wavelength with Hydrogen (or Deuterium) Lamp*

1. Lock the instrument into single beam operation by setting back panel switch to "Flame."
2. Occlude the reference beam with block provided with the instrument.
3. Turn on the hydrogen lamp.
4. Adjust the dynode voltage control until the instrument can show the hydrogen lamp energy "on scale" between 700 and 500 m$\mu$. This can be easily done by moving the wavelength setting by hand rather than by trying to record the scan. Once this dynode voltage range is found, set the 595 m$\mu$ peak to read at a specific %T and use this setting thereafter.

*Continued on page 87*

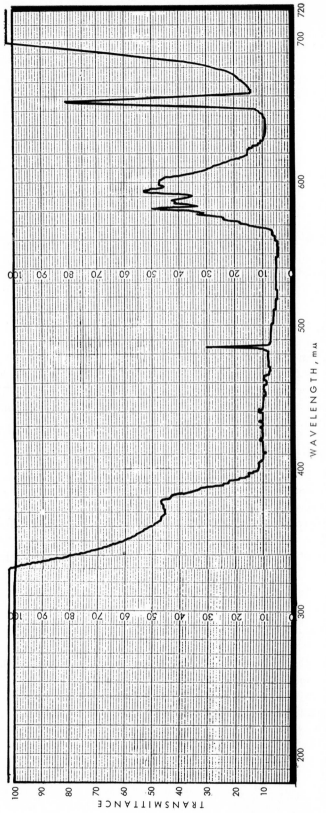

**Figure 2-28.** *Spectral transmittance for deuterium lamp, using Beckman DB spectrophotometer with relatively high dynode voltage adjustment.*

5. Scan 720 to 480 m$\mu$. Record %T for 720, 656, and 595 m$\mu$.
6. Record the m$\mu$ for the peak that occurs at 656.3 m$\mu$.*

---

* For most accurate results, measure the peak manually:
a. Find the 656.3 m$\mu$ peak and check its location several times.
b. Increase voltage to allow the peak to read midscale; the manual slit will be about 0.1 mm.
c. Check the exact position of the peak and read the m$\mu$ from the dial.

Note that the %T values for both the 700 m$\mu$ and 656 m$\mu$ peak are stronger than that of the 595 m$\mu$ range. The scan shown in Figure 2-29 is a prior recording of the same deuterium lamp and shows the differences caused by two changes made between recordings: (1) the dynode voltage on the photomultiplier was increased from 430 to 500 V; and (2) stray light (2%T with Vycor at 210 m$\mu$) was eliminated by changing the collimating mirror. Note the weak 700 and 656 m$\mu$ points of this scan compared to that of the 595 m$\mu$ range. The short 656 m$\mu$ peak of the scan in Figure 2-30 was the result of a tired photomultiplier tube. After replacement of this tube the 656 m$\mu$ peak returned to its normal height. As mentioned earlier, the neutral density filters had not read properly when this PM tube became weak, but they were immediately corrected by the change in the 1P28 tube. No specifications seem possible for response in terms of exact %T readings at specific wavelengths. However, comparison of relative responses for the same components over a period of time is very useful in isolating the cause of the response changes.

The exact contour of the hydrogen lamp spectrum is different from that of the deuterium lamp as shown in Figure 2-31. The wavelength at 656 m$\mu$ is said to be only slightly different for deuterium as compared to hydrogen lamps,[18] but the difference is insignificant for our purposes. The wavelengths we compare for the deuterium lamp response can also be compared for the hydrogen lamp. The scan shown for the hydrogen lamp in Figure 2-31 was taken during our first experience with the Beckman DB. It would have been helpful if we had had enough information at the time to question why that 656 m$\mu$ peak was so short.

## Tungsten Lamp Scan vs. Air

Scanning air with the instrument locked into single beam operation will detect a dirty source, an insensitive area on the detector, dirty or scratched mirrors, or a dead spot on the slit program or the wavelength cam. Any of these defects will cause a complete loss of signal, and the pen will travel toward zero.

---

### Tungsten Lamp

1. Set the switch on the back panel of the instrument to "Flame" to lock the instrument in single beam operation.
2. With the tungsten lamp on, set the meter to 95%T at 590 m$\mu$ using the dynode voltage control and the reference control on the front panel.

*Continued on page* 89

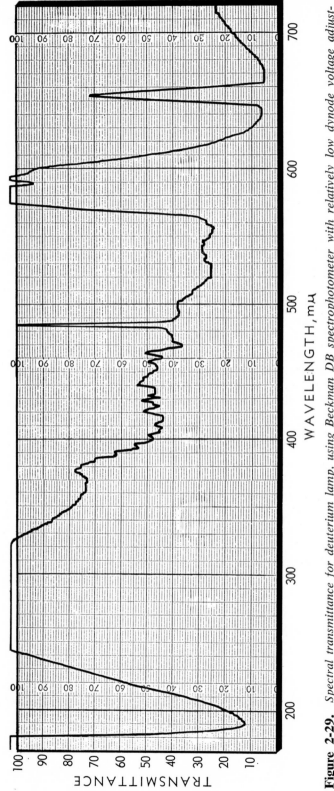
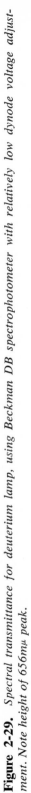

**Figure 2-29.** *Spectral transmittance for deuterium lamp, using Beckman DB spectrophotometer with relatively low dynode voltage adjustment. Note height of 656mμ peak.*

3. Scan from 760 to 320 m$\mu$. Record %T for 700, 595 and 350 m$\mu$.

4. The tracing should be continuous and relatively smooth. If gaps occur in the scan, the cause must be isolated or corrected.

---

The scan for tungsten energy shown in Figure 2-32 has the characteristics we have learned to designate as satisfactory. Note the relatively high energy level in the 700 m$\mu$ range as compared to that in the 595 m$\mu$ area. Incidentally, the entire spectrum cannot be kept on scale and since one must know what happens as the 320 m$\mu$ range is approached, a compromise scan results.

The high energy at 700 m$\mu$ is the direct result of replacing the PM tube. Increasing the dynode voltage on the PM tube (see the discussion of the deuterium lamp above) made no significant difference in the tungsten scan. The tungsten energy scan in Figure 2-33 shows our initial results with the Beckman DB. The energy scans were similar to this for almost three years, until the photomultiplier was replaced. The scan thereafter resembled that of Figure 2-32.

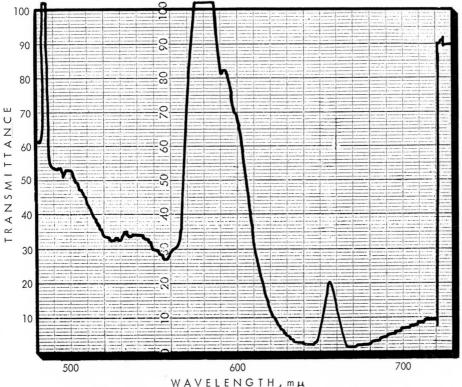

**Figure 2-30.** *Spectral transmittance for deuterium lamp, using Beckman DB spectrophotometer with weak 1P28 photomultiplier. Note height of 656 m$\mu$ peak.*

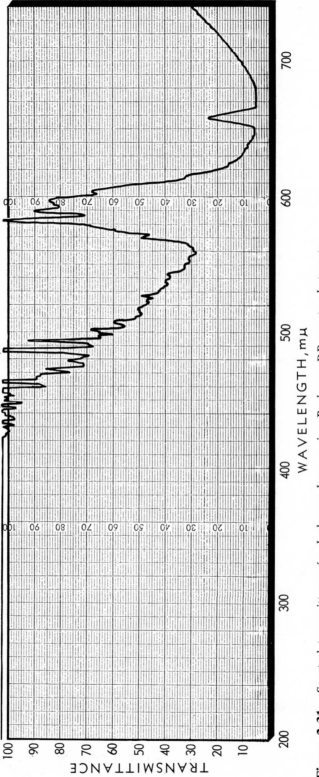

WAVELENGTH, mμ

TRANSMITTANCE

**Figure 2-31.** *Spectral transmittance for hydrogen lamp, using Beckman DB spectrophotometer.*

90

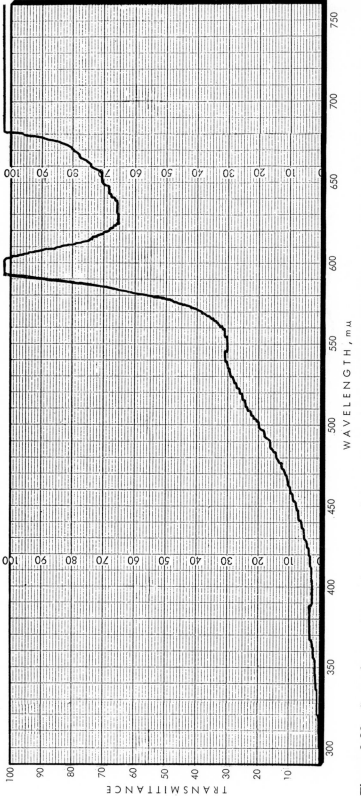

WAVELENGTH, mμ

TRANSMITTANCE

**Figure 2-32.** Spectral transmittance for tungsten lamp, using Beckman DB spectrophotometer. Note high sensitivity in 700 mμ range.

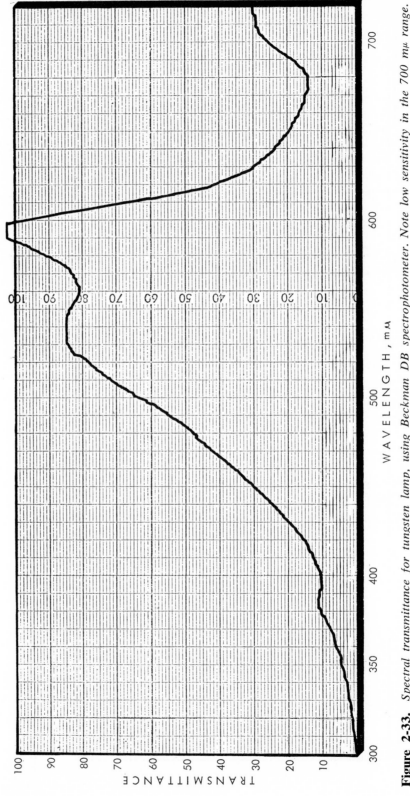

**Figure 2-33.** *Spectral transmittance for tungsten lamp, using Beckman DB spectrophotometer. Note low sensitivity in the 700 mμ range.*

Replacement of the tungsten lamp is required regularly at two to three month intervals. The first indication of defective function is the 100%T falling below specifications in the scan at the 350 m$\mu$ to about 320 m$\mu$ range. With continued use, the aging (or blackening) lamp in the Beckman DB causes the holmium oxide scan to show loss of resolution and even wavelength shifts. These effects of a defective tungsten lamp are shown in Figure 2-34. Initially this lamp was satisfactory, but its performance declined when it was used too long. On this scan note that the resolution of the 637.5 m$\mu$ peak is completely gone and that the peak appears at about 641 m$\mu$.

Another incident of defective lamp operation produced a scan similar to Figure 2-29 except that the 445 to 460 m$\mu$ peaks were not quite as unresolved and the 637.5 m$\mu$ peak also read 641 m$\mu$. The cause was not the lamp itself but a defective capacitor which reduced the voltage to the lamp to 2 volts.

## Daily Scan of Holmium Oxide

If the user conscientiously follows the weekly and monthly checks indicated on the check sheets (Figures 2-18 and 2-19), a scan of holmium oxide appears sufficient for *daily* checking. Observations of the 637.5 m$\mu$ peak can detect defective function of wavelength, resolution, and even stray light. This stray light in our instrument produced poor resolution (but proper wavelength for peak) of the 637.5 m$\mu$ peak which was not corrected by lamp change. In our experience observation of the 445 m$\mu$ peak (pulling away from zero[7]) has not been a satisfactory indication of stray light.

A weak hydrogen lamp produced the jagged curve in Figure 2-35. This alerted us to check the lamp further, and it was replaced.

## CHECK SYSTEM FOR THE BECKMAN DB-G SPECTROPHOTOMETER

The check system for the Beckman DB-G spectrophotometer is basically the same as that shown for the Beckman DB. However, there are different specifications for some of the tolerances, and thus some of the settings for the test procedure are necessarily different. Unless stated otherwise, the test procedures for the DB also apply to the DB-G. Only specific differences will be presented in this section.

Substitution of replica grating (1200 lines/mm at 250 m$\mu$) for the prism in the monochromator makes the DB-G different from the DB in two primary aspects: (1) practically uniform dispersion of about 2.75 m$\mu$/mm is produced, dispersion is slightly increased above 240 m$\mu$, and (2) the wavelength range has been extended to 190 m$\mu$.

The programmed slit cams for this instrument are labeled simply by numbers 1 and 2. Position 1 is used for the 1P28 photomultiplier and position 2 for the R 136. (Since our instrument has the 1P28, designation of programmed slit refers to position 1 throughout the check system).

93

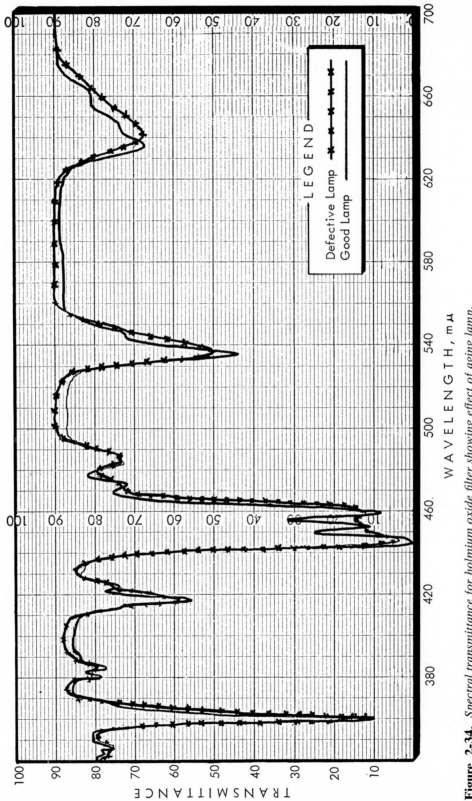

**Figure 2-34.** *Spectral transmittance for holmium oxide filter showing effect of aging lamp.*

94

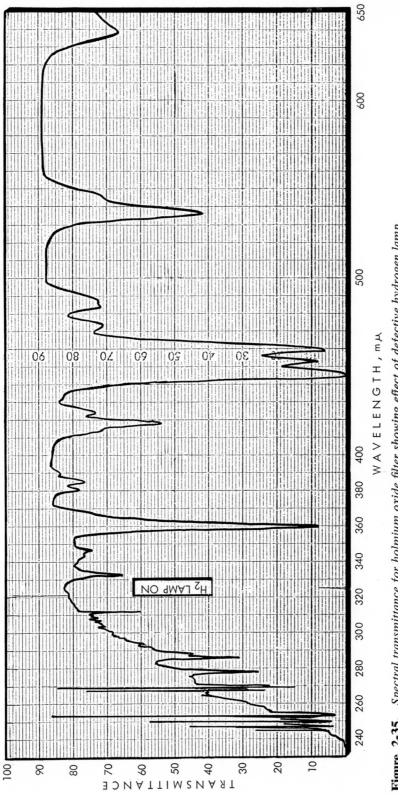

**Figure 2-35.** *Spectral transmittance for holmium oxide filter showing effect of defective hydrogen lamp.*

95

## Double Beam Operation

### Reed Vibration Amplitude

Reeds must have enough amplitude to allow quick adjustment of instrument from "Idle" to "On." When adjusted properly, the reeds appear as a single line in the center of the swing. Unlike the Beckman DB, the sample compartment (cuvette carrier portion) of the Beckman DB-G spectrophotometer can be lifted out, and the reeds then appear below, full length of the compartment area.

---

*Reed Vibration Amplitude*

1. With the power switch in "ON" position, lift the cuvette partition out of the sample compartment.
2. Look at the "line" the reeds make full length and about center in the bottom of the compartment. The line should appear narrow.
3. If the line appears wide (fuzzy) or double, adjust the reeds before using the instrument. Consult the instrument manual for directions.

---

The reed amplitude should not fluctuate from time to time. Although some instruments may need this check less frequently, fluctuation has been a consistent problem with the Beckman DB-G instrument in our laboratory, and we check these reeds every morning before doing anything else on the instrument.

### 0% T

Excessive base line noise has occurred from only two conditions with our Beckman DB-G instrument: (1) reeds not phased properly and (2) an occasional "blip" when the heater turns on in a nearby thermostated waterbath.

---

*0% T*

1. With power control switch in "ON" position, allow instrument to warm up 15 minutes.
2. Set wavelength at 500 m$\mu$; set programmed slit.
3. With sample beam blocked, adjust meter to zero against air, using zero adjustment control.
4. Set wavelength at 700 m$\mu$ and scan to 190 m$\mu$, cutting in the deuterium at 350 m$\mu$.

   Tolerance: $\pm 0.2\%$ T from value at 500 m$\mu$ and must be exactly the same at a single wavelength.

---

**100% T**

The flatness of the 100%T line seems directly related to the precise peaking of the source lamp, provided the source is adequate. The focus of the hydrogen or deuterium lamp is more critical than that for the tungsten lamp. Whenever the line does not appear straight, the ranges below 300 m$\mu$ and above 600 m$\mu$ read higher than 100%T (still within specifications). Considering the spectral energy scan of the tungsten lamp in Figure 2-40 (page 105), we think the curving line is caused by the 100%T having been set in the relatively weaker 500 m$\mu$ area. As the lamp ages, this area seems the first to show the results of further decreasing energy.

---

*100% T, Noise, and Drift*

1. Set programmed slit; set 0%T with sample beam blocked.
2. Set 100%T against air, at 500 m$\mu$.
3. Scan 700 to 200 m$\mu$, cutting in deuterium lamp at 350 m$\mu$.
4. Record readings at 370 and 200 m$\mu$.
   Maximum difference allowable throughout scan is $\pm$ 2.0%T and it must remain exactly the same at any single wavelength. Noise allowed is $\pm$ 0.5%T.

---

## Wavelength with Holmium Glass

A typical scan of the holmium filter on our Beckman DB-G is shown in Figure 2-36.

---

*Wavelength with Holmium Filter*

1. Adjust 0%T and 100%T at 500 m$\mu$ against air, using the linear recording position.
2. Scan holmium glass filter from 700 to 250 m$\mu$ and cut in the deuterium lamp at 350 m$\mu$.
3. Locate and record m$\mu$ peaks for those listed as 279.3 m$\mu$, 360.8 m$\mu$, and 536.4 m$\mu$.
4. Wavelength of peaks must be within the following specifications of those stated for the filter on this instrument:[4]

| | |
|---|---|
| 279.3 m$\mu$ | $\pm$ 0.5 m$\mu$ |
| 287.6 m$\mu$ | $\pm$ 0.5 m$\mu$ |
| 333.8 m$\mu$ | $\pm$ 0.5 m$\mu$ |
| 360.8 m$\mu$ | $\pm$ 0.5 m$\mu$ |

*Continued on page* 98

| | |
|---|---|
| 418.5 mμ | ± 0.5 mμ |
| 536.4 mμ | ± 0.5 mμ |
| 637.5 mμ | ± 0.5 mμ |

If there is a question whether a specific peak meets specifications, it is useful to recheck the wavelength in manual operation. A range of only ± 0.5 mμ is very difficult to maintain for recorded scans. The problem is usually in the recorder lag rather than in instrument maladjustment.

We have never seen the 637.5 mμ peak shift its wavelength when a tungsten source ages, even when the lamp has blackened. Such a response is consistent with the equal dispersion from the grating in this instrument.

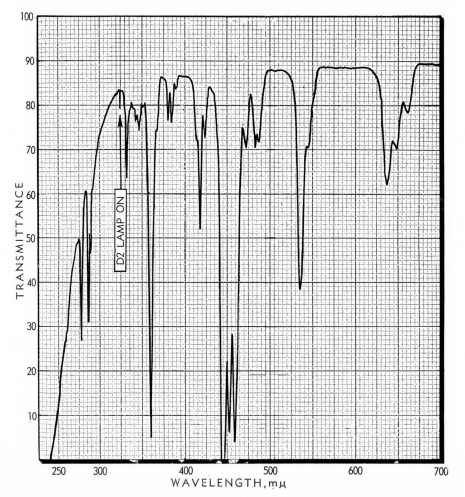

**Figure 2-36.** *Spectral transmittance for holmium oxide filter, using Beckman DB-G spectrophotometer.*

## Reproducibility with Holmium Glass

### *Reproducibility with Holmium Filter*

1. Back up the recorder and repeat scan of the holmium glass filter.
2. The two scan lines must be within 0.5% T of each other. Usually they will superimpose.

## Resolution with Holmium Glass

### *Resolution with Holmium Filter*

1. Using the scan already run with the holmium glass filter, locate the doublet at 382 m$\mu$ and 387 m$\mu$ (The doublet is shown in Fig. 2-37).

**Figure 2-37.** *Scan with holmium filter on Beckman DB-G spectrophotometer.*

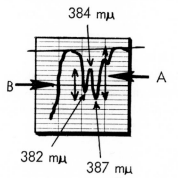

2. Count the height (in spaces on graph) of *A* (the 387 m$\mu$ peak from its base).
3. Count the chart divisions representing the valley *B* (at 384 m$\mu$).
4. Record the value for B/A.
   Tolerance: 0.6 ± 0.05.

## Accuracy with Holmium Glass

### *Accuracy with Holmium Filter*

1. Using the scan already run with holmium glass, locate the 536.4 m$\mu$ peak.
2. Read the %T of this peak and record it on the chart.
3. Compare with the original value for this peak. The current value must be within ± 0.5%T of the original, or ± 1.0%T of the stated value of the filter.

This value for %T reading has remarkedly constant for the same filter. Since filters differ a great deal (5%T to 8%T), the original value must be established for each individual filter.

### Linearity with Neutral Density Filters

Three filters with absorbance (OD) values of 0.3, 0.6, and 0.9 are available from the Arthur H. Thomas Co. (#9104-N25).

---

### *Linearity with Neutral Density Filters*

1. Using the "log" recording position, adjust the zero A against air at 500 mμ.
2. Scan the 0.3 filter from 600 to 500 mμ.
3. Back up the recorder to the starting point and repeat the scan with 0.6 and 0.9 filters on the same graph.
4. Record the A of each at 560 mμ and note their proportionality. Each filter's A at 560 mμ must agree within ± 0.01 of its original value.

---

### Stray Light

The filters used automatically in the Beckman DB-G at specified wavelengths offer some protection against energy of extraneous wavelengths. These filters do not completely rule out the possibilities of stray light in this instrument, but no stray light has been detected in our instrument at the 210 and 580 mμ checkpoints.

---

### *Stray Light*

*Ultraviolet*—using Vycor* filter

1. Using the linear recording position, adjust instrument against blocked sample cell for 0 and against air for 100%T, at 240 mμ.
2. Scan the %T of the Vycor filter from 240 to 200 mμ.
3. Record the %T at 210 mμ on chart.
4. This value must be less than 0.1%T.

*Visible*—using 7 mm didymium filter (Fig. 2-38).

1. Adjust the instrument (linear recording) for 0 with sample blocked, and for 100%T set against air at 360 mμ.
2. Scan the %T for the didymium filter from 360 to 320 mμ.
3. Record the %T at 340 mμ on chart.
4. Set 100%T vs air at 500 mμ and scan the didymium filter from 600 to 550 mμ.
5. Record the %T at 580 mμ on the chart.
6. The value for 340 and/or 580 mμ must be less than 0.1%T.

---

\* Available from Beckman Instruments, Inc., Fullerton, Calif. #95033.

100

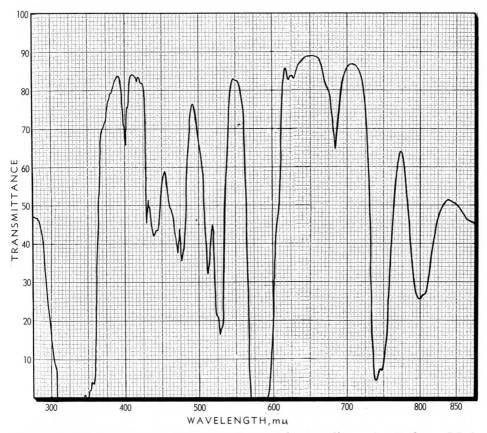

**Figure 2-38.** *Spectral transmittance for 7 mm didymium filter, using Beckman DB-G spectrophotometer.*

## Slit Width of Programmed Slit

The actual slit width of the programmed slit is checked at a given wavelength. The measurement of the slit opening may be done by two methods: (1) slit pickup and (2) equal %T. The slit pickup method is quicker but will give slightly less accurate results for the #1 program. The equal %T method is preferable for both programs but must be used for the #2 program setting.

---

### *Slit Width by Slit Pickup*

1. Set the slit lever in program position #1 (1P28 detector).
2. Set the wavelength at 500 mμ.
3. With the instrument "ON," rotate the micrometer slit control CCW until a drag is felt on the micrometer. This is the manual slit adjustment overriding the programmed slit and indicates the width in operation.
4. Note the width on the micrometer. At 500 mμ the slit should be 0.07 mm.

---

## Slit Width by Equal %T

1. Set the slit selector level in the proper position.
2. Set the wavelength at any desired position.
3. Adjust the meter to read 50%T using the reference control.
4. Change the slit selector level to manual.
5. Open the slit micrometer until the meter again reads 50%T. Read the setting of the micrometer in millimeters. This is the actual slit width of the programmed slit at the respective wavelength.

The program cam follower is adjusted to the slit width value of 0.07 mm at 500 m$\mu$ in both #1 and #2 programs. Other wavelengths may be checked as appropriate. A record of the entire range of the wavelengths of the program is a useful reference if problems arise.

## Manual Slit Opening for Manual Slit Operation

### Manual Slit Opening

1. Set slit selector to manual position.
2. Set the micrometer slit adjustment on the zero stop position and note the background level of meter.
3. Turn micrometer adjustment in a CCW direction until the meter reading begins to increase.
4. The point at which this increase begins is the manual slit zero position and should begin with setting of 0.01 mm or less. (Be sure to return micrometer adjustment back to zero stop before using slit as programmed.)

## Function Tests Using Single Beam Operation

### Slit Zero for Programmed Slit Operation

1. Start with the instrument in double beam mode. Set 0%T with block in sample position; adjust 100%T against air at 500 m$\mu$.
2. Occlude the reference with block and set programmed slit. Switch to single beam.
3. Adjust to 100%T by use of dynode voltage control.
4. Switch to manual slit position with micrometer completely clockwise.
5. Needle should return to 0%T. If it does not, slits are hanging and should be serviced.

### Wavelength with Hydrogen or Deuterium Lamp

The deuterium lamp scan for our Beckman DB-G instrument has a 656 m$\mu$ peak so intense that the whole scan in this area cannot be kept on the recorder graph. It is also impossible to tell the wavelength within 0.5 m$\mu$ from the chart. Therefore, this peak is identified manually, and the recorded scan is used for comparison of the source energy from time to time. Note in Figure 2-39 that the %T is above 100 at 430 m$\mu$. It remained at this level all the way to 190 m$\mu$. We originally included another scan with the gain reduced enough to show the top of the peak in the UV but deleted this step because it added nothing to the interpretation of source strength.

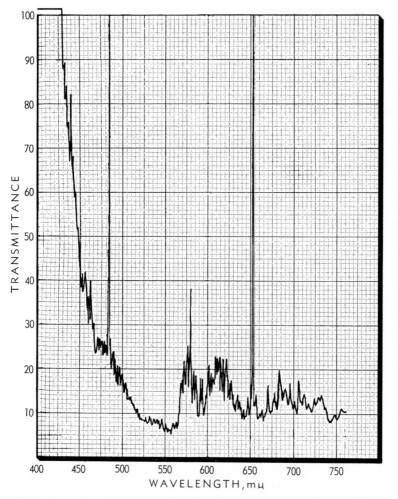

**Figure 2-39.** *Spectral transmittance for deuterium lamp in Beckman DB-G spectrophotometer.*

103

## *Wavelength with Hydrogen or Deuterium Lamp*

1. Lock the instrument into a single beam operation by setting back panel switch to "Flame."
2. Occlude the reference beam with block provided with the instrument.
3. Turn on the hydrogen lamp.
4. Adjust the dynode voltage control until the instrument can show the hydrogen lamp energy "on scale" between 700 and 500 m$\mu$. This is most easily done by moving the wavelength setting by hand rather than by trying to record the scan. Once the dynode voltage range is found, set the 579 m$\mu$ peak to read at a specific %T and use this setting thereafter.
5. Scan 720 to 480 m$\mu$.
6. Record the m$\mu$ for the peak that occurs at 656.3 m$\mu$.*
   Tolerance: 656.3 ± 0.5 m$\mu$.

---

\* For most accurate results, measure the peak manually.

## Tungsten Lamp Scan vs. Air

Scanning air with the instrument locked into single beam operation will detect a dirty source, a dead spot in the detector, dirty or scratched mirrors, or a dead spot in the slit program or the wavelength cam.

---

## *Tungsten Lamp Scan*

1. Set the switch on the back panel of the instrument to "Flame" to lock the instrument in single beam operation.
2. With the tungsten lamp on, set the meter to 15%T at 590 m$\mu$ using the dynode voltage control and the reference control on the front panel.
3. Scan from 760 to 320 m$\mu$. Record %T for 700, 595, and 350 m$\mu$.
4. The tracing should be continuous and relatively smooth. If gaps occur in the scan, the cause must be isolated and corrected.

---

A tungsten scan from our DB-G is shown in Figure 2-40. The %T adjustment for 590 m$\mu$ may differ on other Beckman DB-G instruments and for other lamps. This is the setting that allows us to get the full scan on the graph. The decreased %T in the 500 m$\mu$ region results from the filters in the instrument. As noted earlier, the %T in this range is further reduced as the lamp ages. The 100%T line will fall outside specifications quickly enough to detect aging of the lamp. The main reason for running this scan is to be sure the energy level is satisfactory in the 1P28 weak-response-region from about 600 m$\mu$ upward.

104

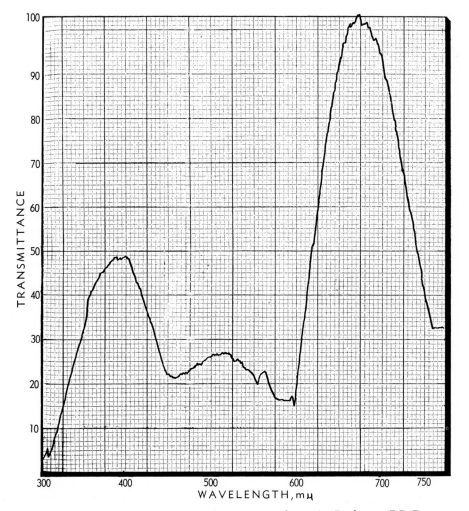

**Figure 2-40.** *Spectral transmittance for tungsten lamp in Beckman DB-G spectrophotometer.*

## REFERENCES

1. Aalund, O.: Adaptation of the LKB flow cell for the Beckman DB Spectrophotometer. Scand. J. Clin. Lab. Invest., *20:*93, 1967.

2. Ayers, G. H.: Evaluation of accuracy in photometric analysis. Anal. Chem., *21:*652, 1949.

3. Beckman Bulletin, 796A: Absorption cells. Beckman Intruments, Inc., Fullerton, Calif., August, 1964.

4. Beckman Instruction Manual, 566-E: Model DB Prism spectrophotometer and Model DB-G grating spectrophotometer. Beckman Instruments, Inc., Fullerton, Calif., June, 1966.

5. Beckman Instruction Manual, 305-A for DU: Beckman Instruments, Inc., Fullerton, Calif., September, 1964.

105

6. Beckman Instructions, 619-B: Laboratory potentiometric recorders. Beckman Instruments, Inc., Fullerton, Calif., July, 1963.

7. Beckman Instruments, Inc., Fullerton, Calif.: Personal communication.

8. Beeler, M. F.: Behavior of photocells. Amer. J. Clin. Path., *32:*140, 1959.

9. Buc, G. L., and Stearns, E. I.: Uses of retardation plates in spectrophotometry. I. Determination of slit shape and slit width. J. Opt. Soc. Amer. *35:*458, 1945.

10. ———: Uses of retardation plates in spectrophotometry. II. Calibration of wavelength. J. Opt. Soc. Amer., *35:*465, 1945.

11. Cahn, L., and Henderson, B. D.: Performance of the Beckman DK spectrophotometer. J. Opt. Soc. Amer., *48:*380, 1958.

12. Cannon, E. G., and Butterworth, I.S.C.: Beer's Law and spectrophotometer linearity. Anal. Chem., *25:*168, 1953.

13. Cary, H. H., and Beckman, A. O.: A quartz photoelectric spectrophotometer. J. Opt. Soc. Amer., *31:*682, 1941; reprinted as Beckman Bull. #6177, February, 1962.

14. Caster, W. O.: Variability in the Beckman spectrophotometer. Anal. Chem., *23:*1229, 1951.

15. Coleman Technical Report #T-198: A procedure for monitoring the performance parameters of Coleman Jr. spectrophotometers. Coleman Instruments, Maywood, Ill., February, 1965.

16. Copeland, B. E.: The National Bureau of Standards' Carbon Yellow filter as a monitor for spectrophotometeric performance. Amer. J. Clin. Path., *49:*459, 1968.

17. Eberhardt, W. H.: Slit-width effects in spectrophotometry. J. Opt. Soc. Amer., *40:*172, 1950.

18. Edisbury, J. R.: *Practical Hints on Absorption Spectrometry, Ultra-violet and Visible.* New York, Plenum Press, 1967.

19. Ewing, G. W., and Parsons, T., Jr.: Intercomparison of Beckman spectrophotometers. Anal. Chem., *20:*423, 1948.

20. Gibson, K. S.: Spectrophotometry (200 to 1000 millimicrons). National Bureau of Standards Circular #484. Washington, D. C., 1949.

21. ———: Standards for checking the calibration of spectrophotometers (200 to 1000 m$\mu$). National Bureau of Standards Circular #LC-1017, Washington, D. C. Reissued January, 1967.

22. ———, and Balcom, M. M.: Transmission measurements with the Beckman quartz spectrophotometer (R.P. #1798). J. Res. N.B.S., *38:*601, 1947.

23. ———, and Belknap, M. A.: Permanence of glass standards of spectral transmittance (R.P. #2093). J. Res. N.B.S., *44:*463, 1950.

24. Goldring, L. S., Hawes, R. C., Hare, G. H., Beckman, A. O., and Stickney, M. E.: Anomalies in extinction coefficient measurements. Anal. Chem., *25:*869, 1953.

25. Gridgeman, N. T.: Reliability of photoelectric photometry. Anal. Chem., *24:*445, 1952.

26. Hartree, E. F., Jones, J. I. M., and Gridgeman, N. T.: Second P.S.G. colllaborative test: potassium dichromate. Photoelectric Spect. Group Bull., *3:*61, 1950.

27. Haupt, G. W.: An alkaline solution of potassum chromate as a transmittancy standard in the ultraviolet (RP #2331). J. Res. N.B.S., *48:*414, 1952.

28. Heidt, L. J., and Bosley, D. E.: An evaluation of two simple methods of calibrating wavelength and absorbance scales of modern spectrophotometers, J. Opt. Soc. Amer., *43:*760, 1953.

29. Henry, J. B., Cestaric, E. S., and Goodwin, A.: A semiautomated system for clinical assays of enzymes. Amer. J. Clin. Path., *40:*252, 1963.

30. Hock, H., Turner, M., and Williams, R. C.: Straylight error in a spectrophotometer. Clin. Chem., 6:345, 1960.

31. Hogness, T. R., Zscheile, F. P., and Sidwell, A. E.: Photoelectric spectrophotometry, an apparatus for the ultra-violet and visible spectral regions: Its construction, calibration and application to chemical problems. J. Phys. Chem., 41:379, 1937.

32. Holiday, E. R., and Beaver, G. H.: Some practical aspects of the effects of stray radiation in spectrophotometry. Phot. Spect. Group Bull., 3:53, 1950.

33. Humes, C.: Personal Communication.

34. Johnson, E. A.: Potassium dichromate as an absorbance standard. Phot. Spect. Group Bull., 17:505, 1967.

35. Keegan, H. J., Schleter, J. C., and Belknap, M. A.: Recalibration of the NBS glass standards of spectral transmittance. J. Res. N.B.S., 67A: 577, 1963.

36. Kemmerer, A. R.: Report on carotene. Assoc. Offic. Agr. Chem. 29:18, 1946.

37. Lee, J., and Seliger, H. H.: Absolute spectral sensitivity of phototubes and the application to the measurement of the absolute quantum yields of chemiluminescence and bioluminescence. Photochem. Photobiol., 4:1015, 1965.

38. Miller, W. C., Hare, G., Strain, D. C., George, K. P., Stickney, M. E., and Beckman, A. O.: A new spectrophotometer employing a glass Fery prism J. Opt. Soc. Amer., 39:377, 1949.

39. McDaniel, J. B. Collodion technique of mirror cleaning. Appl. Optics, 3:152, 1964.

40. McNeirney, J., and Slavin, W.: A wavelength standard for ultraviolet-visible-near infrared spectrophotometry. Appl. Optics, 1:365, 1962.

41. National Bureau of Standards: Optics Metrology fee schedules, photometry. #212.141a. Washington, D. C., June, 1968.

42. O'Connor, R. T., Chairman: *Manual on Recommended Practices in Spectrophotometry,* ASTM Comm. E-13 Report. Philadelphia, Amer. Soc. for Testing and Materials, 1966.

43. Perry, J. W.: Sources and treatment of stray light in spectrophotometry. Phot. Spect. Group Bull., 3:40, 1950.

44. Rand, R. N.: Practical spectrophotometric standards. Clin. Chem., 15:839, 1969.

45. Rawlings, H. W., and Wait, G. H.: Factors affecting the reliability and precision of the spectroscopic determination of Vitamin A. Oil and Soap, 23:83, 1946.

46. Reule, A.: Testing spectrophotometer linearity. Appl. Optics, 7:1023, 1968.

47. Rosenbaum, E. J., Chairman.: Proposed Methods for evaluation of spectrophotometers, Report of ASTM Comm. E-13. Proceedings, Amer. Soc. for Testing and Materials, June, 1958.

48. Royer, G. L., Lawrence, H. C., Kodama, S. P., and Warren, C. W.: Manual and continuous recording attachments for the Beckman Model DU spectrophotometer. Anal. Chem., 27:501, 1955.

49. Sager, E. E., and Byers, F. C.: Spectral absorbance of some aqueous solutions in the range of 10° to 40°C. (RP #2731) J. Res. N.B.S., 57:33, 1957.

50. Saidel, L. J., Goldfarb, A. R., and Kalt, W. B.: False absorption bands in the region of 200-230 m$\mu$ caused by stray radiation in the Beckman spectrophotometer. Science, 113:683, 1951.

51. Service Dept., Scientific Products: Personal communication.

52. Slavin, W.: Optimum photometric range of ultraviolet spectrophotometers. Appl. Spectrosc., 19:32, 1965.

53. ———: Performance evaluation of spectrophotometers in the ultra-violet, visible and near infrared. Presented to Eastern Analytical Symposium, New York, November, 1962.

107

54. ———: Photometric standard for ultra-violet-visible spectrophotometers. J. Opt. Soc. Amer. *52:*1399, 1962.

55. ———: Stray light in ultraviolet, visible and near infrared spectrophotometry. Anal. Chem., *35:*561, 1963.

56. Spruit, F. J., and Keuker, H.: A routine system of maintenance and performance tests for spectrophotometers (Beckman DK2 and DU). Phot. Spect. Group Bull., *16:*468, 1965.

57. Tarrant, A. W. S.: Some comments on the findings of the collaborative test. Phot. Spect. Group Bull., *16:*458, 1965.

58. Tunnicliff, D. D.: Measurement of nearby stray radiation in ultraviolet spectrophotometers. J. Opt. Soc. Amer., *45:*963, 1955.

59. Vandenbelt, J. M.: Holmium filter for checking the wavelength scale of recording spectrophotometers. J. Opt. Soc. Amer., *51:*802, 1961.

60. ———: Investigation of screens as spectrophotometric absorbance standards. J. Opt. Soc. Amer., *52:*284, 1962.

61. Walker, I. K., and Todd, H. J.: Wavelength calibration of spectrophotometers. Anal. Chem., *31:*1603, 1959.

62. Wernimont, G.: Evaluating laboratory performance of spectrophotometers. Anal. Chem., *39:*554, 1967.

63. White, J. M., and Witter, R. F.: Principles of spectrophotometry. U. S. Dept. of Health, Education and Welfare, Public Health Service, NCDC, Atlanta, 1966.

64. Winstead, M.: A check system for proper function of the Beckman DU spectrophotometer. Amer. J. Med. Techn., *32:*35, 1966.

65. ———: Spectral transmittance and the "aging bulb" problem; effect of "frost" on the exciter bulb. Amer. J. Med. Techn., *28:*67, 1962.

# 3

# AutoAnalyzers

The basic AutoAnalyzer* system introduced in 1957 was the first of a series of automated analytical instruments. The continuous-flow concept, using individual modules for specific functions, was originally assigned to single test procedures for batch runs—the single channel unit.[11] The dual channel soon incorporated two test procedures usually requested on the same blood sample. In this use, the AutoAnalyzer system produced sample test values which were read from a calibration curve constructed from several standards. While the curve was not always linear, the accuracy of values usually was better than could be obtained by the same methods run manually.

The SMA* systems, Sequential Multiple Analyzers, use only one standard, and the calibration curve is a computerized comparison to the standard. While the manufacturer introduced these models as screening devices, common use has tended to accept them as replacements for routine quantification methods. With the ever increasing demand for more test values at a faster rate, each laboratory must decide what accuracy it will maintain while attempting to speed up procedures. Many references in the literature indicate that some individual users have chosen to set up their own multichannel systems using combinations of the basic unit. These systems retain the multiple standard calibration curve and usually require only a slightly longer period of time than the SMA.

There is no doubt that the continued demand for more and more test values will cause ever increasing use of automated systems. As Reece has pointed out:

---

* Technicon Corp., Tarrytown, N. Y.

110

"poorly controlled automated methods can turn out spurious results with lightning speed."[9] Properly controlled, each system—the basic single or dual channel, the multi-channel modification of the basic unit, and the single standard multi-channel screening unit—has valid contributions to make. It remains for us, as users, to choose the unit for the use we want to make of it and to monitor the system closely enough to obtain the accuracy level for which the unit is capable.

## BASIC AUTOANALYZER SYSTEM

When a test is run on an AutoAnalyzer, aspiration of the sample for an extended period of time produces a steep rise on the recorder graph from the base line of the curve to a maximum. A steady state response is recorded, and then after the probe has been removed from the sample, there is a characteristic fast fall that returns the pen to the base line. Evaluating the peaks on the recorder graph requires identification of the characteristics of the curve. This basic curve is shown in Figure 3-1, as A. The *rise curve* is the left side of this curve, the *steady state* at the top, and the *fall curve* at the right side. If the sample is aspirated for less time than is required to reach steady state, sharper and lower peaks result for the same sample concentration. Shown as B in Figure 3-1 are the resulting peaks for aspirations of 8, 10, and 15 seconds as compared to the steady state which was reached in 20 seconds. The shape of the rise curve for each is the same, as are the shapes of the fall curves. Only the peak height differs, and this height is directly dependent upon the sampling time.

111

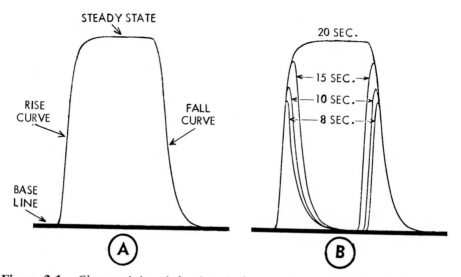

**Figure 3-1.** *Characteristics of the AutoAnalyzer peak curves. (Adapted from Thiers, R. E.: Clin. Chem. 13:451, 1967.)*

## % Steady State

As long as the sampler is able to maintain the exact sampling time for each specimen (*i.e.,* the same % steady state) the sampling rate can be considerably faster than could be used if steady state was attained by each specimen. Note in Figure 3-2D that the steady state for the 250 mgm glucose standard reads 85% T. The three peaks shown as C are the same standard, but the sampling rate of 60/hr causes the peaks to record approximately 77% T. The peaks produced by each test procedure should be checked for their % steady state (%SS) because small variations in sampling time will affect the apparent concentration of samples. If a sampler's cams are improperly made or become worn, the sampling time will vary. Sampling time can also vary as a function of the height of the sample in the cup.[13] For samples well in excess of the nominal amount required, significant errors can occur if the sample height for all specimens and standards is not similar. When small amounts of sample are used, the volumes of samples and standards become critical and they should be identical.

When the %SS is consistently checked, a sudden large difference in the percentage would be sensitive indication of malfunction that requires maintenance or repair.

---

### Calculation of % Steady State (%SS)

1. Read the base line %T and designate as "b."
2. Choose a standard for the test procedure which spans approximately 75% T.

3. Aspirate the standard for 5 minutes. Note the %T of the steady state response and designate as "S."
4. Allow the pen to return to the base line and set the sampling rate at the speed used routinely for the test procedure.
5. Run three consecutive cups of the same standard used for recording steady state. Note the %T for these peaks and designate as "X."

$$\% \, SS = \frac{\text{routine peak response}}{\text{steady state response}} \times 100 = \frac{X - b}{S - b} \times 100$$

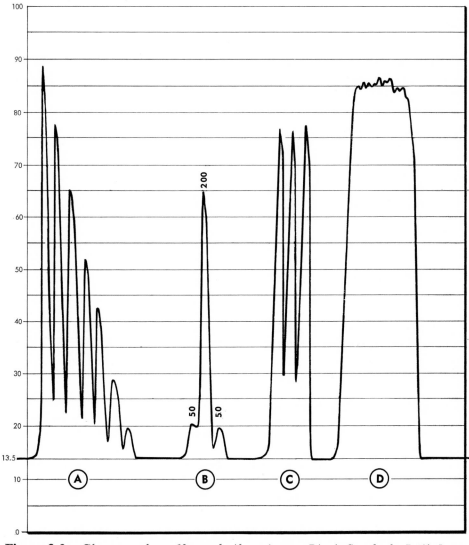

**Figure 3-2.** *Glucose peaks at 60 samples/hour (except D). A. Standards. B. % Interaction. C. % Steady state and reproducibility. D. Steady state and % noise.*

The faster the sampling rate, the lower %SS will be attained by the peaks and the more critical the actual sampling time. Young *et al.* have reported that Sampler I showed little variation in duration of sample aspiration even at 60/hour, while Sampler II showed progressively more variation with increase to maximum sampling rate.[18]

Originally, Technicon Company suggested that a "stat" sample be aspirated continuously in order to interrupt the routine run without causing the operator to get the sampling order for specimens mixed up. With the current use of faster sampling rates that produce peaks at lower %SS, this procedure can no longer be used.

### Noise

The usual allowable limit for noise is ±1%T measured peak to peak along the plateau formed by steady state response. It is convenient to note the noise and calculate it in %, using the steady state response which was run to calculate the routine peak %SS. Figure 3-2 D shows a higher noise level than ideal but still within tolerance.

---

### % Noise

1. Aspirate a standard for 5 minutes to produce a steady state plateau.
2. Note the highest %T traced by any noise (U) and the lowest %T (L). Note the mean between the two(M).

$$\% \text{ Noise} = \frac{U-L}{M} \times 100.$$

Noise level should not exceed about 2%.

---

The frequency and the regularity of the noise pattern should be observed in addition to its magnitude.[14] High frequency noise usually is caused by bubble pattern or pumping variations; low frequency noise can result from an electronic malfunction, *e.g.,* the heating bath on-off cycling.

### Carry-over or % Interaction between Samples

When a high concentration of any test sample precedes a sample of much lower concentration, "swamping" or obvious obliteration of the sample peak occurs. This is not hard to detect because there is no valley between the peaks. However, without washout between samples there is some interaction between all samples, and this often cannot be detected by the graph.[2] The higher the sampling rate, the greater the interaction or %I. The %I usually does not vary widely during any one run and usually remains constant during any one day.[13] Rather wide variations can occur from day to day. The %I is expected to be affected by only the sampling rate and not by the sample aspiration rate.[12] The wash-time

114

between samples greatly decreases the %I with the Sampler II, but the actual amount of interaction should still be calculated each day for each procedure. Bennet *et al.* believe that the degree of interaction should be calculated for each run.[2] A typical example of interaction is shown at B in Figure 3-2.

---

### % Interaction between Samples[2]

1. Choose a low and a high standard for the test procedure, *e.g.*, 50 and 200 mgm% glucose.
2. Using the routine sampling rate for the test procedure, run the standards as low, high, low in consecutive cups. Take their respective concentration values off the calibration curve.

$$\%I = \frac{L_2 - L_1}{H} \times 100$$

---

Interaction can be minimized by careful construction of the manifold.[14] The entire manifold system should be as short as possible, *i.e.*, no excess tubing or coils. The length of any sample stream that is not air-segmented, *i.e.*, the sample pick-up line, should be as short as possible. Connections should be tight, and ends of cut tubing should be straight and snugly fit together. Any dead or irregularly shaped spaces will not be properly cleaned by the air bubbles in the flow stream. In some systems, substitution of all glass tubing for Tygon* will reduce interaction. Frequent changing of the dialyzer membrane also minimizes carry-over.[2] Buildup of a fibrin film on internal surfaces increases interaction in systems using plasma.

### Repeatability

Repeatability is usually defined as the ability to obtain the same response for the same sample within the same run.[6] Reproducibility or precision is calculated from the same sample (or pool) run on different days.

Repeatability is checked by running a single sample in three consecutive cups. With a washout between samples, the AutoAnalyzer should produce peaks within 1% for all three samples. The peaks for replicate standards shown as C in Figure 3-2 demonstrate proper repeatability; if repeatability is checked in this manner, time can be saved by using the replicate peaks to calculate the %SS. We prefer to use a serum sample for this test. We run the same serum sample in three consecutive cups at the beginning of the run and then repeat the procedure at the end of the run.

### Drift

The effect of drift upon the sample values must be considered from two standpoints: base line drift and a change in the chemical sensitivity of the method.[2]

---

* U. S. Stoneware Co., Akron, O.

Drift may continue for long periods in the same direction, or it may change direction in a somewhat random fashion. More often, however, base line drift and method (or calibration) drift are in the same direction.

Base line drift is customarily checked periodically within the run by allowing the pen to return to the base line. The effect of base line drift upon the calibration curve is a shift of constant magnitude. Calibration drift represents a change in the proportional heights of the standard peaks and thus requires repetition of the set of standards periodically within the day's run. The sample values must then be taken from the corrected curve. In order to monitor this drift closely, a single drift-control-standard is repeated in every tenth cup within the run.[13] Since the magnitude of change is not a constant. Bennet *et al.* recommend that a different standard be used in rotation for the drift-control-standard.[2] They also caution that computer interfaced AutoAnalyzer systems must have a separate specific formula for the characteristic curve of each test procedure and that complete drift correction over the whole range of assay values requires drift-control-standards at a minimum of four concentration levels.

Possible causes of drift include: insufficient warm-up period, change in room temperature, or change in speed of an overloaded pump.[2] Frequently, however, the exact cause of drift in individual runs is not identified; often, in these instances, routine maintenance procedures are performed and drift is not detected in the next runs.

## Standardization

With the increasing use of automated methods, standardization has become extremely important if we are to achieve the necessary precision and accuracy for these methods. Standard reference materials* must be used as a base to which routine standards can be compared in order to provide "physiologic interpretations and comparisons of patient data acquired at different times by the same or different laboratories."[17] These materials are just becoming available, but more are being added each year. However, these materials are so costly that clinical laboratories must check secondary standards against them and use the secondary standards routinely. The standards available from the College of American Pathologists are less expensive and more adaptable for smaller laboratories.

Since no primary standards are available for enzymes, the best one can hope to achieve for these tests is reproducibility and clinical correlation. Commercial reference sera for LDH, SGOT, alkaline and acid phosphatase, and amylase have recently been criticized by Dobrow and Amador.[5] They suggest using a large batch of pooled frozen or lyophilized serum whose value has been established by reference methods; periodically this pool should be checked by a reference laboratory for decay of enzyme activity. Our experience with pools and commercial preparations is that we need *both*. The levels for concentration need to be both normal and elevated to detect the problems that arise.

---

* Available from National Bureau of Standards, Washington, D. C.

It is the responsibility of the individual laboratory to determine that the routine standards used for the AutoAnalyzer system do meet their own chosen level of accuracy before and throughout use. On one occasion we found that a commercially prepared standard had a glucose value of 30% in error. Reagents should be checked before being put into routine use. We substitute one reagent at a time and run a calibration curve and five patients' sera of varied concentration levels.

We have found that water used to prepare standards and reagents has significantly affected the test values. [16]

---

### Minimum Specifications for Water Quality

**DEMINERALIZED WATER**

| | |
|---|---|
| Silica | $< 0.1$ ppm |
| Resistance | No less than 1,000,000 ohms |
| Ammonia nitrogen | $< 0.2$ ppm |
| Alicaligenes/pseudomonas | Minimal |
| Sodium | Negative |
| PH | 6.0 to 7.0 |

**DISTILLED WATER**

| | |
|---|---|
| Free carbon dioxide | $< 5$ ppm |
| Hardness | Negative |
| Ammonia, nitrogen | $< 0.1$ ppm |
| pH | 5.5 to 7.0 |
| Metals | $< 0.01$ ppm |
| Resistance | No less than 100,000 ohms |

---

Five to seven concentrations for each standard have been the usual practice with the basic AutoAnalyzer system. Establishment of linearity in this manner is necessary if the test values are to be assigned specific values. Repetition of the set of standards at an interval of 40 cups is necessary because of the usual drift or changes in dialysis due to coating of the membrane. A repeat standard in every tenth cup serves not only to monitor the standard's value but to demonstrate the validity of the assignment of numbered peaks to patients.

The standardization process must include establishing values for precision within run, random duplicates, precision between runs on the same day, precision on consecutive days, accuracy as compared to reference methods, linearity, carryover, drift, stability of sera and reagents, clinical correlation, and establishment of normal values.[6] Each user must choose the details of these procedures to fulfill his own criteria, and the literature has many variations of such reports. We could all profit by attempting to modify the AutoAnalyzer methods to conform to our own choice of reference methods rather than by accepting those given us and making our routine methods conform to the AutoAnalyzer. Using an interfaced

117

computer system, Bennet *et al.* have derived individual formulas for each specific test, depending upon the calibration curve obtained with multiple standards.[2] They point out that correction for drift requires a minimum of standards at four levels of concentration. Hagenbusch, with his own flexible multichannel unit, also bases corrections on a combination of interaction curve and drift curve using a seven point standard curve.[7] Lack of adequate standards of multiple constituents has been pointed out as the major problem in controlling accuracy for the automated battery of tests.[9]

Daily operation for those not using the interfaced computer system should include steady state, % steady state for sampling rate, % noise, % interaction, standard curve, repeatability (3 aliquots), base line drift, repeat one standard every ten cups, repeat the set of standards every forty cups. The work sheet should also include dates for manifold, reagents, and standards; aperture size; setting on potentiometer; base line % T; temperature of dialyzer and heat bath.

## Troubleshooting, Checking and Maintenance by Module

While there is some overlap in symptoms caused by malfunction within different modules, the specific module can usually be isolated by tracing a bubble pattern change or some other specific symptom. Any module containing a motor, chains, or gears has its own characteristic noise that will change when a problem arises. It is highly recommended that the operator become familiar with each module's noise and be able to detect a different sound. White *et al.* use a physician's stethoscope to detect noise levels that are not evident to the ear.[15] By placing the rubber-edged cone to the top or side of the module, an alert operator can determine if there is some foreign noise. The comprehensive discussion by White *et al.* of the mechanical parts of the modules with suggestions for maintenance and repair is of great assistance to both users and institutional service personnel. Only a few of these mechanical problems are included in this troubleshooting section.

Troubleshooting is much easier if adequate records are routinely kept as part of the quality control program. In fact, regulations for Medicare and the Clinical Improvement Act as well as the College of American Pathologists' laboratory accreditation surveys require that a benchbook be kept for each instrument to indicate maintenance and service performed. The information pertaining to Auto-Analyzer Systems should include:

1. Date reagents and standards were made and checked out; reagent base line where applicable.
2. Apertures used in colorimeters for each procedure.
3. Age of manifold—*i.e.*, date made and put into use.
4. Date each module was thoroughly cleaned and oiled if necessary.
5. Date dialyzer bath was cleaned, tubing changed, and water changed; also cycle for on-off of heating element.
6. Temperature of heating bath; cycle of on-off of heating element; date fluid in bath was changed; age of coils and volume capacity of each.

118

7. Date of cleaning and aligning flow cell in colorimeter; date exciter lamps were changed.

8. Date of recorder slide wire cleaning; change in gain if required; date pens were cleaned.

9. Date any module was repaired and details of what was done.

Every laboratory using AutoAnalyzers should have readily available a copy of *Practical Automation for the Clinical Laboratory,* by White, Erickson and Stevens,[15] which has an excellent discussion of operation and maintenance of each module. Information concerning the mechanical parts of the modules is, to our knowledge, not available elsewhere. The illustrations and pictures make this book also useful in teaching students. Unless stated otherwise, the greater part of the modular troubleshooting to follow is abstracted from this book.

## Sampler

The recorder graph shown in Figure 3-3 demonstrates several problems usually associated with the sampler function. The normal function produced A, the set of standards, followed by two satisfactory specimens from patients. Peak B was caused by a hole in the sample cup, which allowed the specimen to leak out until an insufficient amount was present for adequate sampling. Peak C was caused by a partial plug in a reagent line which flushed out; both C and the following sample should be repeated. The base line of such magnitude as is shown in D is usually caused by a change in balance within the electronic system. The exact cause must be isolated, if possible, before running the system again. However, at times a component malfunctions erratically and is extremely hard to isolate. Peak E has been swamped by the extremely high concentration of the previous sample; sample E must be repeated.

---

### *Sampler*

1. Unit inoperative.
    a. Is the unit plugged into power strip and is the general laboratory line live?
    b. Check fuse.
    c. Sampler II has reset button; check.
2. Short sharp peak as shown in B of Figure 3-3.
    a. Insufficient sample in cup.
    b. Misalignment of sample probe into cup.
       (1) Sampler I sometimes pulls sample line upward; or a worn cam lever spring is causing improper crook entrance.
       (2) Clot in sample cup or sample line.
3. Sharp peak but not short, as shown in C of Figure 3-3. Adequate sample but inadequate amount of reagent.

*Continued on page* 120

119

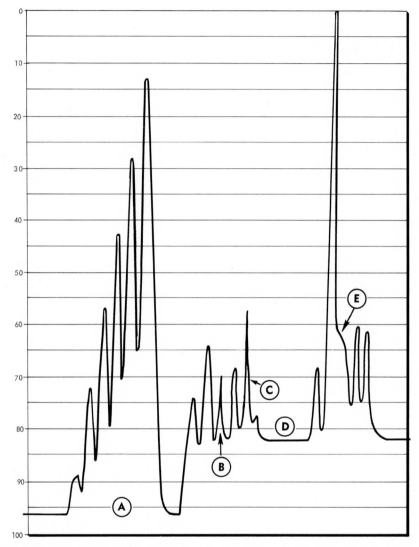

**Figure 3-3.** *Recorder graph for color development showing various unsatisfactory peaks. A. Standards. B. Insufficient sample. C. Insufficient reagents. D. Shift in base line. E. Swamped sample. (Adapted from Technicon Principles of Continuous Flow Analysis. Ardsley, N. Y., Technicon Corp., 1968.)*

4. Irregular peaks on recorder.

    a. Improper washing from empty water well on Sampler II.

    b. Worn analysis cam on Sampler II (widths of peaks different) or debris.

    c. Clot or debris forming plug anywhere in system (peaks will soon not appear at all).

5. Peaks missing on recorder graph, but some peaks appearing.

   a. Wheel lock not secure—can also produce double sampling of same specimen.

   b. Improper seating of analysis cam on Sampler II.

   c. If missing peaks are the last samples on plate, reagent lines may have been put into water too soon. Allow 2 to 3 minutes before putting lines in water after last sample.

6. No peaks on recorder graph.

   a. A plug can be anywhere in the system; check bubble pattern.

   b. Tubing can be disconnected; check flow into colorimeter.

   c. There may be a defect in photocell or recorder.

If the sampler is suspected of incorrect sampling, this may be confirmed in two ways:[15]

1. Fill ten cups properly with pooled serum and process them through the system. If the recorder shows good reproducibility of peaks, the rate of sampling is consistent. If the reproducibility is not good, the problem may be the sampler but it could also be from some other cause. Check further.

2. Verify the sampling ratio with a stopwatch. Time at least ten cycles at speeds of 20, 40 and 60 samples per hour.

---

## Manifold System

Close monitoring of the bubble pattern from the time the sample is picked up until the peaks appear on the recorder is needed to produce valid peaks. Therefore, it is convenient to think of the whole continuous flow as the manifold system. Every bubble does not have identical length, but its flow pattern must be consistent. A break in bubble pattern is a definite indication of trouble and must be investigated. If the pump is left operating, the bubble pattern can be traced backward until the cause of the trouble is found. The following scheme for locating a broken bubble pattern has been adapted from White *et al.*[15]

---

### *Inconsistent Bubble Pattern*

1. Sample and reagent lines joining the pump tubes.

   a. No weight on a reagent line to prevent the tip from curling up out of the fluid.

   b. Empty reagent bottle.

   c. A hole or constriction in either sample or reagent lines.

*Continued on page* 122

2. Good bubble patterns entering the pump lines but changing to erratic ones on exiting.

   a. Snaking of a tube.

   b. Moisture from a split tube.

   c. An old tube that has lost elasticity.

   d. Wrong-sized tube attached to wrong glass connector or nipple.

   e. A connection poorly sealed with cyclohexanone, permitting entrance of air or leaving a gap between tubing ends.

3. A good bubble pattern entering the dialyzer but unsatisfactory upon exiting.

   a. Improper joining of the exterior or interior tubes, nipples, or mixing coils or disconnected tubing. (If the latter, an obstruction in the system may be causing back pressure.)

   b. Precipitate or dirt in the nipples.

   c. Dialyzer not clamped tightly.

   d. Dirty dialyzer plates that cannot be properly paired.

   e. Cracked, leaking dialyzer nipples at the base of the plates.

   f. Rupture of membrane from a clot, dirt, or fibrin.

   g. Unmated dialyzer plates or grooves damaged from rough handling.

   h. Improperly mounted dialyzer membrane.

4. Broken bubble pattern from defect in glass assembly on top of dialyzer.

   a. Incorrect sizes of nipples and glass connections.

   b. A burr inside a nipple.

   c. Nipple connections not flush to the glass.

5. Erratic bubble patterns in the transmission tubing.

   a. Accumulated dirt or particles on the walls of the tubing.

      (1) Clean old tubing with a bleaching solution diluted 1:4 with water or with a detergent solution diluted 1:4 with water (unless a fluorometric method is being carried out).

      (2) Clean new tubing with water containing 2 to 3 drops of Brij-35 per liter. If the bubble pattern continues to break up, milk the tubing by seesawing it over the table edge.

6. Alteration in bubble pattern while passing through a heating bath.

   a. Dirt in the nipples or coils. Clean heating bath coils with Tween 20, a detergent (nonfluorescent), or 10% nitric acid.

   b. A perforated or broken coil.

7. Poor bubble pattern in the mixing coils.

   a. Improper fittings from tube to nipple to coils.

   b. Broken, cracked, or dirty coils. Clean the mixing coils by soaking them in chromic acid solution.

8. Erratic bubble pattern in a colorimeter with erratic recorder tracings.
   a. Improper tilting of the debubbler in the flow cell to carry out the separation of gas and fluids.
   b. Dirt in the flow cell.
   c. A cracked flow cell.
   d. Inadequate removal of waste from the flow cell or an obstruction in the flow cell system.

---

In addition to monitoring the bubble pattern, close attention should be given to the physical condition of the manifold. The pump tubes should be examined daily to be sure they remain clean and undamaged. Since friction is required for efficient pumping, the dull platen should be occasionally rubbed with emery cloth. Among other sources of trouble are the larger pump tubes that tend to break down faster than the smaller ones from the compression of the pump rollers.

---

### *Locating and Correcting Manifold Trouble[10]*

1. A backup of fluids in the lines with an irregular base line on the recorder.
   a. With a new manifold:
      (1) Look for glue in the fittings or leaks in the connections of the manifold.
      (2) Add more wetting agent to the wash water.
      (3) Put helper springs or a number two rubber stopper under the entrance end of the platen.
      (4) *Only as a last resort*—remove the side rails.
      (5) For stiffness of the tubing:
         (a) Run manifold with distilled water containing Tween 20 for about 30 min.
         (b) Always start on the second position.
      (6) Rearrange the lines.
      (7) For irregular pumping that can be caused by an overload of manifold tubing on pump I:
         (a) Remove water well line from Sampler II.
         (b) Use two pumps.
      (8) Be sure the "H" and the cactus are in the right position.
      (9) Check for pinched off lines.
   b. With an old manifold:
      (1) Check for snaking of the manifold lines, a loose manifold, or oil on the manifold or rollers.
      (2) Examine the pump lines for overlaying.

*Continued on page* 124

      (3) Make sure the sample line, the pulse suppressors, the fittings, the transmission tubing, or the coils are not plugged with protein or chemicals.

      (4) Rule out wetting, a big problem in the summer months or when the instrument is left idle.

      (5) Change worn or damaged lines. Never change only one line on the manifold; change all. The sample line is the only exception to this rule.

      (6) Keep a spare manifold on hand.

      (7) Look for pinched off lines.

2. Sensitivity.

  a. Increase the sensitivity by:

      (1) Decreasing the sample rate (not recommended).

      (2) Increasing the sample size.

      (3) Decreasing the diluent size.

      (4) Increasing the chemical reaction time.

         (a) Lengthen the delay coil.

         (b) Decrease the air line to produce a slower rate of flow.

      (5) Dialyzing the sample through two sets of plates.

      (6) Reversing the order of dialysis if a double dialyzer is used.

      (7) Increasing the cuvette size.

  b. Decrease the sensitivity by:

      (1) Increasing the sample rate (not recommended).

      (2) Decreasing the sample size.

      (3) Increasing the diluent size.

      (4) Decreasing the chemical reaction time.

         (a) Shorten the delay coil.

         (b) Increase the air line to produce a faster flow of sample.

      (5) Decreasing the cuvette size.

3. Air entering the cuvette and artifacts appearing on the recorder.

  a. The debubbler C5 fitting is tipped.

  b. The manifold pull off line is too large.

  c. The manifold pull off line is not connected.

  d. The cuvette line is plugged or there is a loose connection.

  e. The pull off line is pinched off.

  f. An improper amount of fluid is entering the cuvette.

4. A worn-out manifold. (A manifold does not always use all of the positions on the end block before it needs to be changed.)

  a. Increase of sensitivity in the lower range; lack of reproducibility in the high range; bending of top half of the curve.

  b. Noise in the base line.

124

  c. Irregular standard peaks.

  d. Fluid backing up into the air lines.

  e. Drift in the base line and the standard curve.

  f. Snaking of the manifold tubing.

5. Wetting agents in distilled water wash and reagents.

  Use only the wetting agent recommended—for example, Tween 20, Brij 35, Levor 4, agent A—to avoid:

  (1) Interaction with the chemical reagents.

  (2) Collection on sides of the tubing that cause plugs in the lines.

  (3) Precipitate in the reagents. Such reagents require frequent filtration.

## Pump

Pump Model I uses a two-speed motor. The second or high speed is available for quickly washing out the lines between procedures. The type C dialyzer membranes, however, are thin enough that they are often ruptured by the high speed pumping. This speed cannot be used for a manifold which has Acid-flex tubing because the pressure separates the tubing from the nipples; nor can it be used with manifolds which contain pulse suppressors.

If the gear head assembly wears enough to cause the internal meshing gears to slip, the driver sprocket cannot maintain a constant velocity. Consequently, a jerking action results, and the manifold tubing has some back movement of the fluid in the tubes. Somewhat the same effect is produced if the springs under the platen become weak. The springs at the entrance end of the platen are stronger than those at the exit in order to force the fluids along the manifold. Extra support springs can be added under the entrance end of the platen to increase the pressure. A new manifold may be stiff enough to require the additional pressure. However, if a #1 rubber stopper is also added under the entrance end of the platen and the manifold does not become "broken-in" in 30 minutes, the springs are too weak and must be replaced. Both entrance and exit springs must be replaced simultaneously. One additional cause of jerky pumping is a loose chain on the roller head assembly caused by worn chain links. In this case, the chain and coupling must be replaced.

Pump II is a heavy-duty module capable of handling 23 tubes on a manifold. A set of ratio gears is used to drive the sprocket which moves the roller chain, thus decreasing one source of slippage. The same considerations for spring tension apply for this pump as with the previous model. The pumps which have a blower underneath require that the blower be operative whenever the pump is used. The motor will be damaged from its own heat if the motor is run even a short time without the blower.

125

A pump that stalls and will not start usually is the result of a blown fuse, misalignment of platen on micro switch, broken switch, loose electrical connection, loose setscrews on gears, or a worn gear head.

## Dialyzer

For the AutoAnalyzer methods using a dialyzed sample, the sensitivity of the response can be greatly affected by the dialysis procedure chosen and the care with which these procedures are monitored. The rate of dialysis is influenced by the concentration of the constituent in the sample, the coefficient of dialysis for the constituent, time, temperature, membrane area, and thickness and porosity of the membrane. Provided the sample and standards have the same relative contribution to the coefficient of dialysis of the constituent being tested (*i.e.,* aqueous standards, blood, or urine), the only factor allowed to vary in a valid determination is the concentration of the constituent. While different constituents vary in their percent of total that dialyzes, the absolute amount dialyzed for each is proportional to its concentration.

Within limits, the percent dialysis of a constituent can be increased or decreased by a change in temperature, time, or membrane area. These factors may be changed by choice to regulate the sensitivity of the method, but they can also be changed by malfunctions. Changing the temperature has a direct relationship upon the percent dialysis; hence, the temperature of the dialyzer bath should be monitored. In addition to reading the temperature itself, the stirrer should be checked to be sure the same temperature exists in the whole bath. We find it useful to time the off-on cycle of the dialyzer heater to detect changes in the efficiency of the heating element. The time the flow stream spends in the dialyzer may be increased or decreased by changing the volume of sample diluent and recipient streams while keeping their ratios constant. From experience we have learned that the glucose value for the standards increases within the run when the dialyzer membrane needs changing. This is an example of an increased time in the dialyzer caused by decreased porosity of a dirty membrane. The membrane area for dialyzing can be increased by using a second set of plates in order to achieve more recovery. We know of no malfunction which increases the membrane area, but a decrease can be produced by mismatched plates or countercurrent stream flow for recipient and sample streams. Both of these errors will produce markedly decreased peak heights compared to those normally seen for the same method.

Matched plates should show only one channel when they are fitted together without a membrane and held up to the light. It is well to check them from time to time, especially when several people work on the AutoAnalyzer and more than one set of plates is used. These plates must always be used as the matched set and never interchanged. Ever so slight a difference in the channels will cause unsatisfactory performance. In addition to the loss in sensitivity of the peaks, the imprecisely defined channel will produce a poor bubble pattern. By contrast, the

126

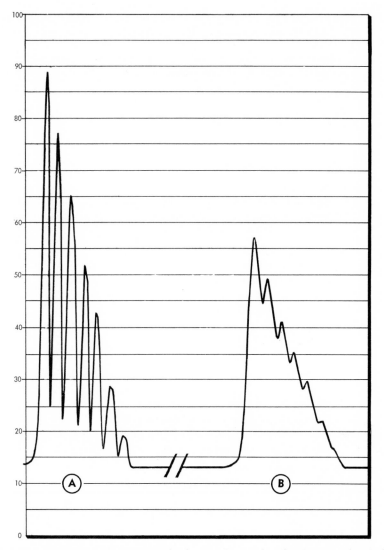

**Figure 3-4.** *Glucose peaks for standards as affected by the flow in the dialyzer. A. Normal concurrent flow. B. Countercurrent flow.*

countercurrent dialysis flow will maintain a good bubble pattern but produce poorly separated peaks. The countercurrent stream effect for glucose is shown as B in Figure 3-4 as compared to the normal peaks (A) for the set of standards. Sooner or later someone in each laboratory will connect the inlet tubing to an outlet nipple in the dialyzer, and it is helpful to be able to recognize this error immediately from the shape of the set of standard peaks. The list of causes of problems in the dialyzer module is drawn from Salancy.[10]

127

## *Problems in Dialyzer Module*

1. Bubble pattern good going into dialyzer; irregular coming out. Recorder: irregular peaks and poor reproducibility.

   a. Leakage in the dialyzer plates.
      (1) Loose nut assembly.
      (2) Misaligned locating pin preventing proper tightening of dialyzer plates.
      (3) Broken or sliced nipples.
      (4) Loosely connected tubing.

   b. Wetting.
      (1) New tubing or membranes in the system.
      (2) Wrong wetting agents or none in the reagents and wash water.
      (3) Changing all the tubing at one time.

   c. Wrinkled or loose membrane.
      (1) Cutting off the membrane hoops before the dialyzer nut is secure.
      (2) Failing to stretch the membrane tightly on the hoop.
      (3) Changing only one membrane on a double dialyzer. Both membranes must be changed at the same time.
      (4) Shifting the dialyzer plate when placing it on top of a membrane.

   d. Dirty membranes or coils.
      (1) Rinse the membranes after they are stretched on the hoop.
      (2) Always check for protein build-up on the coils.
      (3) Change the membranes at least weekly.
      (4) Change the dialyzer coils at least monthly.
      (5) Always clean the nipples of the dialyzer with a wire when changing the membranes.

   e. Hole in the membrane.
      (1) Carelessness when stretching the membrane.
      (2) Chemicals.
      (3) Back pressure from a plug, causing rupture.

   f. Pinched tubes.

2. Loss of sensitivity.

   a. Wrong type of membrane.
      (1) Type "C" membrane required for new tubular flow cell.
      (2) Thicker membrane required for old "standard" flow cell.

   b. Wrong dialysis ratio.
      (1) Pump tube too large for recipient stream.
      (2) Tube too small for sample-diluent stream.

   c. Mismatched plates.

3. Poor separation between peaks—bubble pattern good:
   Check for countercurrent flow of sample and recipient streams.

4. Poor temperature control.
   a. Overheating.
      (1) Split in mercury column of thermoregulator (may usually be rejoined by cooling in ice water).
      (2) Defective thermoregulator.
      (3) Defective relay.
      (4) Low water level.
   b. Underheating.
      (1) Defective heating element.
      (2) Loose electrical connection.

5. Noise.
   a. Chattering relay indicating defective thermoregulator.
   b. Motor in need of oiling. If motor is still noisy after being oiled, have it checked by electrician.
   c. Vibrating stirrer.
      (1) Loose.
      (2) Misaligned.

## Heating Bath

If a problem occurs in the heating bath and it must be torn down, "downtime" can be several hours because of the time required to raise the temperature back to 95°. The most frequent reason for disassembling the heating bath is to replace a broken or leaking glass coil. Davis *et al.* showed that coils used for ferricyanide glucose method become brittle, have the inside glass surface etched away, and eventually develop pin holes.[3] The volume of 40 foot coils of 1.6 mm tubing was 23 cc when new and increased to 34 cc after 32 days when used 24 hours/day, 7 days a week. The increased volume, along with the irregular surface of the interior glass wall, causes a surging exit flow that produces unaccountable variations in the peaks. Davis and his associates recommend that the capacity of the coils be checked and the coil be replaced at a specific volume increase to avoid rupture of the coil causing "downtime" at a crucial time.

### *Capacity of Glass Coil**

1. Connect the barrel of a 50 cc syringe with a short piece of Tygon to the inlet stem of the waterbath coil.
2. Fill the syringe with colored water; clamp the Tygon connection as the water reaches the stem of the coil.
3. Carefully remove the syringe barrel from the Tygon, insert the plunger into the syringe, and adjust the volume of water to 50 cc. Reconnect the syringe to the Tygon.

*Continued on page* 130

4. Inject water into the coil until it flows to the outlet stem of the coil.
5. Record volume and date checked. The volume of water used indicates the capacity of the coil. A new 40 foot, 1.6 mm coil holds about 23 cc. Replacement is suggested when capacity reaches 40 cc.

---

* Davis, H. A., Sterling, R. E., Wilcox, A. A., and Waters, W. E.: Investigation of a potential source of difficulty in the use of the AutoAnalyzer. Clin. Chem. *12:*428, 1966.

Replacement of a single coil that is part of a dual coil bath is difficult, and often one breaks the second coil in the effort. Therefore, it would seem more logical to plan to replace both coils at once and use the double-coil unit mounted on its base as it is received from the company. The glucose-urea dual channel system would receive most efficient use of the coils if they were assigned periodically on a rotation basis between the glucose and the urea. Both coils should then require replacement at approximately the same time. Davis *et al.* reported that the enlarging volume of the coil increased the peak height obtained in the diacetylmonoxime-urea method.[3] The increased sensitivity did not appear to be proportional for all concentrations and was greatest at 70 mgm%. Therefore, if the coils are rotated between glucose and urea, variations should be expected in the urea calibration curve.

The customary check of the coil for leaks is to submerge it in water and, with one end blocked, force air through. Bubbles indicate the hole or crack. However, sometimes one cannot find a  leak and continues to use the coil; more trouble occurs and the coil must again be checked. A more sensitive check for the *small* leak is to submerge the coil in phenolphthalein solution and pump weak sodium hydroxide through the coil.[10] After the coil has been filled and several hours have passed, a pink color will indicate that the coil is leaking.

The only other common problem occurring in the heating bath is poor temperature control. Irregular peaks on the recorder are caused by surging as the stream leaves the bath. As for the dialyzer, the inability to maintain proper temperature can be caused by a split mercury column in the thermoregulator, defective thermoregulator or heater, or low fluid level. Checking the off-on cycle for the heater will often indicate the heater change in efficiency before the problem becomes acute.

## Colorimeter

The ten colorimeter models are all dual-beam systems and differ primarily in their flow cells and photo detectors. Problems associated with the colorimeter usually fall into three types:

1. Dirty optical system.
2. Imbalanced light detector system.
3. Unsatisfactory fluid system.

The cleanliness of the optical system must include the surfaces of lamp, lenses, mirrors, filters, flow cell, and detector. Careful observation and cleaning of these surfaces must be part of a regular maintenance system. Any spillage or fogging from ruptured tube connections will require immediate cleaning of the entire optical system. The older flow cells with portions open to the air caused much more fogging of the optical system than do the newer tubular flow cells.

In addition to its possible contribution to the dirty optical system, the lamp controls the light intensity available to balance the detector system. The signal ratio for the sample and reference sides must remain stable for the recorder tracing to be valid. If the aperture size must be changed several times to retain balance, the operator must find the cause and correct it. If the optical system is not fogged, the lamp is more likely to be at fault than the detector.

After installing the lamp, the operator should wipe off his fingerprints before turning on the lamp. If he does not, the heat will cause these smudges to become permanent on the glass surface, and the amount of light to the two detectors may be altered. With use, the lamp will usually become blackened on one side long before it burns out. It is preferable to change the blackened lamp rather than balance the system by changing aperture sizes. The lamps with blue leads can be used only with photocell colorimeters and have a life expectancy of about 1500 hours. The yellow lead lamps can be used for the phototube or photocell colorimeters but have only 200 hours' life expectancy.

The column of fluid passed through the flow cell must be free of particles and bubbles for the response to be reliable. The newer tubular flow cell avoids many of the problems we had with the previous cells. Occasionally a bubble does lodge in this cell and must be forced out. This can usually be done by momentarily pinching the outlet stream. Proper alignment of this flow cell seems to be the principal point to monitor.

As long as the lamp is burning and fluid is passing through the flow cell, the specific symptoms for malfunction in the colorimeter must be considered from the appearance of the pen tracing on the recorder. For this reason, symptoms for colorimeter and recorder problems are listed together under Recorder.

## Recorder

The recorder is a rugged instrument and is relatively trouble-free. The pen should move freely up and down the scale. If it does not, check the tension on the bull gear first and then look for binding of pulleys, drive cord, or gears.

---

### Recorder

Symptoms with possible causes related to the recorder or the colorimeter include:

1. Repetitious blowing of fuses.[8]

    Excessive line voltage or amperage. Check to see if the line is overloaded.

*Continued on page* 132

2. Pen remains stationary instead of responding to input signals.
   a. Shorted-out line fuse and amplifier fuse.
   b. Defective tubes in amplifier unit.
   c. No signal from colorimeter.
      (1) Is the lamp on and the shield properly positioned?
      (2) Is the flow cell properly aligned—*i.e.*, not blocking the light path?
   d. Synchroverter switch failure.
   e. Defective balancing motor.
   f. Dirty slide wire.

3. Inability to adjust pen on recorder to read zero.
   a. Is the zero aperture in front of sample photocell?
   b. Is the zero control on colorimeter defective?
   c. Is the light shield improperly seated in colorimeter?
   d. Is the pen positioned properly on drive cord?

4. Recorder cannot be set to 100% T.
   a. Improperly seated filters.
   b. Incorrect aperture or filters.
   c. Dirty filters and windows.
   d. Misaligned or incorrectly seated cuvette.
   e. Light guard malpositioned on the gravity cuvette.
   f. Burned out bulb or fuse of either the colorimeter or recorder.
   g. Incorrect reagents.
   h. No fluid entering the cuvette.
      (1) Cuvette tubing disconnected.
      (2) Pull-off line disconnected.
   i. Flow plugged somewhere back of colorimeter.
   j. Wrong size cuvette.

5. Pen responds intermittently—pen travels either to zero or 100% T. If pen goes to zero, check sample side of colorimeter; if pen goes to 100% T, check reference side.
   a. Defective photocell or loose electrical connection.
   b. Defective 100% T potentiometer.
   c. Dirty or defective filters.

6. Pen "hunts" excessively.
   a. Amplifier fuse blown.
   b. Defective amplifier tubes.
   c. Defective amplifier.
   d. Bubbles in cuvette. Check debubbler and the size of the pull-off line of manifold.

7. Excessive jumping of pen when 100%T potentiometer is moved.
    a. Gain too high on amplifier.
    b. Defective photocell in colorimeter (either side).
    c. Defective potentiometer. Could be just dirty; turn firmly from right to left and vice versa and try again before replacing.

8. Excessive jumping of pen when *not* moved.[10]
    a. Dirt trapped in cuvette.
    b. Bubble trapped in cuvette.

9. Irregular artifacts on the recorder with a shift of the baseline toward 100%T.[10]
    a. Sun on the colorimeter.
    b. Fog on the windows of the colorimeter.

10. Drift of the baseline toward 0%T.[10]
    a. Fogging of the windows of colorimeter.
    b. Bulb darkening.
    c. Coating of the cuvette.
    d. Improper warm-up of the bulb.
    e. Manifold trouble.

11. Pen response sluggish.
    a. Gain adjustment too low.
    b. Poor ground connection (neon lamp inside recorder should be glowing if grounding is improper).
    c. Incorrect filters or apertures in colorimeter.
    d. Weak tubes.

12. Pen "hunts" when gain is high but is sluggish when gain is reduced.
    a. Weak or defective colorimeter lamp.
    b. Dirty optical system.
    c. Defective photocells.

13. Recorder drawing a constant result.[10]
    a. Lines disconnected which flow to the cuvette or in the cuvette itself.
    b. Pull-off line pinched off or disconnected.
    c. Drain in the standard cuvette plugged.
    d. Bulb or fuse of the colorimeter burned out.
    e. ⅛ amp fuse of the amplifier burned out.

14. Pen won't trace.
    a. Faulty ink flow.
    b. Carrier too tight.
    c. Paper out of alignment.
    d. Edge of pen worn to sharp point and not touching paper. File down tip.

| | DAILY | WEEKLY | MONTHLY | 3 MONTHS | 6 MONTHS | YEARLY |
|---|---|---|---|---|---|---|
| **A. SAMPLER** | | | | | | |
| Wipe up spillage around modules, under sample tray, etc. | √ | | | | | |
| Clean wash receptacle | | √ | | | | |
| Clean sample probe with wire | | √ | | | | |
| Check sample tubing; replace if dirty | | √ | | | | |
| Move all modules; clean under them | | √ | | | | |
| Routinely replace sample tubing | | | | √ | | |
| Remove bottom of unit; clean, oil motor | | | | | | √ |
| Check for loose electrical connections | | | | | | √ |
| **B. MANIFOLD & PUMP** | | | | | | |
| After daily run is completed, pump water through all lines for at least 15 minutes | √ | | | | | |
| Check pump tubing and fittings; check for leaks | √ | | | | | |
| Check platen and rollers | √ | | | | | |
| Rub platen with fine emery cloth | | √ | | | | |
| Replace pump tubes | | | 2x | | | |
| Replace manifold (average) | | | √ | | | |
| Oil internal chain drive, felt pads, sprockets, blower motor | | | | | √ | |
| Check for loose electrical connections | | | | | √ | |

**Figure 3-5.** *Maintenance schedule for AutoAnalyzer modules.*

| | DAILY | WEEKLY | MONTHLY | 3 MONTHS | 6 MONTHS | YEARLY |
|---|---|---|---|---|---|---|
| **C. DIALYZER** | | | | | | |
| Check water level and temperature | √ | | | | | |
| Change membrane; clean plates and nipples | | √ | | | | |
| Record off-on cycle of heating element | | | √ | | | |
| Clean and refill water bath | | | √ | | | |
| Change coil and tubing (also external transmission tubing) | | | √ | | | |
| Oil motors | | | | √ | | |
| Check for loose electrical connections | | | | √ | | |
| **D. HEATING BATH** | | | | | | |
| Check temperature | √ | | | | | |
| Check off-on cycle of heating element | | | √ | | | |
| Inspect bath fluid: height, odor, color; replace if necessary | | | √ | | | |
| Oil motors | | | | √ | | |
| Clean coils and inside of bath; change bath fluid | | | | | √ | |
| Check for loose electrical connections | | | | | √ | |

**Figure 3-5.** *(Continued) Maintenance schedule for AutoAnalyzer modules*

| | DAILY | WEEKLY | MONTHLY | 3 MONTHS | 6 MONTHS | YEARLY |
|---|---|---|---|---|---|---|
| **E. COLORIMETER** | | | | | | |
| Check alignment of flowcell (*i.e.,* peak the response) | √ | | | | | |
| Remove and inspect filters; clean with lens paper | | √ | | | | |
| Remove housing and inspect for spillage; clean as necessary | | √ | | | | |
| Inspect lamp for blackening; replace when blackened | | √ | | | | |
| Rebuild flowcell assembly | | | √ | | | |
| Clean optical system with lens paper | | | | | √ | |
| Check for loose electrical connections | | | | | √ | |
| **F. RECORDER** | | | | | | |
| Check ink and paper supply | √ | | | | | |
| Flush out pen reservoir and clean pens; flatten pen tip if necessary (sandpaper) | | | √ | | | |
| Check gain (If different filters are used, gain must be checked with change of filters) | | | √ | | | |
| Clean slidewire and lubricate | | | | | √ | |
| Check for loose electrical connections | | | | | √ | |

**Figure 3-5.** *(Continued) Maintenance schedule for AutoAnalyzer modules*

## MAINTENANCE

The test values produced by the AutoAnalyzer can only be as good as the care the operator uses in running the equipment. A great share of the care should be conscientious regular maintenance. Good maintenance is absolutely necessary and neglect sooner or later convinces the operator. The exact time schedule for performing many of the chores will depend upon the amount of use the instrument gets. On the other hand, items such as oiling motors must be done even if the system is used relatively little.

Figure 3-5 represents the usual required procedures for units used eight hours a day, six days a week.

## SEQUENTIAL MULTIPLE ANALYZER (SMA 12/60)

As stated previously, the SMA 12/60 is used in our institution as a screening device and does not replace our routine methods. It is impossible to say whether the answers reported from the routine screen are always used clinically for screening only; hopefully, they are. It has been our experience, however, that the values from this system are much more reliable than were those from the 12/30. Carry-over and drift are much less, and the response curves are more nearly linear for the 12/60.

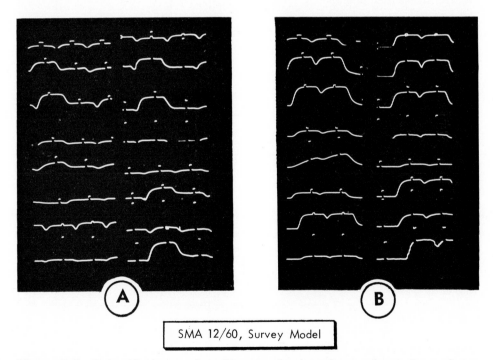

SMA 12/60, Survey Model

**Figure 3-6.** *Polaroid picture of oscilloscope showing plateau shapes for each test (See page 140).*

137

SOUTH BEND MEDICAL FOUNDATION, INC.

Month _____ Year _____

| DAILY MAINTENANCE | Mon. | Tues. | Wed. | Thurs. | Fri. | Sat. |
|---|---|---|---|---|---|---|
| *Beginning of Day* <br> Make daily reagents | | | | | | |
| Change cholesterol pump tubing | | | | | | |
| Clean cholesterol sample line with 1 N Na OH | | | | | | |
| Set base line knobs in 5 turn position | | | | | | |
| Check quantity of reagents | | | | | | |
| Shake all reagents | | | | | | |
| Q.s. cholesterol reagent to 1000 ml | | | | | | |
| Turn all reagent straws up to ceiling | | | | | | |
| Check all sample lines for plugs | | | | | | |
| Check all reagent pump lines | | | | | | |
| *During the Day* <br> Turn on programmer and function monitor | | | | | | |
| Run reagents through system for 20 min. | | | | | | |
| Set reference test and blank energy levels | | | | | | |
| Run two pools to check phasing | | | | | | |
| Check bubble patterns throughout the day | | | | | | |
| *End of Day* <br> Wash out system for 10 min. | | | | | | |
| Discard all used cups | | | | | | |
| Wipe up all spillage | | | | | | |
| Dump all daily reagents | | | | | | |
| Turn off entire instrument | | | | | | |

**Figure 3-7.** *Daily maintenance sheet for SMA 12/60 unit.*

138

SOUTH BEND MEDICAL FOUNDATION, INC.

| WEEEKLY MAINTENANCE | | | | | |
|---|---|---|---|---|---|
| 1. Pump a saline solution through entire system for 30 min; wash with $H_2O$ for 30 min | | | | | |
| 2. With reagent valves in "reagent" position, run alcoholic KOH* through the following reagent lines for 5 min; rinse with $H_2O$ for 5 more minutes:<br><br>  Working biuret<br>  Alkaline iodide<br>  Haba dye<br>  Phosphate buffer<br>  Tartrate buffer<br>  SGOT substrate<br>  Stannous chloride<br>  PMS lines | | | | | |
| 3. Change dialyzer membranes and check bubble patterns before starting | | | | | |
| 4. Clean pump platen with $CCl_4$ | | | | | |
| 5. Clean grease off manifold tubing with $CCl_4$ (quickly) | | | | | |
| 6. Oil the pads on all four pumps | | | | | |
| 7. Check main sample line for any plugs; change if dirty | | | | | |
| 8. Clean all four sample stream-splitters, all sample glass tubing, and any other connections plugged on sample tubing | | | | | |
| 9. Flush the LDH cartridge with alcoholic KOH and rinse in water | | | | | |
| 10. Clean out refrigerator and replace dry towels | | | | | |
| *Colorimeter*<br>1. Remove and inspect filters; clean with lens paper | | | | | |
| 2. Check bulb for blackening or frosting; frost should be wiped off with damp Kimwipe. If bulb is blackened, replace it | | | | | |
| 3. Clean light windows | | | | | |

\* Alcoholic KOH = 4 cc 14 N KOH + 100 cc SDA.

**Figure 3-8.** *Weekly maintenance sheet for SMA 12/60 unit.*

SOUTH BEND MEDICAL FOUNDATION, INC.

| MONTHLY MAINTENANCE | | | | | |
|---|---|---|---|---|---|
| 1. (Every six weeks) Change all manifold tubing | | | | | |
| 2. Check all other tubing for possible changing | | | | | |

**Figure 3-9.** *Monthly maintenance sheet for SMA 12/60 unit.*

Calibration sera must be chosen whose values allow the system to be calibrated at the concentration level of greatest interest to the user. We have chosen values at the upper edge of normal for best separation of normal from abnormal patients. Finley *et al.* pointed out that phosphorus was too high below 2.5 mgm% and too low above 6.2; increasing the stannous chloride does provide linearity somewhat higher.[6] They also found calcium too low below 6 mgm% and too high above 11; SGOT lost linearity above 45 Karmen units. We found glucose to be nonlinear above 200 mgm% when the standard was set at about 100; urea was linear only to approximately 40 mgm%.

Uric acid values appear to vary in their validity from one instrument to another. By modifying the method to dilute the serum in saline and to remove the reaction from the heating bath, we have been able to improve the reproducibility and accuracy.[1] We have also replaced the alkaline phosphatase method with the Babson Phosphastrate.*

Our experience has shown that the sera used for calibrating must be analyzed by reference methods and checked from time to time. Controls should represent the low, normal, and elevated concentration levels. We have found it useful to take a polaroid picture of the oscilloscope weekly (Fig. 3-6).

Figure 3-6 is an example of the comparison of the uric acid plateau. The fifth tracing on the left in both A and B is this plateau. Pattern B was taken two weeks after A. These patterns could be demonstrated by recording each test separately as a steady state on the graph, but the picture gives approximately the same information in much less time.

The bubble pattern in this system must be monitored even more closely than the basic system in order to provide an even line on the graph. For this reason, all connections must be continually checked for cleanliness and snug-fitting joints. Rinsing of all lines and daily special cleaning of some lines becomes very important. The maintenance sheets we use are essentially the recommendations from the manufacturer. These are shown as Figures 3-7, 3-8, and 3-9.

## REFERENCES

1. Ackart, T.: Personal communication.
2. Bennet, A., Gartelmann, D., Mason, J. I., and Owen, J. A.: Calibration, calibration drift and specimen interaction in AutoAnalyzer systems. Clin. Chim. Acta, 29:161, 1970.

---

* General Diagnostics Div., Warner-Chilcott Laboratories, Morris Plains, N. J.

140

3. Davis, H. A., Sterling, R. E., Wilcox, A. A., and Waters, W. E.: Investigation of a potential source of difficulty in the use of the AutoAnalyzer. Clin. Chem. *12:*428, 1966.

4. Department of Health, Education, and Welfare, Social Security Administration: Independent laboratory survey report. Form SSA-1557, February, 1969.

5. Dobrow, D. A., and Amador, E.: The accuracy of commercial enzyme reference sera. Amer. J. Clin. Path., *53:*60, 1970.

6. Finley, P. R., Gillott, L., Peterson, D., Anderson, F., and Boxman, E.: Evaluation of the technical performance of the SMA 12/60. In *Advances in Automated Analysis.* Vol. 1. Chicago Technicon International Congress, 1969, page 145.

7. Hagenbusch, O. E.: Automation and multiphasic screening. Southern Med. J., *62:*1359, 1969.

8. Mabry, C. C., and VanPeenan, H. J.: AutoAnalyzer. In *Workshop on Instrumentation.* Pre-workshop manual. J. R. Schenken, Ed. Commission on Continuing Education, Council on Clinical Chemistry, ASCP, 1967.

9. Reece, R. L.: What you should know about automated chemical screening. Res. Staff Physician, *15:*128, 1969.

10. Salancy, J.: Troubleshooting and preventive maintenance for AutoAnalyzer systems. Workshop Manual. Amer. Soc. Med. Technologists Convention, Detroit, 1970.

11. Skeggs, L. T.: Principles of automatic chemical analysis. In *Standard Methods of Clinical Chemistry.* Vol. 5. S. Meites, Ed. New York, Academic Press, 1965.

12. Thiers, R. E., Cole, R. R., and Kirsch, W. J.: Kinetic parameters of continuous flow analysis. Clin. Chem., *13:*451, 1967.

13. Thiers, R. E., and Oglesby, K. M.: The precision, accuracy and inherent error of automatic continuous flow methods. Clin. Chem. *10:*246, 1964.

14. Westgard, J.: Personal communication.

15. White, W. L., Erickson, M. M., and Stevens, S. C.: *Practical Automation for the Clinical Laboratory.* St. Louis, The C. V. Mosby Co., 1968.

16. Winstead, M., *Reagent Grade Water: How, When and Why?* Houston, Amer. Soc. Med. Technologists, 1967.

17. Young, D. S., and Mears, T. W.: Measurement and standard reference materials in clinical chemistry. Clin. Chem., *14:*929, 1968.

18. Young, D. S., Montague, R. M., and Snider, R. R.: Studies of sampling times in a continuous flow analytic system. Clin. Chem., *14:*993, 1968.

141

# 4

# Densitometers

Quality control of the values obtained by electrophoresis requires three distinctly separate considerations: the method, the technique, and the densitometer. Since serum protein electrophoresis is the procedure most frequently done, the primary focus of this discussion will be that test and the proper monitoring of the instrument. Factors pertaining to method and technique will only be mentioned.

## METHOD FOR ELECTROPHORESIS

The method for serum protein electrophoresis at the South Bend Medical Foundation consists of separation on Sepraphore III* cellulose acetate strips (1″ x 6¾″), using barbital-barbituric acid buffer, pH 8.6, and ionic strength of 0.06. The stain is Ponceau S.

Whether or not the stained fractions can be quantified and the concentration of dye equated to their respective protein content has been argued in the literature for years.[16, 17] The dye-combining capacity of albumin has been noted to be higher than that of the other fractions, no matter what dye is used.[13] Vanzetti states that strips stained with Ponceau S show a dye-binding capacity for albumin which is only slightly larger than that of globulins.[18] Scherr claimed linearity with this dye by the elution method.[15] The dye-binding capacity of Ponceau S for the various fractions is a basic question, as is the degree to which it affects the electrophoresis

---

* Gelman Instrument Co., Ann Arbor, Mich.

142

values. This can only be resolved by establishing normals for the precise method in use in each institution. It is most fortunate when the albumin value obtained by the electrophoretic method closely approximates that obtained by the chemical method.

The amount of serum used and the reading of opaque (uncleared) cellulose acetate strips have been cited as reasons for many of the earlier doubts about the validity of quantification by densitometry.[5] The cellulose acetate membrane itself may be a significant source of error, and, according to Scherr, one type of membrane sometimes gives albumin values as much as 9% higher than other types.[15] Scherr also cites the variation caused by batch-to-batch differences in the membrane as a primary reason to require that a reference serum be used in each run. Luxton compared the cellulose acetate strips from five manufacturers and found the Gelman Sepraphore III superior.[12] None of the others could match the transparency of this material or the uniformity of its wetting property.

## TECHNIQUE FOR ELECTROPHORESIS

Proper technique for serum protein electrophoresis includes use of fresh serum[9,16] and a precise amount of serum applied in a consistent manner to the same position near the cathodic end of each strip. The production of good patterns with smooth, straight areas of stained fractions is an art more than a science. Some

143

facts and suggestions may be given, but the operator's own technique for handling the sample application is equally as important as the settings on the equipment.

The buffer pH should be checked. Its ionic reproducibility may be shown by its resistance on a conductivity bridge. Although many laboratories prefer to use constant voltage, we prefer to maintain current constant. Buffer strength, temperature, and pH may all vary in some degree with time, and these affect current flow more than voltage. Also, when the current is constant, the reading of the voltage can be used as a sensitive means of indicating the cleanliness of the electrode system. For a regularly used system containing the same power pack, tray, and strips, when the current is set to its usual 8 ma for 8 strips, the resulting voltage should be the same at the beginning of the run from one day to the next. If the voltage is considerably lower, dried buffer may have formed around the electrode connections. The connections should then be taken off and cleaned. The electrodes themselves can be kept clean by reversing the current path through them after every two or three runs.

## DENSITOMETER

Evaluating and monitoring the densitometer requires consideration of the same ten characteristics used for the spectrophotometer plus the integration mechanism of the densitometer. Unlike spectrophotometers, however, densitometers are not all constructed to produce a linear response for absorbance. The monitoring of the linear and the nonlinear types will require somewhat different procedures; therefore, this characteristic will be discussed separately. Several characteristics of the two types can be discussed together: zero, integration mechanism, reproducibility, wavelength selection, source lamp, and the slit adjustments.

### Zero and Integration Mechanism

In addition to assuring that the zero setting of the densitometer registers properly, the integration system must also record zero over the period of time it will take to scan patterns. Luxton scans for 100 cm and repeats five times at settings of 0, plus 0.1 cm, and minus 0.1 cm.[10] She checks the integration with scans at 0, 0.1, and 1.0 cm monthly, and checks the integration at $-0.1$, 0, 0.1, 0.2, 0.5, 1.0, 2.0, 5.0, and 10.0 cm at three-month intervals. We have not routinely checked this many integration positions and find it sufficient to make daily checks of integrations at 0, an expected midpoint of about 5.0 cm, and a high point of about 10.0 cm. We allow our scans to run 15 cm, since this adequately covers our pattern length.

For someone who has never closely monitored the zero setting, the error shown in Figure 4-1 should be shocking. On this particular graph, the zero left at 0.2 absorbance units produced an error of 10% for the albumin and 58% for the $\gamma$ globulin because of the width of their respective peaks. This is an error giving high results. An error giving just as significantly low values would occur if the zero were set too low because instruments do not integrate values below the zero setting. We often have students run this kind of graph to demonstrate the error to them.

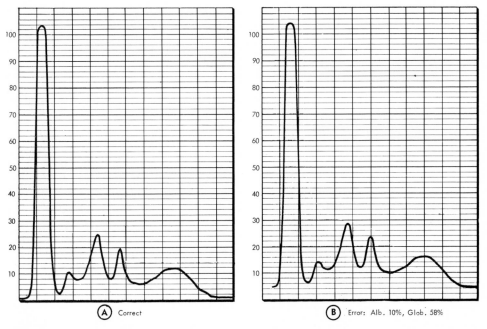

**Figure 4-1.** *Scan of protein patterns showing effect of incorrect zero setting on densitometer.*

## Reproducibility — Day to Day

Under ordinary circumstances, reproducibility is usually described as a scan (or reading) repeated one immediately following the other—*i.e.,* reproducibility of the instrument at any given period. Since many factors can affect the integrated scan of a pattern, particularly with some densitometers, we have used reproducibility to represent the scan of the same reference pattern rerun daily. In our experience such a reference pattern can be kept at least two years if handled and stored carefully.

## Wavelength Selection

In densitometers, filters are used to isolate the wavelength for recording the absorbance of the dyed strip. Choice of the filter for Ponceau S makes a great deal of difference in its absorbance characteristics. A 0.2% solution of Ponceau S in 5% trichloracetic acid has a maximum absorbance at 515 m$\mu$, and when a stained strip is scanned, the maximum occurs at the same wavelength. The spectral transmittance curve for a stained albumin fraction shown in Figure 4-2 was run on a Beckman DB spectrophotometer. Ponceau S has been reported as linear from 475 to 555 m$\mu$ if read on a narrow bandpass instrument, but the linearity decreases about 10% per unit increase in concentration when read on an instrument with a wide bandpass.[11] An interference type filter of 520 m$\mu$ is the filter of choice to provide both linearity and the greatest sensitivity.

145

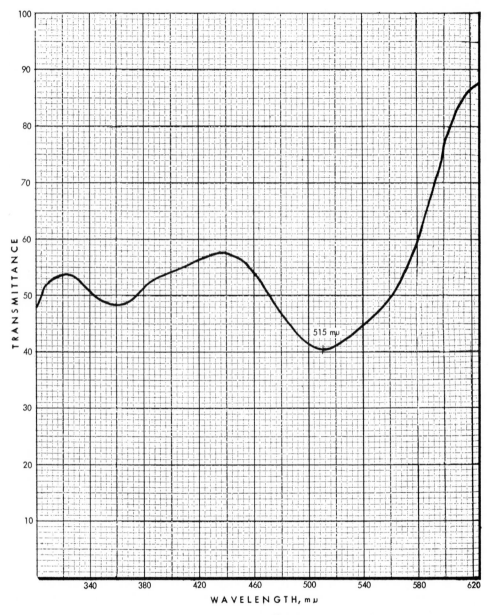

**Figure 4-2.** *Spectral transmittance curve for albumin stained with Ponceau S.*

### Source Lamp

The manufacturer chooses the source lamp for the particular densitometer, and the user can only learn to work within the limitations set. As with other components, the lamp used for replacement should always be the one specified by the

146

manufacturer. With age, all lamps change their output, and this effect is quite marked for some densitometers. It has been our experience that small lamps not only burn out quickly but also change their output long before they actually burn out. This changed light intensity can be detected when the reference pattern is rescanned (this point is discussed later). Each instrument is constructed to use the light from the lamp in a precise focused position. Therefore, when replaced, the lamp must be peaked according to the instruction manual. The outside surface of the lamp should be kept clean; a dirty surface changes not only the intensity of the light but also its focus.

## Slit Adjustments

The slit width and length are restricted by both the instrument and the pattern size. Provided the slit size is proper for either the macro (about ¾ inch) or micro (about ½ inch) pattern being used, the most important consideration becomes the balancing of the optical system of the instrument. In some instances neutral density filters must be used in order to choose the proper slit settings. In general, the narrowest possible slit is preferable, and the slit length should be as long as is practical. This combination provides good separation of peaks and strong photocell response (*i.e.,* high sensitivity).

## Calibration of the Densitometer

In determining how to calibrate the densitometer, one must know whether or not the instrument's absorbance response is linear. The Analytrol Model RB* is an example of the linear type of densitometer, and the Gelscan† is an example of the nonlinear type.

### LINEAR TYPE — ANALYTROL RB

In addition to the current instruction manual,[1] we use two Beckman brochures, *Maintenance of the Model R Analytrol*[2] and *Installing the Nylon Pen Cable in the Analytrol,*[3] when calibrating the Analytrol RB. Nerenberg's *Electrophoresis* includes a very good description of the structure and function of the RB Analytrol.[13] His section on Analytrol troubleshooting appears to be one section from Beckman's Field Service Manual. Table 4-1, a handout sheet from Beckman Instruments, includes references to the current manual for correcting some of the most common problems.

To achieve proper scanning of the Sepraphore III (1″ x 6¾″) Ponceau S stained electrophoretic strips, our RB Analytrol has the following modifications:

1. A Scan-A-Tron† attachment. We have replaced the cam supplied with this kit with a B-2 cam from Beckman Instruments.

2. The slit width is 0.5 mm, and the slit length is 10 mm. We have masked the housing into which the front photocell fits, so that this aperture length is also 10 mm. The

---

* Beckman Instruments, Inc., Fullerton, Calif.

† Gelman Instrument Co., Ann Arbor, Mich.

**Table 4-1. Analytrol Operator's Troubleshooting Guide**

Troubles that occasionally disrupt the operation of the Analytrol can often be corrected easily by the Operator. Consult this troubleshooting guide prior to calling your Beckman Field Engineer—it may save you time and the cost of a service call.

| SYMPTOM | POSSIBLE CAUSE | REMEDY |
|---|---|---|
| 1. No pen response, lamp and fan off, chart paper does not pull through. | Power cord disconnected at wall plug. Defective 3 amp fuse at rear of instrument. | Plug power cord into wall receptacle. Replace fuse. (Buss. AGC 3) |
| 2. No pen response, lamp and fan on, chart paper pulls through. | Amplifier gain too low. Defective ½ amp Slo-Blo fuse on amplifier. Loose plugs to amplifier. | Increase gain (page 3-4, RB-IM-6). Replace ½ amp fuse. (Littelfuse 313, ½ amp Slo-Blo) Tighten plugs to Servo amplifier. |
| 3. Lamp off, fan on. | Lamp burned out. | Replace lamp (page 4-2, RB-IM-6). |
| 4. Pen deflects to chart top and stays. | Obstructed light path to front photocell. Loose connections on front photocell. | Check light path and remove obstructions. Tighten connections to photocell. |
| 5. Pen deflects to chart bottom and stays. | Light shield obstructing light path to rear photocell. Loose connections on rear photocell. | Re-position light shield. Tighten connections to rear photocell. |
| 6. Pen response sluggish. | Low amplifier gain. | Increase gain (page 3-4, RB-IM-6). |
| 7. Pen response sluggish with gain control full clockwise. | Defective tubes in amplifier. | Set gain to proper point (page 3-4, RB-IM-6) and if pen response is still sluggish, check amplifier tubes. Replace those found defective. |
| 8. Pen response erratic. | External light influencing front photocell. Defective chopper. | Check position of light guard over strip guide. Replace chopper. |

| Symptom | Probable Cause | Remedy |
|---|---|---|
| 9. Unable to calibrate properly. | Loose cam. Cam installed backward. | Tighten cam nut. Install cam correctly (p. 5-2, **RB-IM-6**). |
| 10. Calibration difficult with dark or small slit. | Too much light reaching rear photocell. | Add neutral density filters to rear filter holder. |
| 11. Calibration difficult with light or clear strip. | Too much light reaching front photocell. | Add neutral density filters to front filter holder. |
| 12. Pen will not zero or reach calibration set point. | Wrong calibration set point value used. Front slit not centered. Obstructions in front and/or rear light path. Calibration filter out of position in holder allowing dark band between clear and filter area to obstruct light path. | Use correct calibration set point. Center front slit. Clear light path of obstructions. Re-position calibration filter in its holder. |
| 13. Pen oscillates | High amplifier gain. | Decrease gain (page 3-4. **RB-IM-6**). |

strip carrier likewise has a limiting slit length of 10 mm. These carriers are part of the Scan-A-Tron kit. We scan each carrier in order to use only those that do not add error to the integration. We have found the edges of the cut-out portions of some of these carriers rather irregular.

3. The 520 m$\mu$ interference filter used in front is the Beckman #328066. The back filter can be the 500 m$\mu$ interference filter which comes with the instrument, but this sometimes requires inclusion of a 0.3 neutral density filter to balance the photocells. We have also alternately chosen a 550 m$\mu$ interference filter for the back which balanced the system without use of the neutral density filter.

4. The clear lamp is a 100 watt GE #PH-100T8-108 SC.

5. *Digital counter for integration.** A digital counter attached to the integration system constantly counts the "saw marks." The operator notes and records the total on the counter as each valley appears between the fractions. Originally we scanned the strips, marked the intersection points, and rescanned in order to identify the valley precisely. When it became apparent that the operator could detect these valleys on the first scan, we eliminated the rescanning.

According to Beckman Instruments proper calibration of the Analytrol is still done with the B-5 cam and a continuous gradation optical wedge made by Kodak. Since their set point readings have never been correlated to the B-2 cam we use, and the Kodak wedge is not available, we devised the following procedure.

To calibrate our Model RB Analytrol densitometer, we use three neutral density filters: 0.3, 0.6, and 0.9.† Their exact values we determine on a Beckman DB-G spectrophotometer, but because they are $10 \times 25$ mm, they can be read on any spectrophotometer that will accommodate a 10 mm square cuvette. These are the same filters we use for checking the Beckman DB and DB-G spectrophotometers for reproducibility. Their size is such that when used each can be carefully taped to the Analytrol housing between the housing and the front photocell. We have taped the top and bottom of this housing aperture to a length of 10 mm to provide a controlled area in which the light from the lamp is focused for reading the strips. The filter fits neatly over this aperture.

Before starting the calibration procedure of the Analytrol optical system, we read the neutral density filters and from them assign a value to the Analytrol's calibrating filter as given below. (The readings are an example and are not intended as precise values for other individual filters of even the same type.)

1. The neutral density filters read: I = 0.340, II = 0.635, and III = 0.935 on the Beckman DB-G.

2. As a starting place, set the pen to zero on the graph and put the calibration filter into the optical path. With the calibration control knob adjust the pen to the 9 cm mark on the graph and integrate for 5 cm. Total integrations = 449. Remove the calibrating filter from the optical path.

3. Tape the III filter to the housing and scan its integration for 5 cm. Total integrations = 468.

---

* Don Dalke, South Bend Medical Foundation, Inc., South Bend, Ind.

† Neutral Density Filters #9104 N25, Arthur H. Thomas Co., Philadelphia, Pa.

4. The absorbance of the calibrating filter, under our conditions, may now be determined as follows:

$$\frac{449}{468} \times 0.935 = 0.905$$

## Calibration with Neutral Density Filters

Calibration of the Analytrol with neutral density filters is a straightforward, relatively easy procedure, but it will not prove valid unless all the components of the instrument are functioning properly. Refer to the components as identified in

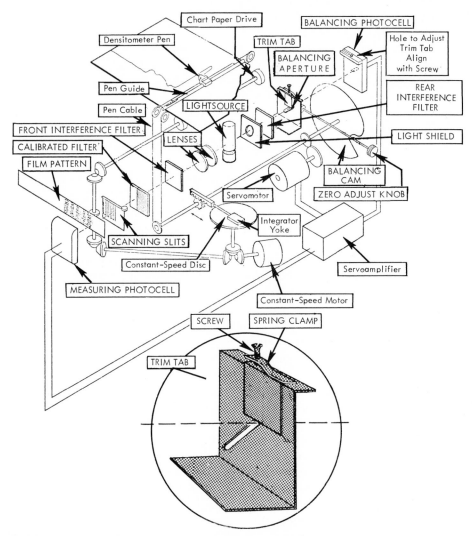

**Figure 4-3.** *Function diagram of components of RB Analytrol. (Modified from Beckman Instruction Manual RB-IM-6, March, 1966.)*

151

the functional diagram of the RB Analytrol shown in Figure 4-3. When an un-stained portion of the cellulose acetate is in position for its absorbance to be read, the pen is at zero on the graph and the large notch of the balancing cam is at the top. This setting allows the light from the lamp to traverse frontwards and backwards to strike both photocells. The voltages from the two photocells is equal under these circumstances. As the stained portion of the strip is positioned into the optical path, the decreased light on the front photocell produces a lower volt-age. The difference in the voltage between the two photocells is amplified and fed to a servomotor which rotates the balancing cam until enough light has been cut from the back photocell to again make the voltages equal. The pen is linked to the balancing cam so that the more the cam has to turn to balance the voltages, the higher the pen moves on the graph.

When the Analytrol is first calibrated using the B-2 cam, clear lamp, and 520 m$\mu$ filter, it is not always easy to set the zero. Check the lamp first and be sure its outside surface is clean; focus the light with the lenses so that the sharp beam strikes the central portion of the slit. Now check the light from the lamp to the back photocell; be sure the light shield is in place between the lamp and the rear filter. With a very small slit, a neutral density filter may have to be inserted in the rear filter holder to reduce the light sufficiently to the back photocell to allow the instrument to reach a zero setting. An alternative would be to use a slightly larger slit width, but under no circumstances should the slit width chosen be as wide as the narrowest stained fraction of the pattern to be scanned.

Only after the zero setting has been attained can the absorbance be calibrated. The diagram in Figure 4-3 shows the balancing aperture, balancing cam, and balancing photocell spread apart for easy identification. Actually the balancing cam has just enough room to turn between the other two components, and the photocell is fastened by a flange on top of the housing of the balancing aperture. Also fastened to the top of this housing is the spring clip which governs the position of the trim tab. The trim tab is a small plate riding behind the top portion of the aperture and shutting off part of the opening. The height of this tab is regulated by slightly turning the screw in the spring clip. As the light travels from the lamp toward the back photocell, the beam through the balancing aperture is cut from the bottom by the balancing cam and from the top by the trim tab. The area of the light beam which strikes the photocell is precisely controlled by these adjust-ments to the balancing aperture. Thus the limit for the amount the cam turns to balance the light is determined by the trim tab setting. If the tab is too high (area of slit is too large) the cam will turn through a greater angle in order to balance the output of the two photocells. In this case the pen will move a greater vertical distance to cause the tracing to be too steep. On the other hand, if the trim tab is too low, the cam will not turn enough, and the pen will produce a tracing that is too short. Since the pen travel is directly controlled by the turning of the cam, the establishment of linearity becomes the precise setting of the trim tab.[3] To make the trim tab adjustment screw more accessible we have bored a small hole, as indicated in Figure 4-3, in the flange of the photocell.

152

The trim tab adjustment is a very sensitive setting, and a small change makes a large difference in the pen travel. For our cellulose acetate patterns the albumin peak for a Versatol* control value of 4.5 gms extends to about 12.5 cm on the graph when the trim tab is set at its lowest position. In the highest position of the trim tab the same peak far exceeded the top edge of the graph.

The zero adjust (position of balancing aperture), the calibration set point knob (amplification of voltage from rear photocell) and the trim tab adjustment are all inter-related. The zero setting and the trim tab adjustments for linear calibration with the neutral density filters are therefore trial and error settings until the proper combination has been reached. Once determined, however, these settings have usually remained constant for at least a year.

---

## Calibration of the RB Analytrol with Neutral Density Filters

1. Place a cleared portion of the cellulose acetate strip (blank) in the strip holder and position it properly to set the zero point for the instrument. Leave this strip holder in place throughout the following procedure.

2. Slide the calibrating filter into position to read in the instrument and set the pen to record 9.1 on the graph. Pull the calibrating filter out of the optical path.

3. Remove the front photocell and carefully tape the 0.3 filter to the housing so that it covers the aperture at the front (measuring) photocell. Replace the photocell to its proper position. Read and record the absorbance of this filter. For our Filter I this value is 0.340, and it should read close to 3.4 in the Analytrol.

4. With the 0.3 filter still in place, pull the calibrating filter into the optical path and record the value of the combined filters. For example, the value should be 0.340 + 0.906 or 1.25 (*i.e.,* 12.5 on the Analytrol).

5. If the value of the combined filters does not read within ± 0.2 of the proper value, make the necessary correction by adjusting the trim tab.

6. Recheck all values for zero, the neutral density filters and the combination of the 0.3 and the calibrating filter.

7. Once the overall calibration is proved linear, daily use requires only that the zero and calibrating filter be properly adjusted. Daily checking of the linearity is done with a Kodak Step Tablet as described below.

---

## Daily Check of Analytrol Linearity

The easiest way we have found to monitor the linearity of the Analytrol is to daily scan a Kodak Photographic Step Tablet, #2.† This neutral density strip has 21 steps ranging from approximately 0.05 to 3.05. Each strip is individually

* General Diagnostic Division, Warner-Chilcott Laboratories, Morris Plains, N. J.
† Eastman Kodak Co., Rochester, N. Y.

calibrated by the Kodacolor Processing Division of Kodak and the data sheet is provided with the Step Tablet.

We find it convenient to set the #1 step (0.04 density) to record 0.4 using the zero adjust knob and to adjust the pen with the calibration potentiometer knob to read 13.8 for Step #10 (1.38 density). We then scan the strip and allow each step to record on the graph. See Figure 4-4. In our experience, the values for each step through #11 (1.53 density) have checked within ± 0.2 cm on the graph. It is gratifying to find the instrument readings close to the company's calibration for this strip because the size of the strip and its steps make it impossible to check its absorbance on our DB-G spectrophotometer.

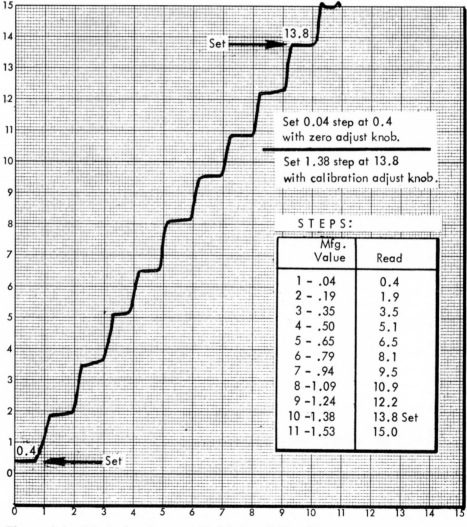

Set 0.04 step at 0.4 with zero adjust knob.

Set 1.38 step at 13.8 with calibration adjust knob.

STEPS:

| | Mfg. Value | Read |
|---|---|---|
| 1 - | .04 | 0.4 |
| 2 - | .19 | 1.9 |
| 3 - | .35 | 3.5 |
| 4 - | .50 | 5.1 |
| 5 - | .65 | 6.5 |
| 6 - | .79 | 8.1 |
| 7 - | .94 | 9.5 |
| 8 - | 1.09 | 10.9 |
| 9 - | 1.24 | 12.2 |
| 10 - | 1.38 | 13.8 Set |
| 11 - | 1.53 | 15.0 |

**Figure 4-4.** *RB Analytrol scan of Kodak Step Tablet #2.*

154

## NONLINEAR TYPE — GELSCAN

The Gelscan we used was a model #39365 with a slide holder to accommodate the 1 inch wide Sepraphore III strips. This instrument has three filters so arranged that the user chooses the light "color" by positioning a filter selector. These filters are thin plastic disks, but the transmittance of the green one is well suited for use with the Ponceau S. The maximum transmittance of the filter occurs about 512 m$\mu$, as shown on the DB-G scan (Fig. 4-5). The settings for slit width and length are screwdriver adjustments A and B on the left side of the densitometer. The terms *width* and *length* were reversed in the manual published in 1968, but we chose to maintain the original terminology because it represents more closely the same terms for the spectrophotometer slit. Figure 4-6 identifies the slit length and width as it is used to pass the light through a stained serum protein strip. The choices available for slit length are 1, 3, and 10 mm and for slit width from 0 to 2 mm. For quantification we counted the horizontal boxes traversed rather than using their nomogram. The Gelscan densitometer was said to record true optical density,

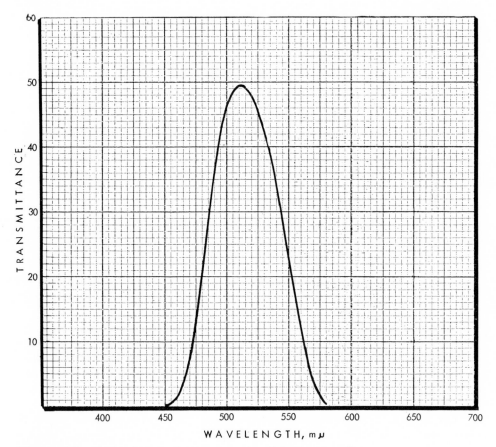

**Figure 4-5.** *Spectral transmittance curve for Gelscan green filter.*

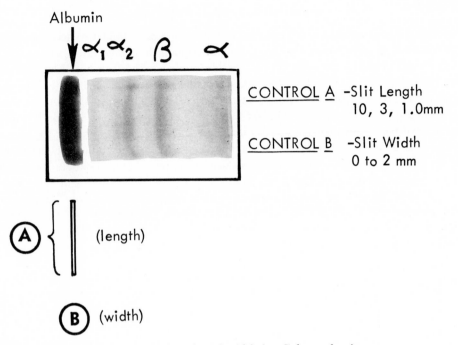

**Figure 4-6.** *Definition of slit length and width for Gelscan densitometer.*

and the paper was marked in increments from 0 to 2. The albumin peak for our usual Versatol control (albumin value 4.1) reached about 0.6, and the total scan for all the fractions gave about 90 to 100 integrations.

In 1969 after Gelman offered a modification (model #39372) which converted the log to linear response before the signal was fed to the recorder, we had our unit converted. The paper for the unit was marked 0 to 100, and the operator was instructed to set the absorbance of the albumin peak of each scan to read 90 on the paper. The increased sensitivity now provided a total integration of about 225 to 275 for our same electrophoretic patterns.

In order to calibrate this instrument (either the original or after modification) one must scan a pattern whose albumin value is already known.[6] Then by trial and error settings of the slit dimension controls A and B, the instrument is made to quantify the desired albumin value. During our entire use of this instrument we left control A set on 3 mm. Table 4-2 shows the values obtained with various settings for control B. These values were obtained on reference pattern #1 for a particular lot number of Versatol. Our total protein value was 7.2 gm, and the albumin was 4.3 by our chemical method.[7] Therefore we chose 0.50 as the final setting for slit control B.

The concept of the Gelscan instrument seems somewhat unique in that it is constructed so the user can change the value of the albumin-globulin ratio to

156

Table 4-2.  Determination of Proper Setting for Gelscan Slit Width (Control Knob B)

| Slit Width Control B Setting mm | Total Integrations | Albumin gm | γ Globulin gm |
|---|---|---|---|
| 0.4 | 253 | 3.90 | 1.44 |
| 0.45 | 236 | 4.1 | 1.4 |
| 0.50 | 212 | 4.3 | 1.26 |
| 0.70 | 205 | 4.4 | 1.16 |
| 0.8 | 187 | 4.73 | 1.03 |

suit his own preference. As can be seen from the values in Table 4-2, the albumin value increases as the setting for the B slit control is set larger. This functional characteristic appears acceptable under two conditions: (1) that once set, the A/G would remain stable and (2) the same reference pattern scanned daily would give reproducible quantification.

The degree of change for the A/G is clearly denoted in the two scans from the same pattern shown in Figure 4-7. Scan #1 gave an albumin value of 3.6 and the γ globulin was 1.6 with slit settings of 3 x 0.5 mm. The bulb was changed and properly peaked; scan #2 gave an albumin of 5.2 and γ globulin of 0.86 for the same slit settings. By changing the slit settings to 3 x 0.3 mm, the albumin became 3.6 and the γ globulin was 1.5. This incident happened to us before we understood the necessary daily monitoring or the variation in the lamp intensity within relatively short periods of time.

The lamp in this instrument is the GE #313, a small bulb that ages rather rapidly. As it ages, the intensity and the focus change so that some means of continual monitoring is absolutely essential. We found this could be done with neutral density filters in the following manner:

1. Set the zero in the usual manner.
2. Set the albumin peak of the Reference Pattern #1 to read 90. This is the permanent reference point also used for scanning the same reference pattern daily as the quality control measure of the instrument itself.
3. Tape neutral density filters into the strip carrier and read them.

A permanent record of these neutral density readings should be kept for the slit control B settings as related to the value for albumin. While not linear, the neutral density readings can be reproduced by changing the control B slit adjustment. A new bulb with full light intensity requires a small setting for control B; as the bulb ages, the setting must be increased. Not all lamps require the same setting even when new. Thus, one must monitor the neutral density filter readings daily and adjust control B as necessary. It is much quicker to adjust the control B

157

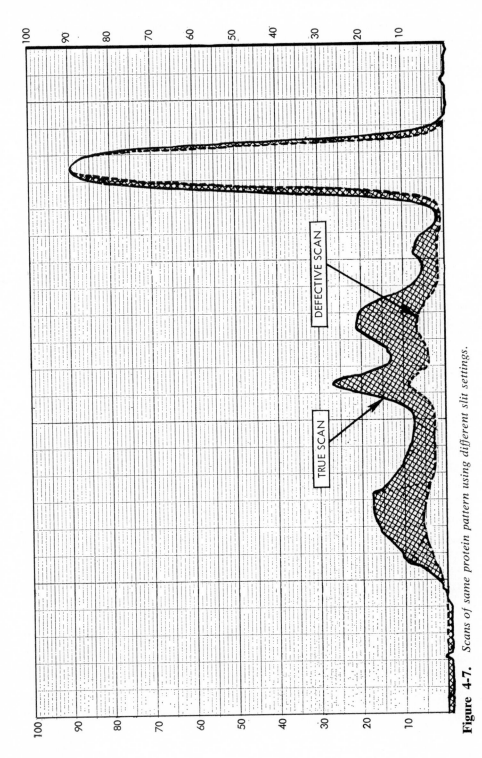

**Figure 4-7.** *Scans of same protein pattern using different slit settings.*

for the desired optical density reading than to scan the reference pattern repeatedly until the proper setting has been determined. Once the neutral density filter readings have been set to their usual reading, the reference pattern should then be scanned.

When the same reference pattern #1 was used for scanning on both the Analytrol and the Gelscan, the albumin values were about the same, but the γ globulin Gelscan values were always about 0.5 higher than those on the Analytrol. This clearly demonstrates again that each institution *must* establish its own normal values with the exact procedure being used.

## Quality Control for the Gelscan Densitometer

We found the following procedures necessary to maintain consistent quantification of the serum protein fractions using the Ponseau S stained Sepraphore III strips:

A. *Original Calibration*

1. Install a new lamp in the densitometer, and peak its light output as indicated by Gelman instruction sheet.

2. Choose a very good stained pattern to use as a permanent reference pattern. We prefer to use Versatol for this pattern, and the albumin value assigned to it is established by our chemical method.

3. Zero the pen on the graph with the clear portion of the pattern in position and then set the pen to read 90 for the albumin peak.

4. Scan the pattern. If necessary, adjust the slit control screws A and B until the scan will produce the proper albumin value. As mentioned previously, we leave A at 3 and adjust only B. Record the settings for A and B. Without changing the pen settings, remove the stained strip from the carrier and read the neutral density filters. Record the value for each. As long as this reference pattern is maintained in satisfactory condition, the filter values serve as reference points.

The normal range must now be established for the entire electrophoresis method as run in one's own institution. These values should be calculated only after the precise details of the entire system have been established, including the standardization of the densitometer.

B. *Daily calibration check*

1. Using the reference pattern, zero the pen and set 90 for the albumin peak.

2. Read the neutral density filters and record their values. Compare these values with their reference point readings as obtained above. If the filters do not check within ± 1 of their reference point readings, adjust control B as necessary. Some adjustment is expected to be required from week to week.

3. Retain a scan of the reference pattern as the assurance that the densitometer is properly adjusted for that day.

4. Include a control sample in the electrophoresis run and retain its scan for the check of the entire system.

159

In conclusion, although the procedures differ for each type of densitometer, technologists must daily assure themselves of the following:

1.  The calibration of the instrument is valid (*e.g.*, readings on Kodak Step Tablet #2).
2.  The electrophoretic system is reproducible as demonstrated by values for the control sample's separate fractions falling within ± 2 SD for this method.

## REFERENCES

1.  Beckman Instrument Inc.: Instruction manual RB-IM-6. *Model RB Analytrol Recording Densitometer.* Fullerton, Calif., Beckman Instruments, Inc., 1966.
2.  ———: Field Service Manual. *Maintenance of the Model R Analytrol.* (Reproduced in Manual for Regional Seminar on Instrumentation, ASMT-ASCP, Chicago, March, 1966.)
3.  ———: Technical Bulletin TB6125. *Installing the Nylon Pen Cable in the Analytrol.* Palo Alto, Calif., Spinco Div., Beckman Instruments, Inc., May, 1962.
4.  Biere, R. O., and Mull, J. D.: Electrophoresis of serum protein with cellulose acetate. Amer. J. Clin. Path. *42:*547, 1964.
5.  Grunbaum, B. W., Zec, J., and Durrum, E. L.: Application of an improved micro-electrophoresis technique and immunoelectrophoresis of the serum proteins on cellulose acetate. Microchem. J., *7:*41, 1963.
6.  Haer, F.: Personal communication.
7.  Henry, R. J.: *Clinical Chemistry. Principles and Technics.* New York, Hoeber Med. Div., Harper Row, 1964.
8.  Lange, C. F.: Advances in electrophoretic and chromatographic technics. In *Progress in Clinical Pathology.* Vol. 3 M. S. Stefanini, ed. New York, Grune & Stratton, 1970.
9.  Lubran, M.: Problems of electrophoresis. Hosp. Topics, *45:*61, 1967.
10. Luxton, G. C.: Serum protein electrophoresis. Evaluation and modification of the micro-zone system, Part I. Canad. J. Med. Techn., *30:*4, 1968.
11. ———: Serum protein electrophoresis. Evaluation and modification of the micro-zone system, Part II. Canad. J. Med. Techn., *30:*55, 1968.
12. ———: Serum protein electrophoresis. Evaluation and modification of the micro-zone system, Part III. Canad. J. Med. Techn., *30:*83, 1968.
13. Nerenberg, S. T.: *Electrophoresis. A Practical Laboratory Manual.* Philadelphia, F. A. Davis, 1966.
14. Ritts, R. E., Jr., and Ondrick, F. W.: Electrophoresis of serum proteins on cellulose acetate. Amer. J. Clin. Path., *41:*321, 1964.
15. Scherr, G. H.: Cellulose acetate electrophoresis in microbiology and immunology. Trans. N. Y. Acad. Sci., *23:*519, 1961.
16. Strickland, R. D., Podleski, T. R., Gurule, F. T., Freeman, M. L., and Childs, W. A.: Dye-binding capacities of eleven electrophoretically separated serum proteins. Anal. Chem. *31:*1408, 1959.
17. Sunderman, F. W., Jr., and Sunderman, F. W.: Studies on the serum proteins, IV. The dye-binding of purified serum proteins separated on continuous-flow electrophoresis. Clin. Chem., *5:*171, 1959.
18. Vanzetti, G., Palatucci, F., and Cosci, G.: Automatic analysis of electrophoretic strips by means of a cyclic electronic scanner. Clin. Chim. Acta, *20:*215, 1968.
19. Williams, F. G., Jr.: Microzone electrophoresis of serum proteins. In *Serum Proteins and the Dysproteinemias.* F. W. Sunderman and F. W. Sunderman, Jr., eds. Philadelphia, J. B. Lippincott Co., 1964.

# 5

# Flame Photometers*

The flame photometer is basically a photometer in which the flame replaces the source lamp. Assignment of the same checking functions used for the spectrophotometer is easy to rationalize. The operator still must check the flame characteristics, noise and drift, zero and maximum response, reproducibility, sampling, linearity, the optical system, and the electronic system. In the spectrophotometer the stability of the source lamp has been controlled so effectively by the manufacturer of the instrument that the user almost takes this function for granted. In the flame photometer, however, the operator must control the stability of the flame during the entire operation of the instrument.

The clinical values obtained by flame photometry should be more accurate and more uniformly comparable between laboratories than are those from other chemical tests. The instruments available are capable of producing reliable answers. Pure standards are used to set the instrument before reading the test samples. Test procedures don't vary much from one laboratory to another. Gambino has stated that sodium values should be accurate within $\pm 1.8\%$ and potassium $\pm 7\%$.[18] His values are consistent with Tonks' estimate:[38]

$$\text{Allowable error in}\% = \frac{\frac{1}{4} \text{ normal range}}{\text{mean of normal range}} \times 100$$

* Most of this material appeared in Quality Control for Flame Photometry in the American Journal of Medical Technology (*34*:305-333, 1968) and is reprinted with permission of the publisher.

The allowable error for a sodium value of 145 mEq would be 2.6 or 3 mEq. Reference laboratories listed in Gambino's report agreed within ± 4 mEq.

The values shown in the College of American Pathologists' survey for 1968, set 3, list the reference laboratories within ± 4 mEq for sodium values of 145 and 124. Participants' values were ± 6 for 1.5 SD and ± 7 for 2 SD for the 145 mEq sample and 6 and 8 for the 124 mEq sample.

Recently the Standards Committee of the College of American Pathologists reported the accuracy deemed necessary for medical significance as compared to the "state of the art achievements" (*i.e.,* good performance) for the more common laboratory tests.[2] By comparing the performance to medically significant levels of accuracy, tests were noted which did not meet the physicians' needs. This evaluation was intended as provisional, but the comparison of accuracy levels points clearly to those tests that must be improved as rapidly as possible. A sodium value of 150 mEq is shown to require ± 2.6% accuracy (± 2 CV) and the present performance is given as ± 4%. These calculations were done from the values of the 1967 CAP survey and by this standard 19.4% of the participants' values would be excluded by the ± 2.6% specification. Potassium values of 3 and 6 mEq were listed as requiring ± 16.6 and ± 8.4% accuracy respectively. Performance was ± 7.4 and ± 6.6%.

Wide variations between clinical chemistry values for different laboratories are usually rationalized as being caused by systemic constant differences in methodology. The normal range established for a single laboratory is thus expected to accommodate these differences. The danger of wide variations in flame photometer test values is that the variations are not constant. Since changing flame conditions cause the fluctuations to vary from day to day and even from hour to hour, variations in sample values cannot be related to an individual laboratory's normal range.

In our experience, the 125 mEq range of sodium is the most difficult to control. Between-laboratory values can be as much as $\pm$ 12 mEq different, and within the same laboratory the values may differ by only $\pm$ 2 mEq. This situation can be corrected to $\pm$ 4 mEq between laboratories by carefully monitoring the flame photometers. Allowable error of $\pm$ 4 mEq at the 125 mEq range (2 CV = 3.2%) is slightly over the specification of the College of American Pathologists. The same allowable error of $\pm$ 4 mEq at the 150 mEq range closely approximates the current goal. The desired accuracy for potassium is easily attained.

The most important parameters dictated in instruments will be discussed in relation to the Coleman 21,* the Beckman 105† and the Instrumentation Laboratory 143‡ flame photometers. The theoretical information describing each parameter is followed by directions for performing the routine check procedures. These procedures are numbered for clarification; the numbers indicate the order in which the procedures occur on the check sheet for the specific instrument.

The first consideration in determining the necessary quality is whether the instrument is a direct measurement or an internal standard type. The direct measurement type will be discussed first, since the function of this instrument is subject to all the interacting factors that influence the stability of the flame and hence the emission values for test samples.

## DIRECT MEASUREMENT FLAME PHOTOMETER

The Coleman 21 flame photometer is a direct measurement instrument with a total-consumption burner. The fuel can be line gas, propane, or butane; the oxidant is oxygen. The glass filters are chosen to allow use of the 589 m$\mu$ sodium line, the 766 m$\mu$ potassium line, and the 622 m$\mu$ calcium line. The detector is a 1P39 phototube. The readout may be done with any stable galvanometer, but the Coleman Jr. spectrophotometer is convenient. A check sheet for this instrument is shown in Figure 5-1.

### Burner

Details of the Coleman total consumption burner are shown in Figure 5-2. The insert shows a diagram of the cross section of the atomizer as it fits into the burner body. Oxygen enters the atomizer around the atomizer orifice, D. As the oxygen passes D, it causes pneumatic aspiration of the sample, through C. The fuel enters through B, passes up through the holes in the burner baffle plate, E,

---

* Coleman Instruments, Maywood, Ill. Division of Perkin-Elmer Corporation.

† Beckman Instruments, Inc., Fullerton, Calif.

‡ Instrumentation Laboratory, Inc., Lexington, Mass.

# DAILY CHECK SHEET FOR COLEMAN FLAME PHOTOMETER, MODEL 21

Hospital _____   Instrument # _____   Month _____   Year _____

| | 1 | 2 | | | | 3 | | | 4 | 5 | | 6 | 7 |
|---|---|---|---|---|---|---|---|---|---|---|---|---|---|
| | | Burner | | | | Flame | | | | $H_2O$ Contam | | | Control |
| Date | $O_2$ tank # | Top | Screen | $O_2$ # | Max K | Size | Cone | Color | Sound | Asp rate cc/min | vs NaO | vs KO | Elect Ck ±%T | Na: VA# _____, mfg. _____<br>K: VAA# _____, mfg. _____ |
| 1 | | | | | | | | | | | | | | Na |
| | | | | | | | | | | | | | | K |
| 2 | | | | | | | | | | | | | | Na |
| | | | | | | | | | | | | | | K |
| 3 | | | | | | | | | | | | | | Na |
| | | | | | | | | | | | | | | K |
| 4 | | | | | | | | | | | | | | Na |
| | | | | | | | | | | | | | | K |
| 5 | | | | | | | | | | | | | | Na |
| | | | | | | | | | | | | | | K |
| 6 | | | | | | | | | | | | | | Na |
| | | | | | | | | | | | | | | K |

**Figure 5-1.** *Daily check sheet for Coleman flame photometer, Model 21.*

165

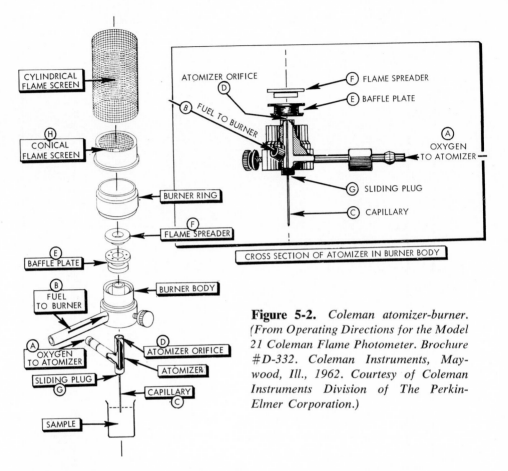

**Figure 5-2.** *Coleman atomizer-burner. (From Operating Directions for the Model 21 Coleman Flame Photometer. Brochure #D-332. Coleman Instruments, Maywood, Ill., 1962. Courtesy of Coleman Instruments Division of The Perkin-Elmer Corporation.)*

and around the outside edge of the flame spreader, F. The fuel and oxygen are mixed at the burner tip. The entire aspirated sample is sprayed into the flame through the atomizer orifice, D. The oxygen canal should be frequently flushed free of trapped particles by pushing upward on the sliding plug, G, with the cleaning tool.

## 2. Check Procedures for Coleman Burner

Before the flame is turned on:

a. Take the screen off and look at the top of the atomizer-burner. If encrustation is present, clean it off.

b. Look for discolored rings on the screen's surface; if present, wash the screen.

c. When the burner is turned on, flush the oxygen passage by pushing upward on the atomizer plug with the tool provided. Record the pressure of the secondary oxygen gauge.

d. See page 171 for check procedures for maximum potassium emission.

The gas burns at the bottom of the conical screen (H, Fig. 5-2) and may be seen as a little mound at the base of the main flame. This burning base forms a pilot flame to maintain the faster turbulent flame at gas flow speeds which otherwise would extinguish it.[39] Atomizer-burners of this type are said to be totally free of flame flashback even when used with combustible solvents.[29] This burner will flash, however, if the gas flow rapidly decreases while the burner is lit; such a flash melts the plastic parts and singes the chimney lining. The chimney lining may then drop particles into the flame, causing erratic emission. Total-consumption burners produce turbulent, ill-defined diffusion flames whose emission intensity varies in different parts of the flame.[29]

## Flame Characteristics

The flame and control of its characteristics are the basic consideration for all flame photometers. Measurement of the element's emission and assignment of a concentration value therefore require that the flame remain absolutely stable or constant during the process. Stability is the primary goal of flame control: stability of flame position, size and shape, composition or character, and temperature is necessary before consistency in sample excitation can be achieved.[39] A few factors such as gas, oxidant, and filters are predetermined by the instrument itself. Among the many other factors influencing the stability of the flame are the user's adjustments of fuel and oxygen pressures and aspiration. Most of the factors interact and therefore must be considered together.

The choice of gas and oxidant is dictated by the instrument; therefore, the maximum flame temperature and limit of excitable elements is predetermined for the user. The Coleman 21 flame photometer, which uses line gas or propane with oxygen, provides a flame temperature of about 2700°C.[42] Maximum flame temperatures for various fuel and oxidant combinations are shown in Table 5-1.

Table 5-1. Maximum Flame Temperatures*

| Fuel | Flame Temperature °C | |
|---|---|---|
| | In Air | In Oxygen |
| Illuminating gas | 1700 | 2700 |
| Propane | 1925 | 2800 |
| Butane | 1900 | 2900 |
| Hydrogen | 2100 | 2780 |
| Acetylene | 2200 | 3050 |
| Cyanogen | 2330 | 4550 |

* From Willard, H. H., Merritt, L. L., and Dean, J. A.: *Instrumental Methods of Analysis,* 4th ed. New York, D. Van Nostrand Company, Inc., 1965, p. 319.

In general, sodium and potassium are best determined at a temperature of about 1800°C. Sodium excitation increases about 15% with a 1% increase in temperature. Potassium excitation is affected even more by temperature changes because its excitation potential is lower; ionization of potassium also increases with increased temperature so that the net excitation is variable.

Adjusting the fuel/oxidant ratio can raise or lower the temperature somewhat,[12] but what is more important, the mixture of gases, and therefore the flame character, varies with different ratios. The fuel/oxidant ratio is classified as stoichiometric, lean, or rich in terms of the fuel content. A stoichiometric mixture is one in which the amount of oxygen is just sufficient to burn the fuel;[29] the flame appears blue with a white inner cone whose height is about one-fourth the overall flame height. As oxygen is added to this flame (*i.e.,* flame becomes lean), the inner cone becomes shorter and brighter until an excess of oxygen causes the inner cone to flare yellow and then white streaks perpendicular to the flame. For the optimum lean flame, addition of oxygen is stopped just short of flaring. A rich mixture gives a flame whose inner cone is taller and eventually, with a small amount of oxygen, can become soft and sooty. Figure 5-3 shows the temperature distribution in the flames of rich, stoichiometric, and lean mixtures. Sodium can be measured satisfactorily in any of these mixtures; potassium is best determined in a mixture slightly more lean than stoichiometric; calcium is best determined in a lean mixture.[24]

Since it is not practical to regulate the flame by measuring its temperature, the appearance of the flame must be used to judge the gross adjustment of the fuel/oxidant ratio. The cone size as related to the flame size and the color of the cone indicate proper adjustment of fuel and oxygen.[41] (See Fig. 5-4.) An experienced operator instinctively notes these flame and cone characteristics and makes the proper adjustments before using the instrument. The operator should check the following flame characteristics before he starts to aspirate any samples.

---

### 3. Flame Characteristics (See Fig. 5-1, Coleman.)

After the flame has burned about 5 minutes, observe and record in the proper space on the check sheet:

1. *Size and Shape of Flame.* The height should be 3½″ to 4″ and the width about ⅜″. If outside these limits, the flame must be trimmed to size with gas regulation and then readjusted for maximum potassium emission.

2. *Cone Height.* The cone should be between ¼″ to ⅜″ high; if it is higher, increase the oxygen as dictated by maximum potassium emission.

3. *Color of Flame.* A yellow or white flare at the base of the flame indicates too much oxygen; readjust flame for maximum potassium emission. If the whole flame appears a color other than clear blue, there is general air contamination. If there are erratic flares through the flame, try to find

Continued on page 170

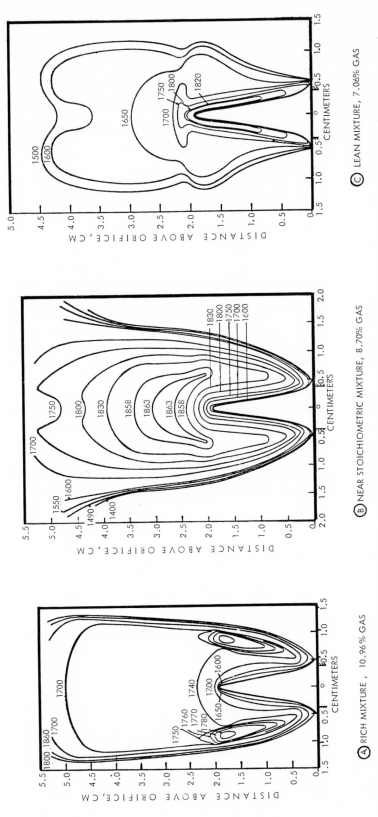
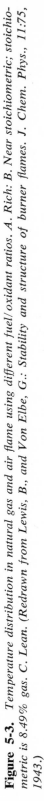

**Figure 5-3.** *Temperature distribution in natural gas and air flame using different fuel/oxidant ratios. A. Rich; B. Near stoichiometric; stoichiometric is 8.49% gas. C. Lean. (Redrawn from Lewis, B., and Von Elbe, G.: Stability and structure of burner flames. J. Chem. Phys., 11:75, 1943.)*

the cause of airborne particles. If possible, remove such cause; if not possible, read the galvanometer with caution and ignore erratic fluctuation.

4. *Sound.* Aspirate water and listen to the sound. If the noise is a steady buzz of its usual tone, mark the check sheet "satisfactory" (S). If the sound is raspy, the flame needs oxygen. If the sound is shrill, the oxygen pressure is too high. Recheck the flame for maximum potassium emission.

---

To obtain satisfactory clinical values by flame photometry, fuel/oxidant ratio and atomization rate must be controlled within 1%,[24] which means that fuel and oxygen pressures must each be kept to less than 1% variation. Such precision cannot, in practice, be obtained with the Coleman 21 flame photometer, and probably not with most other instruments.

The technologist can, however, find and work with the fuel/oxidant ratio that produces maximum emission for any particular element. Small changes in gas and/or oxygen flow then have less effect on the emission being measured. Figure 5-5 illustrates these relative areas for sodium and potassium.

As shown in Figure 5-5, sodium emission varies little with as much as a ± 25% change in sample atomization rate. Potassium emission, by contrast, is greatly affected by ± 25% change in sample atomization rate. The oxygen giving maximum emission was just under 15 inches. This produces a cooler flame than that for the maximum sodium emission.

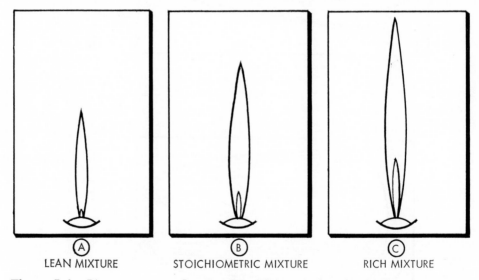

(A) LEAN MIXTURE  (B) STOICHIOMETRIC MIXTURE  (C) RICH MIXTURE

**Figure 5-4.** *Line gas oxygen flames using different fuel-oxidant mixtures. A. Lean. B. Stoichiometric. C. Rich. (After Mavrodineau, R., and Boiteux, H.: Flame Spectroscopy. New York, John Wiley & Sons, Inc., 1965.)*

170

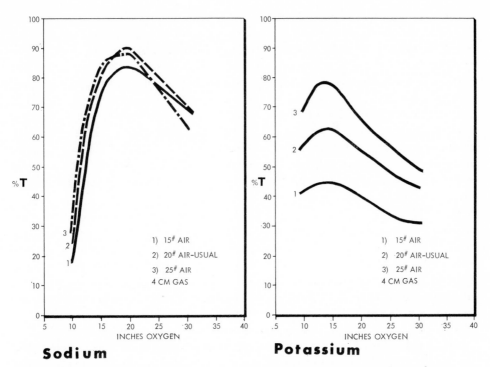

**Figure 5-5.** *Maximum emission curves obtained on a Beckman 9200 flame photometer. (From Mosher, R. E., et al.: The use of flame photometry for the quantitative determination of sodium and potassium in plasma and urine. Amer. J. Clin. Path., 19:461, 1949. Reprinted by permission of The Williams & Wilkins Co., Baltimore, Md.)*

The maximum emissions for sodium and potassium with the Coleman 21 flame photometer are similar to those shown in Figure 5-5 but are compromised on two points. The optical system of the Beckman 9200, on which the values in Figure 5-5 were obtained, can be adjusted by mirrors; the optical system of the Coleman 21 is fixed. The Coleman flame is adjusted to one fuel/oxidant ratio, and both sodium and potassium are read without readjustment of the flame. Since potassium requires the more critical adjustment, the flame is adjusted to a height of 3½ to 4 inches with the fuel regulator. The approximate oxygen regulation is judged by gross inspection of the flame, and the final adjustment in oxygen is made as required for maximum potassium emission.[25]

---

*2d. Maximum Potassium Emission (See Fig.5-1 Coleman.)*

1. Trim the flame to a height of 3½ to 4 inches with the fuel regulator.
2. While aspirating a midrange potassium standard, adjust oxygen-mixing valve until maximum emission is indicated by the highest obtainable %T.

---

171

The composition of line gas may vary somewhat in different locales, but the pressure is likely to vary considerably from place to place and even during different periods of the day. In South Bend, for example, this pressure may vary sporadically as much as 3 inches. A stable flame cannot be maintained with line gas whose pressure is fluctuating. A check for fluctuation may be done by attaching a water column to the line between the gasline outlet and the instrument. A Coleman booster pump installed between the gas outlet and the instrument greatly reduces the fluctuation. Even with the pump, however, the pressure may not be absolutely constant, and continual adjustment may be required to maintain relatively reproducible atomizing rates. Occasionally differences in fuel/oxidant ratio can be traced to defective oxygen gauges, but almost always the cause is fuel fluctuation.

## Atomization

The atomizer has been described earlier as part of the total-consumption burner (Fig. 5-2). The pneumatic aspiration of the sample is controlled entirely by the flow rate of the oxygen through the atomizer. As the aerosol enters the flame and the mist is vaporized, each drop is excited separately; consequently, the emission of light from the flame cannot be entirely uniform.[24] The most constant emission is produced from many fine droplets. Droplet size decreases proportionally with increases in oxygen pressure and with decreases in the atomizer diameter.[5, 9, 24]

To obtain optimal emission in the flame of the Coleman 21 flame photometer, the oxygen pressure is set as high as possible (between 12 to 14 pounds) while maintaining an aspiration rate of 1 to 2 cc/min and an overall flame height between 3½ to 4 inches.[25] An aspiration rate less than 1 cc/min sprays insufficient sample into the flame for proper sensitivity, and a rate greater than 2 cc/min lowers the flame temperature too much. These adjustments for fuel/oxygen ratio must be consistent with the adjustment to maximum potassium emission previously discussed.

Even though the fuel and oxygen pressures are kept constant, the aspiration rate may change due to encrustation of salts on the burner tip,[10, 24, 40] viscosity of the sample,[12, 15, 24] slow buildup of protein film on the atomizer capillary wall,[31] or a plug in the atomizer. The burner tip becomes encrusted with dried salts over a period of time; excessive sample flow rates cause encrustation to form faster than usual. The burner must be regularly inspected and cleaned.

Viscosity of the sample can be affected not only by protein and bile salts,[5] but also by temperature differences.[15] If standards or sample dilutions are refrigerated, they must all be allowed to come to room temperature before atomization. Natelson reported a 10% emission decrease during a one-hour period, caused by accumulation of protein film on the capillary wall at the atomizer orifice.[31] Viscosity differences and film buildup can be minimized by working at reasonably high dilutions and by adding a wetting agent to all solutions.[12, 15] Surface tension does not affect the atomization into the total-consumption burner.[12, 15]

An alert operator can detect changes in the aspiration rate by noticing the time interval between aspiration of the sample and brightening of the flame or by hearing a difference in the sound of the spraying.[24] A stable atomization produces

172

a steady, moderately rapid deflection of the galvanometer needle.[21] Since the signal readout on the Coleman is not integrated, small changes in emission normally cause slight fluctuation of the needle. A drift downward in the transmittance reading suggests clogging of the atomizer.[30] However, immediately after rinsing the atomizer with water, the operator can usually obtain the original reading again without any adjustment of the instrument. Fluctuation can also be caused by air bubbles entrapped on the capillary surface and then escaping into the flame. Quickly raising and lowering the sample frees such bubbles. Attention to these small details can save an operator much time and frustration by avoidance of unnecessary fluctuation.

### 4. Aspiration Rate (See Fig. 5-1 Coleman.)

1. Adjust the flame, using the current gas and fuel adjustments that have been providing an overall flame height of 3½ to 4 inches and maximum potassium emission.

2. Allow the atomizer to aspirate for 2 minutes from a beaker containing 10 cc of water. Measure the water left and calculate the cc/min aspirated. The proper rate is 1 to 2 cc/min.

3. If the aspiration rate is not proper, the gas and oxygen may be adjusted within the flame height and maximum potassium emission limitations. If the aspiration rate cannot be satisfactorily adjusted, try a different atomizer.

4. Continue to use this oxygen regulation for this particular atomizer and check it at least weekly. Check it at any time the %T of a sample drifts downward.

Because atomizers vary in diameter, it is practical to keep several on hand and choose the one most compatible with the maximum emission of a particular instrument at a specific time.

A 2000 pound oxygen tank, fitted with two-stage regulators, will have a relatively constant delivery rate until the pressure falls below 500 pounds.[12] For this reason the tank pressure should be recorded when the oxygen is turned on, and the tank should be changed when the pressure reaches 500 pounds.

### 1. Oxygen Tank Pressure (See Fig. 5-1, Coleman.)

When the oxygen pressure has been adjusted for the poundage dictated by the particular atomizer, notice the tank pressure and record it on the check sheet. If the pressure is close enough to 500 pounds to go below this figure during the run, change the tank before starting the run.

## Optical and Electronic Systems

The operator can do little to change the optical system of the Coleman 21 flame photometer. The flame height is restricted to 3½ to 4 inches to allow the desired area of the flame to be focused through the lens upon the phototube. As shown in Figure 5-6, the maximum emission for aqueous solutions occurs in an area approximately two thirds up the flame from its base.[11]

The location of the potassium maximum between those for sodium and calcium is another reason for our choice of potassium as the maximum emission adjustment for the fuel/oxidant ratio. The calcium maximum emission is very close to the inner cone, and emission decreases markedly as measurement is made upward in the flame.[12]

The lens holder of the Coleman 21 flame photometer is bent at an angle that will allow the lens to pick up the area of maximum emission for the aqueous solutions. This focused beam of light can be seen by lifting the chimney and looking at the lens and entrance window from the side. If the light does not center well, the lens holder can be adjusted somewhat. This alignment may not be critical, but it may make a difference in calcium emission.[25]

Filter leaks (*i.e.,* insufficient selectivity) can be detected by reading potassium and calcium solutions of different concentration through the sodium filter, or sodium and calcium through the potassium filter.[45] The inherent enhancement of potassium by sodium is adequately obviated by the recommended addition of 25 mEq/1 sodium to the potassium standards.[28] No calcium effect on potassium or sodium occurs with the line gas and oxygen flame.[15, 45]

The portion of the Coleman signal detection system, which is called the "electronics," consists of the power supply and the amplifier circuit. An electronics technician would approach the problems with a systematic tracing to the cause, but operators of flame photometers can only recognize certain symptoms and then replace a few parts.

Since the most common symptoms, causes, and corrections are well outlined in the manual,[33] they will not be repeated here. We can add a few observations.

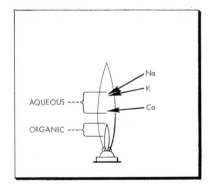

**Figure 5-6.** *Distribution of emission in flame. Potassium position added from own experience. (After Buell, B. E.: Use of organic solvents in limited area flame spectrometry. Anal. Chem., 34:635, 1962. Adapted by permission of the American Chemical Society.)*

174

By far the most frequent problem is fluctuation of the galvanometer needle. The cause of fluctuation may be isolated between the electronics and the flame emission by checking for stability of the instrument with a filter inserted upside down.

---

### 6. Electronics Check (See Fig. 5-1, Coleman.)

With the flame burning:

1. Insert a filter upside down in the filter slot.
2. Adjust the needle to 50%T and observe for 60 seconds.
3. If fluctuation continues ($\pm$ 2 divisions), the cause is in the electronics; if needle is steady, the cause is in the atomizer burner.

---

Once the electronics check has ruled out the flame as the cause, either the spectrophotometer or the electronics of the flame unit could be the offender. The spectrophotometer should be checked for stability after it has been disconnected from the flame unit. Electric circuits in the laboratory are often overloaded; addition of a special line for the spectrophotometer solved these problems in our laboratory. Large erratic fluctuations can be caused by coarse or fine galvanometer potentiometers if they are either dirty or defective. Particles of dirt can sometimes be knocked off by turning the adjustment several times clockwise and then counterclockwise with quick but firm movements.

Fluctuation can be caused by several parts of the amplifier circuit. Repairs to this circuit—the part inside the "black box"—are beyond the competence of the user. Several possible causes can, however, be eliminated by the operator. One problem, sometimes overlooked, is overhead or bench lighting that shines into the chimney and strikes the phototube; such lights must be turned off while using the flame photometer.[25] Another possible cause is a light leak into the electronics box itself. Once in one of our units the lid fell off the box and rested on top of the tubes; the galvanometer needle wavered whenever a hand moved across the top of the chimney.

The defective component of an electronics system that does not respond to emitted light can sometimes be isolated by observation of the following symptoms. If the ballast lamps are lit and the controls affect the galvanometer but the galvanometer will not move off zero with emitted light, the problem is likely the amplifier tube or the phototube.

The phototube, a 1P39, (A in Fig. 5-13) is comparatively insensitive in the potassium emission range of 766 m$\mu$. For this reason, potassium zero standard becomes hard to set as the tube deteriorates; adjusting the bias corrects the problem for a short time but then the phototube requires replacement.

The technologist can replace some parts of the power supply. If the ballast lamps light and the controls affect zero but the galvanometer index is any place other than pegged at zero, an $OD_3$ or an $OA_3$ voltage regulator tube may be defective. If the lamps do not light and the controls do not affect the galvanometer, one or both of the lamps may be burned out, the rectifier may be defective, or excessive moisture may be causing a short circuit in the power supply. Changing the lamps and/or the rectifier tube will eliminate these causes of malfunction.

The flame unit can be functioning properly and then suddenly appear to be as dead as if the electric plug had been disconnected. This may be due to shorting as a result of excess moisture.

Before removing the power supply for troubleshooting, it is wise to unplug the instrument in order to avoid a shock. When the power supply has been taken out of the flame unit, damp insulation under the base of the power supply will indicate excess moisture. Sometimes the lamp or the rectifier tube becomes shorted by the moisture; if the instrument does not function after it has dried, try replacing these parts.

The power supply in our Coleman 21 flame photometer has shorted from moisture absorbed after samples were spilled in the chimney housing. Once defective air-conditioning caused condensation of moisture on the walls of the laboratory; the flame photometer in this room required 2 days to dry out and become operative.

The Coleman flame photometer depends upon the heat from the ballast lamps to keep it free of moisture under ordinary circumstances. Therefore, this unit should be left on continuously; the flame alone should be turned off when the instrument is not in use.

## Standardization

Standardization of the routine procedure with calibration curves requires some preliminary consideration of the emission characteristics of the excited elements. Whether the sodium emission plot is curved or straight depends upon the final sodium concentration in the flame. Using a mixture of illuminating gas and air, Barnes, *et al.* found a loss of linearity at sodium concentrations above 10 ppm[1] (Fig. 5-7).

At the same concentrations line gas and oxygen would give a relatively more curved line because of the increased flame temperature. In concentration ranges of 12 to 20 ppm, such as the usual 1:200 dilution of a serum sodium determination provides, the calibration plot is therefore not ordinarily a straight line.

Our chief problem in trying to control the Coleman flame photometer has been to maintain a consistent calibration curve for sodium. The calibration is sometimes linear, but at other times, for the same gas and oxygen adjustments, the convex line is 8 mEq/1 high at the 125 mEq/1 range. Based on 9 standards between 75 and 160 mEq sodium, the calibration curve, when convex, *always* shows the greatest increase at the range of approximately 125 mEq. Therefore, a *control that has a value near 125mEq/1 must be run.*

An error in adjustment may cause inconsistent calibration. One time the booster pump of an instrument in our laboratory was accidentally set to deliver 12 inches

176

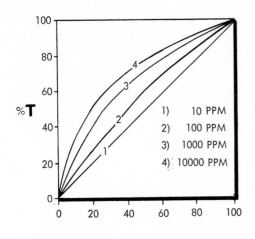

Na CONCENTRATION AS % OF FULL SCALE

**Figure 5-7.** *Typical curves for sodium emission. (From Barnes, R. B., et al.: Flame photometery—a rapid analytical procedure. Industr. Engin. Chem., 17:605, 1945. Reprinted by permission of the American Chemical Society.)*

water column gas pressure instead of 6 inches. An excessively curved sodium calibration plot resulted; it returned to a straight line when the pressure was corrected. The diaphragm regulator in the instrument is supposedly capable of producing a preset constant pressure to the atomizer, regardless of great increases in the inlet pressure.[25] If the inlet hose frequently pops off and/or the atomizer bubbles into the sample beaker, increased gas pressure may be reaching the atomizer.

When individual instruments are adjusted properly, the sodium calibration curves are almost identical. The standards are made from reagent grade sodium chloride and also contain 0.02% Sterox SE.* The %T for a typical curve (Table

**Table 5-2. Typical Sodium Calibration Curve for Coleman Model 21**

| mEq/1 Standard | %T |
|:---:|:---:|
| 0 | Set 0. |
| 150 | Set 65.0 |
| 75 | 38.5 |
| 90 | 44.0 |
| 100 | 48.0 |
| 115 | 53.0 |
| 125 | 56.5 |
| 135 | 60.0 |
| 140 | 62.0 |
| 150 | 65.0 |
| 160 | 68.0 |

* Sterox SE is obtainable from Hartman-Leddon Co., Philadelphia, Pa.

177

5-2) is within $\pm 0.5\%\,T$ of the readings to be generally expected.[25] These statements are not meant to imply that the Coleman flame photometer can be used with a precalibrated scale panel or a single standard calibration line. To avoid the shifting sodium curve requires precise fuel/oxidant adjustments and frequent calibration checks using several standards.

The sodium calibration curve is routinely checked at the beginning of every run by reading the 100, 125, and 135 mEq/1 standards against the 150 mEq/1 standard set at 65%T. If any one of the standards does not read within $\pm 0.5\%\,T$ of its value from the linear calibration curve, any test sample in the same range is read against its closest standard. Controls with values near 140 mEq/1 are out of range only when gross changes in fuel/oxidant ratio occur. A control in the 125 mEq/1 range will detect slight shifts in the calibration curve. In each run a commercial control* should be included in this range. The same operator may reread his own diluted control throughout a single day.

---

### 7. Sodium Control (See Fig. 5-1, Coleman.)

1. Run the Versatol A control with each batch of test samples. This value must be $\pm 4$ mEq/1 of manufacturer's value.
2. The same diluted Versatol A is reread during the day and recorded on the check sheet under "Control." Values on the same dilution should not vary more than $\pm 2$ mEq/1.

---

The potassium calibration curve usually is a straight line; tendency toward concavity at low concentrations is linearized by sodium present in the standards and in the patient's serum.[24] However, the line can become convex at higher concentrations and at higher flame temperatures. A problem with potassium values may be caused by temperature changes due to fuel fluctuations.

In the past our potassium values for our flame photometers were frequently high on commercial controls by as much as 0.8 mEq/1 at the 5.0 mEq/1 level. Our standards, as recommended by the Coleman manual,[33] contained the usual 25 mEq/1 sodium and 0.02% Sterox SE. We found that the potassium elevation was proportional and that it could be corrected by adding an ion-free serum** to the standards. Since such standards containing protein cloud on standing, freshly diluted Versatol† is a more convenient standard. The test is controlled with a commercial product,‡ at the 3.5 mEq/1 level.

---

\* Versatol A (Abnormal), General Diagnostics Div., Warner-Chilcott Laboratories, Morris Plains, N. J.

\*\* Chem.-Varion. Registered trademark for ion-free serum. Clinton Laboratories, Los Angeles, Calif.

† Versatol. General Diagnostics Div., Warner-Chilcott Laboratories, Morris Plains, N. J.

‡ Versatol AA (Abnormal Alternate). General Diagnostics Div., Warner-Chilcott Laboratories, Morris Plains, N. J.

---

### 7. Potassium Control (See Fig. 5-1, Coleman.)

1. Run a Versatol AA control sample with each batch of patient's serum. This control must check within ± 0.3 of manufacturer's value.

2. The same dilution may be reread during the single day. Repeat reading should not give values different by more than ± 0.2 mEq/1.

---

Routine calcium determinations were run on the Coleman flame photometer for about 8 months. During the standardization of the method, all the booster pumps for the Coleman flame instruments were accidentally adjusted to 12 inches gas pressure with the oxygen pressure proportionately higher as necessary for maximum potassium emission. Parker's[34] procedure was modified so that 6 mEq/1 sodium was present in the calcium zero standard and the diluent. Versatol was used as the standard and commercial controls* at the 3.5 and 6.5 mEq levels. Controls were good, recovery of added calcium was good, and the values correlated well with our former EDTA titration method.[17]

After the error in gas pressure was discovered and corrected, the 6.5 mEq control values were low by at least 10%, sometimes more. Comparisons by EDTA titration confirmed that patient's values in the range over 5.5 mEq/1 were also low by the flame method. Comparison of calcium values was again made using the Coleman flame photometer, the EDTA titration method, and atomic absorption. In spite of concentrated effort to find a constantly satisfactory fuel/oxidant ratio, the Coleman values were not only low in the 5.5 to 6.5 mEq/1 range but also high in the 3.0 to 4.0 mEq/1 range. We therefore concluded that calcium determinations could not be run on the Coleman flame photometer.

## Contamination

So many concomitants have been reported to effect the sodium, potassium, and/or calcium emission that no attempt will be made to list them here;[24, 35] various releasers and protectors have also been reported for interferents.[20]

Significantly elevated sodium and potassium values occur when the samples are diluted with water contaminated by an *Alcaligenes-Pseudomonas* organism.[43] Frequently this bacterium has been cultured from deionized water and also from distilled water. The organisms do not precisely fit any single bacterial species.

Although quantitative data relating to interferences cannot be transferred directly from one instrument to another,[24] several metals may be interferents. Addition of $Ca^{++}$, $Fe^{+++}$, $Mn^{++}$, and $Sn^{++++}$ elevates sodium and potassium values. $Ni^{++}$, $ZN^{++}$, $Mg^{++}$, $NO_3^-$ and $PO_4^\equiv$ elevate sodium values but do not affect potassium values. Sometimes the emission value of a solution containing protein is affected more by the contamination than is an aqueous solution; $Cu^{++}$ effect on sodium is such an example. The converse is observed for $Fe^{+++}$ effect on potassium. Such

---

* Versatol A and Versatol AA.

179

observations illustrate the complex nature of contamination that may make patient values appear *increased* in relation to an aqueous standard and vice versa. Iron contamination may cause this situation. Cholesterol[30] and globulin[12, 23] have been reported to cause clouding of diluted patient samples; this clouding has been noticed in water contaminated with $Cu^{++}$ and $Zn^{++}$. Sometimes the sodium or potassium value of a clouded solution may seem changed, but usually no significant difference in emission is detected.

As a consequence of our experience with contaminated water, a daily check of the water used for diluent has become routine procedure.

---

### 5. Water Contamination (See Fig. 5-1, Coleman.)

1. Set the sodium zero standard and read the water to be used for the day's diluent. If the water reads more than $1\%T$ higher than the sodium zero, substitute a different water.

2. Repeat the procedure using potassium zero. The water will normally read about $3\%T$ less than the potassium zero because of the added sodium in the latter. If the water reads the same as, or higher than, the potassium zero, substitute a different water.

---

Contamination of sodium and potassium solutions by containers is reported less likely when bottles are chosen in the following order: Jena glass < polyethylene < Pyrex < medicine glass < stoppered bottle.[45] We have successfully used No-Sol-Vit* bottles for Coleman standards but not for solutions containing lithium.

Air contamination, which can be a factor in interference, usually is not detected during use of the Coleman flame photometer if smoking is not allowed in the room while the instrument is in use and the room is well ventilated and air-conditioned. Smoke has often been reported to increase significantly the potassium;[3, 7, 28, 32, 37] dust, soap powder, and ocean winds pollute the air with sodium for hours.[7] Proposed air-cleaning devices have included an electrostatic precipitator[32] and a glass chimney to enclose the flame[37] in a fashion similar to that currently used on the Instrumentation Laboratory flame photometer, IL 143.

Airborne particles will cause erratic $\%T$ fluctuations in the galvanometer needle, but are also detectable as small bright flares scattered throughout the flame. Visual inspection of the flame for overall coloration and flares is important in detecting general air contamination, as has been indicated on the check sheet.

In handling pipettes and sample cups or pouring solutions, the operator must avoid touching a surface diluted material will contact. Sodium values obtained in our laboratory have been elevated by about 4 to 20 mEq/1 and potassium values by 4 mEq/1 from finger contact; potassium will vary more when the finger belongs to a smoker.

---

\* Scientific Products Co., McGraw Park, Ill.

180

DAILY CHECK SHEET FOR BECKMAN FLAME PHOTOMETER, MODEL 105

Hospital _____  Instrument # _____  Month _____  Year _____

| Date | | 1 Flame | | | | 2 Atomizer | | 3 Readout | | 4 Contamination | | 5 Control | | | | | | | | |
|---|---|---|---|---|---|---|---|---|---|---|---|---|---|---|---|---|---|---|---|---|
| | Ht. | Color | Cones | Gas # | Air # | Asp Rate cc/min | Drain | Meter Zero | Integ. Time Sec | H$_2$O | Air | | V# ___ mfg. ___<br>VA# ___ mfg. ___<br>VAA# ___ mfg. ___ | | | | Na | K | | |
| | | | | | | | | | | | | | V | VA | VAA | V | VA | VAA | V | VA | VAA |
| 1 | | | | | | | | | | | | Na | | | | | | | | | |
| | | | | | | | | | | | | K | | | | | | | | | |
| 2 | | | | | | | | | | | | Na | | | | | | | | | |
| | | | | | | | | | | | | K | | | | | | | | | |
| 3 | | | | | | | | | | | | Na | | | | | | | | | |
| | | | | | | | | | | | | K | | | | | | | | | |
| 4 | | | | | | | | | | | | Na | | | | | | | | | |
| | | | | | | | | | | | | K | | | | | | | | | |
| 5 | | | | | | | | | | | | Na | | | | | | | | | |
| | | | | | | | | | | | | K | | | | | | | | | |
| 6 | | | | | | | | | | | | Na | | | | | | | | | |
| | | | | | | | | | | | | K | | | | | | | | | |

**Figure 5-8.** *Daily check sheet for Beckman flame photometer, Model 105.*

181

# DAILY CHECK SHEET FOR IL FLAME PHOTOMETER, MODEL 143

Hospital _____  Instrument # _____  Month _____  Year _____

| | 1 | | | | 2 | | | | 3 | 4 | 5 | | | | | | | | |
|---|---|---|---|---|---|---|---|---|---|---|---|---|---|---|---|---|---|---|---|
| | Flame | | | | Atomizer | | | | Readout | Contam | Control | | | | | | | | |
| Date | Screen | Color | Cones | Tuning | Air # | Asp Rate cc/min | Drain | Red Plug | Roll off mEq/1 | H$_2$O | | V# _____ mfg. _____ Na K | VA# _____ mfg. _____ | VAA# _____ mfg. _____ | | | | | |
| | | | | | | | | | | | V | VA | VAA | V | VA | VAA | V | VA | VAA |
| 1 | | | | | | | | | | | Na | | | | | | | | |
| | | | | | | | | | | | K | | | | | | | | |
| 2 | | | | | | | | | | | Na | | | | | | | | |
| | | | | | | | | | | | K | | | | | | | | |
| 3 | | | | | | | | | | | Na | | | | | | | | |
| | | | | | | | | | | | K | | | | | | | | |
| 4 | | | | | | | | | | | Na | | | | | | | | |
| | | | | | | | | | | | K | | | | | | | | |
| 5 | | | | | | | | | | | Na | | | | | | | | |
| | | | | | | | | | | | K | | | | | | | | |
| 6 | | | | | | | | | | | Na | | | | | | | | |
| | | | | | | | | | | | K | | | | | | | | |

## INTERNAL STANDARD FLAME PHOTOMETER

Both the Beckman Model 105* and the Instrumentation Laboratory (hereafter designated IL) Model 143 flame photometers are internal standard instruments and both have chambers to premix the propane and compressed air. Because of their similarity, the instruments will be discussed together and differences will be pointed out.

The directions for check procedures related to each parameter are numbered to identify them by instrument to their respective check sheets. The Beckman check sheet is Figure 5-8, and the IL check sheet is Figure 5-9.

The internal standard, lithium, is added to the diluent, and a sufficient quantity is made to last about a week. Both Beckman Instruments and Instrumentation Laboratory sell a lithium concentrated solution, and we find it more convenient to buy the liquid than to weigh the deliquescent salt.[22] Although the exact lithium concentration in the diluent is not critical, it *is* critical that standard and unknown be diluted in the same solution and in exactly the same manner.[4, 26]

The diluent containing lithium provides a constant amount of internal standard to be excited in the flame along with each test element. The light emitted by the lithium and the test element is measured, and the ratio of the two intensities is used to calculate the concentration of the test element.[6]

The use of lithium as internal standard is not a perfect solution to all the problems of flame photometry.[39] Lithium can be used successfully with the low-temperature propane-air flames but not with hot flames; for example, at 2800°C potassium ionizes almost five times as much as lithium.[15]

In the propane-air flame, sodium emission characteristics are very similar to those of lithium; potassium differs slightly; calcium differs more. These errors in the internal standard method due to emission differences, however, are far less than those caused by atomization and flame fluctuation in the direct measurement method (Fig. 5-10).[5] A 40% decrease in gas pressure causes no error in the internal standard method; decrease in air pressure and increase in viscosity causes much less error in the internal standard method than in the direct measurement method. The errors in the internal standard method shown for differences of air pressure and viscosity occur in the atomization and vaporization processes.

### Atomizer and Spray Chamber

The atomization rate is a compromise between factors affecting the mist that eventually enters the flame.[24] When the sample enters the spray chamber, the large droplets in the spray fall out, and only the finer droplets enter the flame. The faster the sample enters, the more uniform the droplets will be; a greater percentage of the larger droplets will be thrown against the wall of the chamber by increased air pressure. In general, since the particles entering the flame are uniformly small, high analytical precision can be achieved with this system.[39] The usual efficiency of the atomizer (fraction of atomized sample entering the flame) is only 1% to

---

* The Beckman Model 105 is currently not being marketed in this country. Its advantages are important enough that the author is still using the instrument.

183

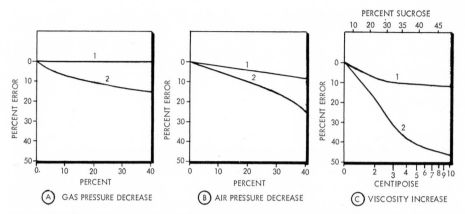

**Figure 5-10.** *Effect of variation in gas pressure, air pressure, and viscosity: (1) internal standard method; (2) direct measurement method. (After Berry, J. W., Chappell, D. G., and Barnes, R. B.: Improved method of flame photometry. Industr. Engin. Chem., 18:19, 1946. Reprinted by permission of the American Chemical Society.)*

6% but may be raised to 10% to 15% by decreasing the suction rate with a longer or finer capillary.

Increased surface tension of the diluted sample markedly increases the droplet size and therefore decreases the atomizer efficiency; it also causes fluctuation in emission.[12] Salts, such as the lithium, or wetting agents, minimize the surface tension differences between aqueous standards and serum dilutions.

In both the Beckman and the IL flame photometers, the orifice of the pneumatic atomizer is located just inside the spray chamber at right angles to the inlet for the compressed air. In the IL 143, the adjustment of the aspiration rate is made by changing the height of the atomizer tip in relation to the stationary air stream. Moisture in the air line must be removed daily before the air pressure can be assumed constant. In the IL photometer, moisture is removed by turning on the instrument, allowing the air pressure to purge the line, and then turning the instrument off again. After the pressure has bled off, the gas and instrument are turned on to allow flame ignition. The aspiration rate of the Beckman 105 is controlled by changing the air pressure. The optimal aspiration rate for both instruments is approximately 1 cc/min.

A beaker of diluent must be aspirated when these instruments are first turned on to equilibrate the chamber temperature, to rinse the chamber well, and to wet the chamber walls to prevent adherence of droplets. A spray chamber increases the probability that one sample may contaminate the next and that the zero base line may gradually increase.[39]

---

### 2. Aspiration Rate (See Fig. 5-8, Beckman; Fig. 5-9, IL.)

When the flame has been burning for about 5 minutes:

1.  Record the air pressure on the check sheet.

184

2. Calculate the aspiration rate by atomizing from a 3 cc sample for 2 minutes and measuring the liquid remaining. If the rate is less than 1 cc/min or more than 1.5 cc/min, adjust to within this range.

3. Check the spray chamber drain to be sure it is free running and has the proper amount of water present in the column.

---

Efficient draining of the spray chamber is very important. In the IL flame photometer, the air space immediately below the chamber should be ⅛ inch; this is midway between the bottom of the bowl and the drain elbow. Less space risks flooding the chamber, and a water level below the bend in the column causes erratic aspiration. In the Beckman flame photometer, flooding of the chamber can occur from the drain hose being only slightly elevated on a table top or from the hose outlet being under water. The drains must be consistently rinsed well to avoid obstruction from protein buildup or bacterial growth. After the run has been completed, copious amounts of water must be aspirated, not only to rinse the atomizer thoroughly but also to clean out the burner system. Partial obstruction of the burner orifices or salt deposits of the Meker grid can cause fluctuation of emission.[10, 16] Operators accustomed to total-consumption burners, which require no such precautions, sometimes neglect these steps.

Provided the air pressure remains constant, a change in the aspiration rate is proof of a plugging atomizer and must be quickly detected. A dropping lithium indicator on the IL photometer signals plugging. However, even though the lithium indicator is still within the bounds of its two lines, more than $\pm 1$ mEq/1 sodium difference can often be obtained on repeat readings. Furthermore, values for sodium and potassium serum dilutions have decreased markedly while aqueous standards have remained constant and the lithium indicator has not changed. After the atomizer has been flushed by moving the sample beaker up and down, the same cups of serum dilutions read properly. Throughout episodes of atomizer plugging the sodium digital readout fluctuates much more than usual. This fluctuation may be the first indication of an atomizer plugging in the IL instrument.

The Beckman 105 flame photometer produces an integrated signal in a given period of time as regulated by a sensitivity adjustment on the photomultiplier. If the atomizer plugs and less sample is excited, a longer integration is required to produce the predetermined lithium signal. Since the excitation potential of potassium is lower than that for lithium, increase in the integration time after calibration causes high potassium values. The excitation potential for sodium is reasonably close to that for lithium and therefore very little increase in sodium values is detected. These unequal elevations are only detectable on samples of known value. *Whenever* the atomizer begins to plug, the integration time *always* increases and can be measured. With experience, the operator senses increased times and can prevent inaccuracies. When protein samples were interspersed with rinse water after every fifth sample and when standards were repeated at about this same interval, values were consistent on both instruments.

185

**Burner**

The intimate mixing of propane and air in a spray chamber before the mixture enters the burner produces a homogeneous flame. This flame is so nearly in thermo-dynamic equilibrium that it may be characterized by merely stating its temperature.[24] The 1750°C temperature for the IL flame photometer[13] is somewhat below 1925°C for propane and compressed air as was shown in Table 5-1. One can only surmise that the heat loss occurs in the dissipation at the grid of the Meker burner. Both instruments use this exceedingly stable burner;[39] the small orifices in the grid prevent flashback.[19] Flame height should be kept constant, since a fixed optical system is used. This parameter is not as critical however, as it is for the total-con-sumption burner because of the homogeneous nature of the premixed flame. The inner cones should be smooth, upright, and sharp in outline.[39]

In the IL 143 flame photometer, an approximate 1:3 fuel/air ratio is con-tinually controlled by a double pancake regulator which adjusts the propane in proportion to the air present.[13] Air pressure may be checked by inserting a pressure gauge in the line at the chamber inlet. Flame height is adjusted with a needle value, and the height is kept so that a cherry discoloration the size of a quarter is formed on the screen above the chimney. This is only a gross adjustment, and the flame should be "tuned" to peak lithium response.

---

*1. Flame Height, Color, and Cones (See Fig. 5-9, IL.)*

After the flame has been burning about 5 minutes, carefully slide the chimney cover up enough to check the flame visually.

A. Note the size of the cherry discoloration on the chimney screen. If larger or smaller than a quarter, decrease or increase the flame height as in-structed in the instrument manual. Check the flame "tuning."

B. Note the overall flame color; it should be clear blue. If it is tinged with some other color, look for possible contamination.

C. Note the size, position, and sharpness of cones. If they must be adjusted, consult instruction manual. Check the flame "tuning."

---

Usually it should be sufficient to check the flame "tuning" monthly, but the flame must be checked any time reproducibility or stability becomes questionable. IL flame photometers manufactured before 1968 had four digits in their serial num-bers; those in 1968 were given five digit numbers. The stability stated for four-digit instruments was $\pm 2$ mEq for sodium and $\pm 0.25$ for potassium. For five-digit instruments the stability is $\pm 0.5$ mEq and $\pm 0.25$ mEq respectively. These stability specifications refer to the values obtained while continually aspirating the 140/5 standard.

186

### *"Tuning" the IL Flame (See Fig. 5-9, IL.)*

1. Aspirate any solution containing lithium (Li).
2. Turn fuel adjustment control (inside left panel) CCW until Li indicator reaches a maximum upward indication.
3. Set Li indicator with Li set control to top black line on Li meter.
4. Turn fuel adjustment control CW until indicator drops down to lower black line.
5. Four-digit IL flame photometers (models from 1964 to 1968) may require a slightly leaner flame.

A change in the fuel/air ratio for the IL instrument is detected by the "roll-off" of the sodium digital counter and is described under the readout discussion. The fuel/air ratio for the Beckman 105 instrument is regulated by setting the pressure gauge for air first and then the fuel. The proper air pressure is the amount required to maintain an aspiration rate of 1.0 to 1.5 cc/min. The optimal propane/air ratio is established by reducing the fuel flow rate until the "carbon veil" just disappears from the flame.[4] The flame height can be conveniently oriented if the tip of the flame is barely visible over the chassis bar just above the peephole. If the fuel tank depletes while a sample is being recorded, the sodium emission is elevated off scale; potassium and calcium values are also elevated to a lesser degree. Forewarning of the incident occurs as a change in the flame's appearance.

### *1. Flame Height, Color, and Cones (See Fig. 5-8, Beckman.)*

1. After the flame has been burning about 5 minutes, note the flame height. Adjust if it is more than ¼ inch below or 1 inch higher than the chassis bar.
2. Note the overall flame color; if not clear blue, look for possible contamination.
3. Note size, position, and sharpness of cones. If they must be adjusted, consult instruction manual.
4. Record the gas pressure.

The air compressors used on both these instruments require that the accumulated water be drained out; the specifications for the pump of the IL flame photometer quote "daily."[26] The hole in the red bleeder plug at the rear of the IL instrument must be checked weekly. Likewise, the filters for the intake line to this pump must be faithfully changed according to the manufacturer's instructions to assure continued freedom from air contamination.

## Optical System and Readout

Though the optical systems of both instruments are fixed, they are quite different because of the plan for the emission detection. The Beckman photometer uses a single photomultiplier detector with filters arranged to synchronize with the commutator disk picking off the signal. The IL photometer uses individual photo-tubes to detect sodium, potassium, and lithium emission. (Compare the block diagrams in Figures 5-11 and 5-12.)

Filters isolate the 589 m$\mu$ sodium, the 671 m$\mu$ lithium, and the 766 m$\mu$ potassium lines.

The IL 143 flame photometer uses phototubes: 922 (S-1) for lithium and potassium, and 926 (S-3) for sodium. The spectral sensitivity curves for these

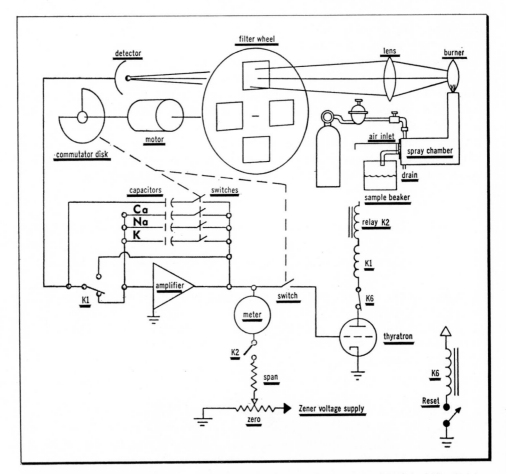

**Figure 5-11.** *Block diagram of Beckman flame photometer, Model 105. (From Beckman Model 105 Flame Photometer Instructions. Beckman Instruments, Inc., Fullerton, Calif., 1965.)*

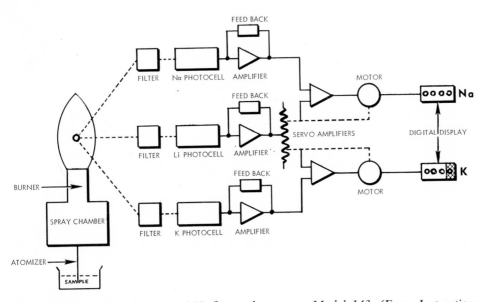

**Figure 5-12.** *Block diagram of IL flame photometer, Model 143. (From Instruction Handbook for the Model 143 Flame Photometer. Instrumentation Laboratory Inc., Lexington, Mass.)*

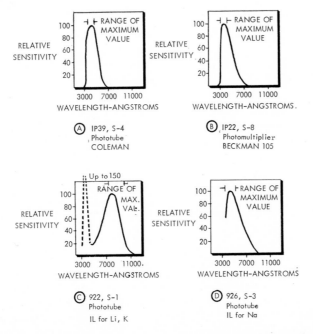

**Figure 5-13.** *Spectral sensitivity curves for various detectors. (From Phototubes, Photocells. Brochure #IG1018. Radio Corporation of America, Harrison, N. J.)*

189

tubes (Fig. 5-13) show good sensitivity in the wavelength range for detection of the specific lines of the elements.[36]

Since each element's emission is detected by a separate phototube, no use can be made of cause-effect relationships between sodium and potassium values obtained on any single sample. An advantage to the separate detectors is that amplification circuit boards can be interchanged in troubleshooting.[26]

The single photomultiplier tube of the Beckman 105 flame photometer is type 1P22 with an S-8 response. The sensitivity curve for this tube is comparatively weak in the 766 m$\mu$ range, but its inherent amplification is great. The single detector is useful in troubleshooting.

The signal readout in the IL flame photometer is direct, through a servocounter. Such a readout is extremely fast but fluctuates (or "hunts") within $\pm$ 0.5 mEq/1.

As the sample cup is removed from the atomizer, the operator should note the amount of "roll-off" on the sodium digital counter. If it is more than 10 mEq/1, the fuel/air ratio or the aspiration rate may be at fault. The correction made for the ratio balance, however, is a correction of the lithium zero.

---

### 3. "Roll-off (See Fig. 5-9, IL.)

Aspirate a sodium standard and note the "roll-off" when the cup is removed from the atomizer. If it is more than 10 mEq/1, rinse the atomizer and repeat. If the "roll-off" is still high, check the aspiration rate. If the aspiration rate is within the correct range, check the flame "tuning" and/or adjust the Ratio Control according to the instruction manual.

---

The readout in the Beckman flame photometer is an integrated signal; therefore the needle remains quite stable. The integration time is kept between 22 and 28 seconds by adjusting the sensitivity control. This adjustment regulates the amplification of signal from the photomultiplier tube. This parameter should be checked at least daily and more frequently if the atomizer is plugging. The meter zero is also checked daily.

---

### 3. Meter Zero and Integration Time (See Fig. 5-8, Beckman.)

1. While atomizing water, hold in the reset button. Note if the meter needle stops on zero. If it does not, while holding the reset button in, adjust the needle to zero with the Balance Control.

2. Aspirate the "sodium-potassium zero standard" and clock the integration time. If outside a range of 22 to 28 seconds, adjust the sensitivity control. Recheck this time; repeat adjustment as necessary to bring the time within range.

---

## Standardization

The calibrated curve for sodium in the IL instrument is almost linear.[8, 18] Linearity, originally described as electronic correction, is actually accomplished by selective choice of electronic components.[13] However, the electronic components of some instruments provide a more linear curve than do those of others. The sample dilutions on both the IL and the Beckman instruments can be read if a lithium concentration of 13 mEq/l is used as the diluent. Both of these instruments give essentially the same sodium values for the same sample dilutions when the instruments are calibrated to a single midscale standard (150 sodium and 5.0 potassium). As was noted for the Coleman instrument, 125 mEq/l sodium range on these instruments is also the portion of the calibration curve most likely to show nonlinearity.

Routine standardization can be achieved with a midrange standard for sodium and potassium, but commercial controls should cover three different ranges.* Values for these controls must agree with the manufacturer's values within ± 4 mEq/l for sodium and ± 0.3 mEq/l for potassium.

---

### 5. Sodium and Potassium Controls (See Fig. 5-8, Beckman; Fig. 5-9, IL.)

1. Run a Versatol, Versatol A, and Versatol AA control with each batch of test samples. Values for sodium must be ± 4 mEq/l of the manufacturer's value and for potassium ± 0.3 mEq/l.

2. The same diluted control samples can be reread during the day and recorded on the check sheet under "control." If the values for the reread dilutions gradually increase, make new dilutions.

---

The calcium values obtained with the Beckman 105 instrument in our laboratory have been satisfactory when compared to atomic absorption values. The lithium-lanthanum diluent tends to precipitate on the inside of the chamber and can become a problem. The chamber should be taken out and cleaned regularly after about 200 hours of use with the diluent. The quality of the lanthanum seems to vary from time to time even from the same company. Usually the calcium content can be verified, but the other contaminants may not be easily identified. Before a new lot number of lanthanum is put into use, the new diluent should be used to check a complete set of standards and controls. Standards, both intermediate and working, seem to pick up sodium after a variable period of time. When this happens, the sodium and calcium values on the controls become low. New standards made from fresh diluent solve this problem. It is practical, therefore, to adapt a two week period for use of standards and/or diluent. The calcium emission appears more sensitive to changes in fuel/oxidant ratio than either sodium

---

\* Versatol, Versatol A, and Versatol AA or similar controls.

191

or potassium. As long as this parameter is carefully regulated, commercial controls*
from 3.5 to 6.5 mEq remain within ± 0.3 of the manufacturer's value.

### Contamination

Contamination, especially of the diluted specimen, is a major consideration
when lithium is present in the diluent. Even polyethylene bottles cleaned with
nitric acid have contaminated standards. New polyethylene bottles should be used
for diluent and standards only and for no other purpose.

Contamination of glassware can be proved by rinsing the piece with a small
amount of water and then aspirating the rinse water into the flame; discoloration of
the flame is indicative of contamination. Aspiration of the pure water itself is
checked the same way but cannot be read in %T as on the Coleman instrument.

---

### 4. Water Contamination (See Fig. 5-8, Beckman; Fig. 5-9, IL.)

1. Aspirate the water into the flame and note the color of the flame. Rarely
   will the flame remain pure blue, and darker shades of orange will soon
   become discernible as contamination.

2. If contamination of water is observed, use different water.

---

Contamination of the air or spray chamber will also be indicated by a discolored flame when no liquid is being aspirated. The operator should make a habit
of noticing the color of the flame at various times during the run.

---

### 4. Air Contamination (See Fig. 5-8, Beckman.)

1. While standardizing the instrument, and at intervals during the run,
   notice the color of the flame when no liquid is being aspirated.

2. If the flame color is not clear blue, stop the run; rinse the atomizer and
   spray chamber with copious amounts of water. If the intensity of the
   color does not lessen, the contamination is in the air in the room.

3. If the room is contaminated, try to find the cause and remove it. If this
   is not possible, proceed cautiously with the run; frequently check
   standards and zero between samples.

4. Indicate any of these observations on the check sheet.

---

### REFERENCES

1. Barnes, R. B., Richardson, D., Berry J. W., and Hood, R. L.: Flame Photometry—a
   rapid analytical procedure. Industr. Engin. Chem., *17*:605, 1945.
2. Barnett, R. N.; Medical significance of laboratory results. Amer. J. Clin. Path., *50*:671,
   1968.

---

* Versatol, Versatol A, and Versatol AA or similar controls.

3. Beckman Bull. 259-A, Instructions for the Beckman flame spectrophotometer (DU attachment 9200). Beckman Instruments, Inc., Fullerton, Calif.

4. Beckman Model 105, flame photometer instructions. Beckman Instruments, Inc., Fullerton, Calif., 1965.

5. Berstein, R. E.: Correction of sources of error in the estimation of sodium, potassium and calcium in biological fluids and tissues by flame spectrophotometry. Biochim. Biophys. Acta, 9:576, 1952.

6. Berry, J. W., Chappell, D. G., and Barnes, R. B.: Improved method of flame photometry. Industr. Engin. Chem., 18:19, 1946.

7. Bills, C. E., McDonald, F. G., Nierdermeir, W., and Schwartz, M. C. Reduction of error in flame photometry. Anal Chem. 21:1076, 1949.

8. Boling, E. A.: A flame photometer with simultaneous digital readout for sodium and potassium. J. Lab. Clin. Med., 63:501, 1964.

9. Britske, M. E.: Turbulent flames as light sources for the analysis of solutions by flame photometry. [Transl. from Russian] Zarodski. Lab., 30:1465, 1964.

10. Brown, D. E.: Flame photometry. Amer. J. Clin. Path., 26:807, 1956.

11. Buell, B. E.: Use of organic solvents in limited area flame spectrometry. Anal. Chem., 34:635, 1962.

12. Dean, J. A.: *Flame Photometry*. New York, McGraw-Hill Book Company, 1960.

13. Fleischman, M.: Personal communication.

14. Ford, C. L.: A short method for the flame photometer determination of magnesium, manganic, sodium and potassium oxides in Portland cement. Beckman reprint #R-6169, Beckman Instruments, Inc., Fullerton, Calif.

15. Foster, W. H., and Hume, D. N.: Neutral cation interference effects in flame photometry. Anal. Chem., 31:2033, 1959.

16. Fox, C. L., Jr.: Stable internal standard flame photometer for potassium and sodium analyses. Anal. Chem., 23:137, 1951.

17. Freier, E.: Calcium, EDTA-Calcein method. Microchem. Workshop for Med. Techn., U. Colo. School Med., Denver, 1961.

18. Gambino, R.: Critique for CC #31. Council Cont. Educ., Amer. Soc. Clin. Path., Chicago, 1965.

19. Gaydon, A. G., and Wolfhard, H. G.: *Flames, Their Structure, Radiation and Temperature*. London, Chapman and Hall, 1953.

20. Gilbert, P. T., Jr.: Advances in emission flame photometry. Beckman reprint #-6217, Beckman Instruments, Inc., Fullerton, Calif.

21. Hald, P. M., The flame photometer for the measurement of sodium and potassium in biological fluids. J. Biol. Chem. 167:499, 1947.

22. Harley, J. H., and Wiberley, S. E.: *Instrumental Analysis*. New York, John Wiley and Sons, Inc., 1954.

23. Henry, R. J.: *Clinical Chemistry, Principles and Technics*. New York, Hoeber Medical Division, Harper & Row, 1964.

24. Hermann, R., and Alkemade, C. T. J.: *Chemical Analysis by Flame Photometry*. New York, Interscience Publications, 1963.

25. Humes, C., Personal communication.

26. Instruction handbook for the Model 143 flame photometer. Instrumentation Laboratory, Inc., Lexington, Mass.

27. Lewis, B., and Von Elbe, G.: Stability and structure of burner flames. J. Chem. Phys., 11:75, 1943.

28. Manual of operation and maintenance for Weichselbaum-Varney universal spectro-photometer. Fearless Camera, Los Angeles, Calif.

29. Mavrodineau, R., and Boiteux, H.: *Flame Spectroscopy*. New York, John Wiley and Sons, Inc., 1965.

30. Mosher, R. E., Boyle, A. J., Bird, E. J., Jacobson, S. D., Batchelor, T. M., Iseri, L. T., and Myers, G. B.: The use of flame photometry for the quantitative determination of sodium and potassium in plasma and urine. Amer. J. Clin. Path., *19:*461, 1949.

31. Natelson, S.: The routine use of the Perkin-Elmer flame photometer in the clinical laboratory. Amer. J. Clin. Path., *20:*463, 1950.

32. Olney, J. M., and James, A. H.: An air-cleaning apparatus for the flame photometer. Science, *115:*244, 1952.

33. Operating directions for the Model 21 Coleman flame photometer. Brochure #D-332. Coleman Instruments, Maywood, Ill., 1962.

34. Parker, D. M.: Method for micro-calcium using the Coleman flame photometer. Amer. J. Med. Techn., *26:*19, 1960.

35. Parks, T. D., Johnson, H. O., and Lykken, L.: Errors in the use of a Model 18 Perkin-Elmer flame photometer for the determination of alkali metals. Anal. Chem., *20:*822, 1945.

36. Phototubes, photocells. Brochure #IG1018. Radio Corporation of America. Harrison, N. J.

37. Sims, A. H., and Kaplow, L.: Exclusion of air-borne contamination in flame photometry, J. Lab. Clin. Med., *41:*303, 1953.

38. Tonks, D. B.: Quality control systems in clinical laboratories. Postgrad. Med., *34:* No. 4, A-58, 1963.

39. Vallee, B. L., and Thiers, R. E.: Flame photometry. *In,* Kolthoff, I. M., and Elving, P. J., eds., *Treatise on Analytical Chemistry,* Vol. 6. New York, Interscience Publications, 1965, p. 3463.

40. West, A. C., and Cooke, W. D.: Elimination of anion, interferences in flame spectros-copy—use of (ethylenedinitrilo) tetraacetic acid. Anal. Chem., *32:*1471, 1960.

41. White, J. U.: Precision of a simple flame photometer. Anal. Chem., *24:*394, 1952.

42. Willard, H. H., Merritt, L. L., and Dean, J. A.: *Instrumental Methods of Analysis.* 4th ed. New York, Van Nostrand Company, Inc., 1965.

43. Winstead, M.: *Reagent Grade Water: How, When and Why?* Amer. Soc. Med. Technolo-gists, Houston, 1967.

44. Winstead, M.: Quality control for flame photometry. Amer. J. Med. Techn. *34:*305, 1968.

45. Woldring, M. G.: Flame photometric determination of sodium and potassium in some biological fluids. Anal. Chim. Acta, *8:*150, 1953.

# 6

# pH METERS

Until fairly recently pH meters for aqueous solutions were rather haphazardly used in the clinical laboratory. When blood pH values necessitated values discriminated to $\pm$ 0.005 pH unit, the natural reaction was then to be more critical of the aqueous values. Still more recently the appearance of ion-selective electrodes has forced the conscientious user to review the whole theory and application of pH measurements. Assignment of significance to a $\pm$ 0.05 mV response from an ion-selective electrode[56] is frightening to those of us comfortably accustomed to our usual pH meters. The forecast that such measurements may be just around the corner causes us to try now to improve our current use of these meters. An adequate check system to be applied to the use of pH meters for aqueous solutions must include careful notation of specific component choices, an understanding of how each contributes to the measurement, and some degree of alertness as to how the addition of other ion-selective electrodes will fit into the same scheme.

Measurements with the pH meter are made by determining the potential (or electromotive force) developed by an electrical cell. This cell consists of two electrodes: an *indicator electrode* (usually the glass electrode) and a *reference electrode* (usually the saturated calomel electrode)immersed in a solution. When the meter (*i.e.,* electrode response) has been calibrated by reading a standard buffer solution in the electrical cell, the response given by reading a test solution in the same cell may be read from the meter. The operator may take the meter reading in potential or mV response or in pH units assigned for the specific temperature prevailing.

However, what seems to be a straightforward measurement is limited by uncertainties within the electrical cell, so that, at best, pH can be defined only in operational terms rather than in absolute ionic activity values. Furthermore, the magnitude of the uncertainties must be monitored by the operator and noted in order that values may be comparable from one time to another and between one laboratory and another.

The following definition of pH was endorsed by standardizing groups in the United States, Great Britain, and Japan.[3, 9]

$$pH\ (x) = pH\ (s) + \frac{(E_x - E_s)\ F}{RT\ \ln 10}$$

where pH (x) is the pH of the test sample related to the pH of a standard buffer, pH (s). $E_x$ and $E_s$ are the electromotive force values for test sample and standard buffer; F is Faraday or 96,487.0 coulombs equivalent $^{-1}$; R is the gas constant or 8.3143 joules degree $^{-1}$ mole $^{-1}$; T is Kelvin temperature ($°C + 273.15$); and the ln, or natural log of 10, is 2.30259.

The buffers necessary for determining the pH values by the operational definition equation are standardized by the National Bureau of Standards and their values are assigned from measurements on a hydrogen-silver, silver-chloride cell, a cell without liquid junction. The response of the hydrogen cell is assigned zero potential at all temperatures.[3] The established values for $pa_H$ [or $p(a_H\ \gamma_{Cl})$, the acidity

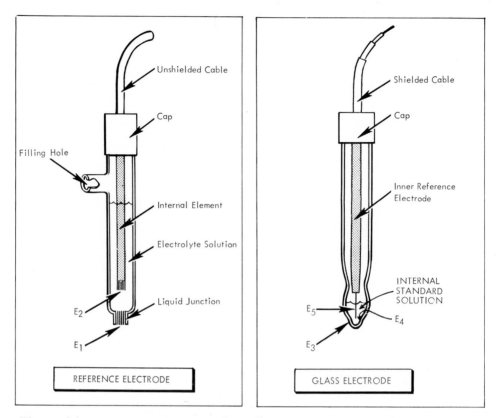

**Figure 6-1.** *Diagram of electrical cell usually used for pH measurement.*

function for buffers extrapolated to zero concentration of chloride] have been provided at temperatures from 0° to 95°C.[7] These values are given later under Buffers.

The electrical cell ordinarily used in pH measurements is shown in Figure 6-1. It consists of a reference half-cell, an indicating half-cell, and the salt bridge between them. The reference half-cell is the saturated calomel electrode whose potential is logarithmically related to chloride activity, and the indicating half-cell is the glass electrode whose potential is logarithmically related to the hydrogen ion activity. As can be seen from the diagram, several separate potentials exist in this system, some of which are not present in the hydrogen cell used by the National Bureau of Standards to establish the values of the standard buffers. Herein lies part of the uncertainties mentioned earlier. The emf of the cell is the sum of all these separate potentials. The equation usually used to express this relationship is:

$$pa_H = \frac{E - (E^{0\prime} + Ej)}{0.05916}$$

where E is the total emf of the cell, $E^{0\prime}$ is the standard potential of the cell, and Ej is the potential across the liquid junction. In order for the operational definition

198

to give meaningful pH values "the values for ($E^{o'}$ + Ej) must remain unchanged when the standard solution is replaced by the unknown. These conditions are approximately fulfilled only when the unknown is a fairly dilute aqueous solution of simple solutes and its acidity matches closely that of the standard solution selected. Unfortunately, the great majority of test solutions will not meet these stringent requirements, and the measured pH cannot then justifiably be regarded as an approximate measure of the (conventional) hydrogen ion activity of the test medium."[3] These restrictions, therefore, limit the accuracy of the pH value to within approximately ± 0.03 pH units even if the measurement is made using an instrument capable of precision to 0.1 mV.[50] As long as we understand that the pH values are "assigned numbers," our chief concern becomes faithful reproducibility. It follows that assignment of significance to small *changes* in pH values is valid when these values are obtained by a combination of good operator technique and a pH meter with excellent precision. The validity and also the limitation of the significance of the measurement are directly controlled by the operator's technique —and this is the challenge!

## REFERENCE ELECTRODES

Both the calomel and silver-silver chloride reference electrodes are used in aqueous pH measurements, but the former is the more common. Use of the silver-silver chloride electrode is usually in combination electrodes at temperatures over 80°C[4] or at elevations of both temperature and pressure.[45]

The structure of the calomel electrode is shown in Figure 6-2. Usually the cable lead wire can be seen to go into the mercury but cannot be seen beyond this point. The mercury forms a solid interface with the mercurous chloride—potassium chloride paste. The level of the potassium chloride solution is best kept just below

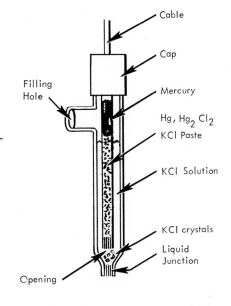

**Figure 6-2.** *Diagram of calomel reference electrode.*

the air vent so that there is ample potassium chloride present in the mercurous chloride column. The opening in the bottom of the column container makes this equilibrium possible. It is important that the column of paste does not break up and allow "pockets" to form. Even if the pockets are filled with potassium chloride, the temperature effect is different and the electrode may have erratic or drifting potentials.[45] If the KCl solution level is low, the pockets will contain air and the electrode response becomes so erratic that it cannot be controlled.

The properties of the calomel electrode have been listed by Mattock:[45]

1. *Stability with Time.* When freshly prepared, this electrode may take several days to settle down. During this period fluctuations of potential occur in the order of several millivolts. The saturated calomel electrode, once stabilized, should remain constant within ± 0.02 mV for several months if thermostated.

2. *Temperature Effects.* The potential values of the calomel electrode decrease markedly with temperature. As the KCl concentration increases, the magnitude of the decrease in potential increases; saturated KCl shows the greatest effect at all temperatures. (Wright has shown that for the pH measurement to be better than 0.001 unit, the temperature stability of the reference electrode must be better than ± 0.05°C.[64]) The saturated KCl calomel electrode has a temperature coefficient of − 0.7 to − 0.8 mV per degree C.

   The thermal effect of most concern with calomel electrodes is hysteresis. The lag for the saturated calomel electrode can be several hours, depending upon the temperature changes. Mattock found that commercially prepared electrodes containing saturated KCl solution in contact with the calomel inner element stabilized to within 1 to 2 mV after 5 to 10 minutes. For values within ± 0.1 mV, several days were required for equilibration. He also found that for temperatures above 70°C, the potentials drifted or oscillated.

3. *Effect of Atmospheric Oxygen.* The potential of calomel cells using HCl as the electrolyte are seriously affected by dissolved oxygen forming in the electrode. The calomel reference cell using neutral KCl is much less affected. Since the requirement for the calomel cell in measuring pH is to provide *stability* (and not necessarily a constant standard mV value) the atmospheric oxygen causes no problem.

4. *Effects of Chemical Impurities.* Chemical substances to be avoided in the salt bridge include acids, cyanides, sulphides, complex-forming agents, silver, and perchlorates. Back diffusion into the reference electrode must be prevented by maintaining the outward gravity flow of the KCl. Aside from the possibility of chemical reaction, back diffusion should not be allowed because of the instability it produces.

5. *Polarization.* If the calomel electrode is accidentally allowed to take appreciable current, polarization will occur with a concomitant rise in resistance. A considerable time lag may occur before the potential returns to its original value. The maximum anodic current density tolerable without significant polarization is 15 $\mu A/cm^2$ for about 5 hours.

The calomel half-cell of fixed potential uses a neutral potassium chloride solution, and the exact potential depends upon the strength of the solution and

**Table 6-1. Standard Calomel Half-cell Potentials as a Function of Temperature in Absolute Volts***

| Temperature (°C) | Saturated[a] | 3.5 $N$[b] (at 25°C) | 1 $N$[c,e] (at 25°C) | 0.1 $N$[d,e] (at 25°C) |
|---|---|---|---|---|
| 0 | 0.2602 | — | 0.2854 | 0.3338 |
| 10 | 0.2541 | — | 0.2839 | 0.3343 |
| 15 | 0.2509 | — | — | — |
| 20 | 0.2477 | — | 0.2815 | 0.3340 |
| 25 | 0.2444 | — | 0.2801 | 0.3337 |
| 30 | 0.2411 | — | 0.2786 | 0.3332 |
| 35 | 0.2377 | — | — | — |
| 38 | 0.2357 | — | — | — |
| 40 | 0.2343 | 0.2466 | 0.2753 | 0.3316 |
| 50 | 0.2272 | 0.2428 | 0.2716 | 0.3296 |
| 60 | 0.2199 | 0.2377 | 0.2673 | 0.3229 |
| 70 | 0.2124 | 0.2331 | 0.2622 | 0.3236(?) |
| 80 | 0.2047 | 0.2277[f] | — | — |
| 90 | 0.1967 | 0.2237[g] | — | — |
| 100 | 0.1885 | — | — | — |

* By permission from Hills, G. J., and Ives, D. J. G.: The calomel electrode and other mercury-mercurous salt electrodes. In *Reference Electrodes: Theory and Practice*. D. J. G. Ives and G. J. Janz, Eds. New York, Academic Press, 1961, p. 161.

[a] At room temperatures, the variation with temperature is represented approximately by the equation $E'' = 0.2444 - 0.0025(t - 25)$ where $t$ is temperature in °C; at higher temperatures, the form of the variation differs from that predicted by the more accurate equation for $E'$, i.e.,

$$E' = 0.2412 - 6.61 \times 10^{-4}(t - 25) - 1.75 \times 10^{-6}(t - 25)^2 - 9.0 \times 10^{-10}(t - 25)^3$$

[b] Directly determined, i.e., $E''$ value.

[c] Expressed by $E'_{1N} = 0.2801 - 2.75 \times 10^{-4}(t - 25) - 2.50 \times 10^{-6}(t - 25)^2 - 4 \times 10^{-9}(t - 25)^3$.

[d] Expressed by $E'_{0.1N} = 0.3337 - 8.75 \times 10^{-5}(t - 25) - 3 \times 10^{-6}(t - 25)^2$.

[e] Both sets are $E'$ values and where a salt bridge is used, the corresponding $E''$ value may be approximately found by adding the quantity $(E'' - E')$ at 25°.

[f] At 79.9.

[g] At 89.9°C.

the temperature. See Table 6-1. The most commonly used reference cell is the *saturated* calomel. If the concentration of potassium chloride used in the calomel half-cell is equal to that in the salt bridge, the junction potential shown as $E_2$ in Figure 6-1 is eliminated.[30] Variability in the junction potential, shown as $E_1$ in Figure 6-1 is less when the concentration of the KCl is high,[1, 48] but the electrode form using saturated KCl is subject to serious hysteresis on changes of temperature.[8] For this reason the use of 3.5 KCl is considered preferable, and crystallization of the salt is avoided. The accumulation of solid salt at the bridge-solution interface impedes the establishment of reproducible liquid junction potentials and increases the resistance of the cell.

Variation in liquid junction potential has been stated to be the most important source of error in pH measurements.[47] If pH discrimination to better than 0.02 pH unit is required, consideration must be given to the causes of junction potential errors. A potential from differences in ionic transport across the boundary layer always exists between two solutions of differing compositions and strengths. Potassium chloride satisfies the requirement for equal transference of ions and therefore is commonly used as the bridge solution. Since the National Bureau of Standards buffer scale is based on measurements made without a liquid junction, use of cells with a liquid junction introduces an error into the measurement, an error variable under several circumstances.

Factors affecting the junction potential include pH (mobility) effects, ionic strength effects, colloidal effects, temperature effects, and geometry of the junction.[47] Hydrogen and hydroxyl ions, both being highly mobile, cause increased differences in liquid junction potentials. With 3.5 M KCl and 1M HCl the $E_j$ is 16.6 mV, with 3.5 M KCl and 0.1 M NaOH the $E_j$ is $-2.1$.[47] Standardization with only one buffer at the range of pH 7.0 usually can provide values $\pm 0.02$ between pH 3 and 10. Outside this range, however, standardization at pH 7.0 alone is not sufficient to maintain this accuracy. Mattock further points out that the slope (i.e., in mV theoretically 0.198T) must be determined in the region over pH 9 for measurements of high pH. Measurements in the 3 to 10 pH range require that the standard buffer be within a pH unit of the unknown if values better than $\pm 0.01$ pH unit are required.[44]

The ionic strength of the standard buffers is less than 0.1, and test solutions whose ionic strengths differ by even 0.1 from the buffer give significant differences in liquid junction potentials if pH values of $\pm 0.005$ are required.[47]

Temperature changes affect both ionic mobilities and activity coefficients, thus making comparisons difficult.[47] In accurate measurements, therefore, it is advisable to adopt a uniform temperature throughout.

The physical structure of the liquid junction and the effective flow of potassium chloride through the port are both within the control of the user. Several types of junction are shown in Figure 6-3. Leakage from the salt bridge solution should be low, but satisfactory performance depends upon continuous, unimpeded, positive flow through the junction.[63]

The *free diffusion junction,* first classified by Guggenheim,[31] allows two solutions to meet at an initially sharp boundary with subsequent free diffusion. $A_1$ and $A_2$ of Figure 6-3 are both of this type. In $A_1$ the 3-way tap rotates, allowing the sample salt bridge boundary to form as shown in (c). Reproducibility for a cell using this junction is reported to have been $\pm 10$ $\mu$V (or 95% confidence level of $\pm 0.005$ pH unit).[48] The $A_2$ junction in which plates slide to allow the sample

202

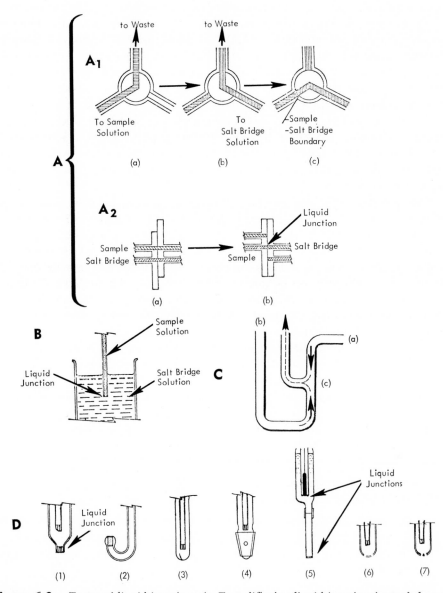

**Figure 6-3.** *Types of liquid junction. A₁. Free diffusion liquid junction formed through a three-way tap. A₂. Free diffusion junction formed with two sliding faces. B. Simple dipping form of free diffusion liquid junction. C. Flowing junction. D. Restrained flow junction: (1) ceramic plug; (2) J-type with ceramic plug; (3) fiber wick; (4) glass sleeve; (5) porous stone; (6) palladium annulus; (7) controlled crack.*

salt bridge mixture is cited by the same author to have a reproducibility of $\pm 30\mu$V. The free diffusion junction is the type normally used in most precise measurements and in attempts to obtain fundamental data. The capillary tube containing the sample may be dipped into the salt bridge, as shown in B of Figure 6-3. This was originally called the "indefinite" type of junction by Guggenheim because it did not precisely conform to the free diffusion junction. This junction is capable of giving highly reproducible results both with simple aqueous solutions and with complex biological fluids.[48]

The *flowing junction,* shown as C in Figure 6-3, is said to produce a potential difference of about 1 mV from the free diffusion type.[3] All of the junctions shown as A, B, and C have a confined cylindrically symmetrical junction which is more stable than junctions allowing a streaming flow of concentrated bridge solution to go into the test solution.[3]

The *restrained flow junction* has a device to control the flow of salt-bridge solution into the test solution. The examples shown as D of Figure 6-3 are: ceramic plug, fiber wick, J-type incorporating ceramic plug (this arrangement allows the heavier salt solution to come from below the test solution to avoid turbulence), small fiber, glass sleeve, and one using porous stone. Palladium annulus is a wire surrounded by concentric space through which the salt solution flows. Controlled crack is also a similar type of junction. Although the fiber junction was previously the most commonly used, the trend now is to favor the ceramic diaphragm or the ceramic plug.[5] This junction is highly reproducible and easy to establish. Intermediate range pH reproducibility is said to be $\pm 0.2$ mV; with 1 M HCl, $\pm 0.8$ mV and with 1 N NaOH, $\pm 0.4$ mV. The corresponding figures for the ground glass sleeve, according to Mattock and Band, are $\pm 0.2$ mV, $\pm 3.2$, and $\pm 2.0$ mV.[48] These authors also highly regard the controlled crack and palladium annulus junctions.

The type of sample should be considered when selecting the liquid junction for the reference electrode. These recommendations have been made:

1. The palladium annulus is preferable for microtitration and application under high pressure or vacuum.

2. The asbestos fiber is satisfactory for general use but tends to clog in some media.

3. The ground glass sleeve is better for precipitate titrations, titrations in non-aqueous solvent systems, and handling of colloids and suspensions.

4. The ceramic plug junction is recommended for precise work, especially at either high or low pH ranges.[45]

Having chosen the reference electrode liquid junction of appropriate type, the user must continually monitor details of technique and good maintenance:

1. Carefully inspect the calomel element of the electrode. The calomel should be silver-gray, not brown. No air bubbles should be present in the column. Air bubbles can sometimes be removed by gentle evacuation of the salt bridge chamber or by warming the electrode in water.[3] (Bubbles get into the column if the KCl level in the bridge is too low.)

The drop of mercury at the top of the calomel column must be intact and must make good contact with the wire which dips into it. The wire may not even be visible if the mercury is in its proper position.

2. Maintain electrolyte in the reference electrode at sufficient level to make the proper contact with the calomel inner column and also to sustain a slight pressure head above the sample solution when the electrode is immersed into the solution. One to two centimeters is sufficient for the latter.[49] If the pressure head is not maintained, the sample solution can flow back into the reference electrode.

3. If the calomel cell is using saturated KCl (and most of them are) check to see that a few crystals of KCl are present. Avoid an excess of crystalline KCl, which leads to cake formation. (Slower and less reproducible results are traceable to caked KCl hindering the flow.) Prewarming the KCl before adding it is a convenient way to provide the crystals.

4. Be sure the air vent is uncovered while making readings so that the flow of salt bridge solution is not slowed; close when not in use.

5. Avoid contamination of the porous junctions. Relatively large fluctuations in potential have been observed when these junctions were not adequately rinsed between measurements.[3] Rinsing the reference electrode (as is also true of the glass electrode) with the next sample solution would be preferable but is often impractical. Thorough rinsing with pure water is satisfactory, and the excess should be shaken off or touched off with nonfibrous paper. Change the KCl frequently to avoid the possibility of contamination. The KCl should be purer than the usual reagent material off the shelf. In our laboratory we prefer to buy a neutralized, saturated KCl prepared for use with pH meters.

6. Store the reference electrode so that the KCl concentration is maintained and the junction is kept from plugging. For short storage periods, the saturated KCl calomel electrode can safely be left in water if the KCl level inside the electrode is well above the water level.[45] Feldman cautions that prolonged storage in water can change the junction potential enough that the potentiometer cannot be balanced with a standard buffer.[27] Therefore, the safest prolonged storage is the use of a tight-fitting rubber cap over the tip of the electrode. When the cap is removed, a moist spot on the inside of the cap at the port will indicate that the junction has not dried. Reference electrodes using unsaturated KCl must be stored in the same solution which forms the salt bridge.[45]

## GLASS ELECTRODES

The bulb type glass electrode shown in Figure 6-1 is that typically used in the clinical laboratory for measuring pH of aqueous solutions. The tip of the bulb is made of pH sensitive glass, and the potential shown as $E_3$ (the potential between the outer surface and the test solution) is the only potential, hopefully, that varies proportionately with the hydrogen ion activity of the solution.

The other contributions to total potential of the electrode come from $E_5$, the metallic terminal of an inner reference electrode which contacts the internal standard solution, and $E_4$, the potential between the internal standard solution and the inner surface of the glass membrane.

Details of the interior of this and other configurations of glass electrode structure are shown in Figure 6-4. The same sources of potential appear in each of these, including the combined reference and indicating electrode shown as (C).

From the discussion of check systems for glass electrodes it will be seen that attention must be given to what can cause the various potentials to change as measurements are being attempted. In the operational definition of pH:

$$pH(x) = pH(s) + \frac{(E_x - E_s) \, F}{RT \ln 10}$$

we have already noted that pH measurements are made in terms of the difference in electromotive force (emf) measured by the indicator electrode for a standard buffer solution and the test solution, $E_s - E_x$. The value in pH units was an assigned one for the standard buffer solution. The calculated pH of the test solution depends upon this standard and the ability of the glass electrode to respond in a linear fashion to the change in hydrogen ion activity (or emf). This linear response of the electrode must, in reality, be proven by the operator every time the instrument is used. The instrument is calibrated or standardized by setting the scale to read a midrange buffer and then checking the readings for a buffer on each side of the calibration buffer. If the mV response between these buffers is not correct, then the operator must correct the "slope" of the instrument.

*Slope* is defined as the mV response per pH unit. Since $H^+$ activity of the buffer and the solution changes with temperature, the mV difference between them will be different at different temperatures; the proportion of their mV response per 1 pH unit, however, remains the same for any one given temperature. Let's assume that

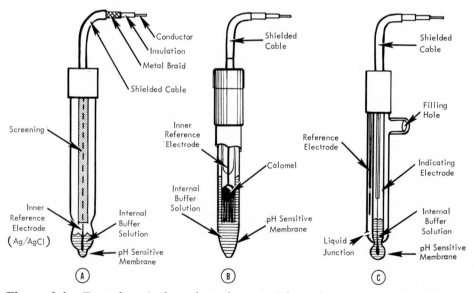

**Figure 6-4.** *Examples of glass electrodes. A. Silver–silver chloride. B. Calomel. C. Combination.*

at 25° three standard buffers were read in mV and their assigned pH values at this temperature plotted against the respective mV responses. This plot is shown as Figure 6-5. If the pH 7.0 buffer is set at 0 mV on the meter, the pH 10 buffer will read — 177.48 mV, and the pH 4.0 buffer will read + 177.48 mV. The difference of 177.48 in both cases represents a change of 3 pH units or 59.16 mV per pH unit. The 59.16 mV/pH can be called the slope of the mV response-pH unit line for 25°; at 30° this slope would be equal to 60.15 mV as shown in Table 6-2.

The slope of any line representing mV response per pH unit can be expressed by

$$\frac{\text{mV response span}}{\text{pH unit difference}}$$

This is commonly related to the Nernst or theoretical response. The Nernst response in mV per pH unit, defining the slope of the mV response line at a particular temperature in Kelvin units, is taken from the Nernst equation:[4]

$$E_x = \frac{2.3026RT}{F} \, pH$$

where:

$$\frac{2.3026RT}{F} = \text{slope factor}$$

Another expression often used for the slope factor is mV = 0.198T, where T is in Kelvin units (273.15 + °C). This same slope factor is present in the operational definition equation which is often shown as

$$pH(x) = pH_s + \frac{(E_x - E_s)}{k}$$

where:

$$k = \frac{2.3026RT}{F}$$

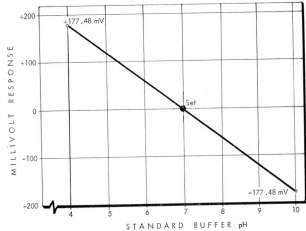

**Figure 6-5.** *Millivolt response for three standard buffers at 25°C.*

**Table 6-2. Slope or mV Response per pH Unit at Various Temperatures***

| °C | Slope† $\dfrac{2.3026\ RT}{F}$ millivolts |
|---|---|
| 0 | 54.197 |
| 5 | 55.189 |
| 10 | 56.181 |
| 15 | 57.173 |
| 20 | 58.165 |
| 25 | 59.157 |
| 30 | 60.149 |
| 35 | 61.141 |
| 38 | 61.737 |
| 40 | 62.133 |
| 45 | 63.126 |
| 50 | 64.118 |
| 55 | 65.110 |
| 60 | 66.102 |
| 65 | 67.094 |
| 70 | 68.086 |
| 75 | 69.078 |
| 80 | 70.070 |
| 85 | 71.062 |
| 90 | 72.054 |
| 95 | 73.046 |
| 100 | 74.038 |

\* By permission from Bates, R. G.: *Determination of pH: Theory and Practice.* New York, John Wiley & Sons, Inc., 1964.

† Slope factor $\dfrac{2.3026\ RT}{F}$ or $\dfrac{RT\ \ln 10}{F}$ is the same as 0.198T expressed in mV.

The efficiency of the electrode in terms of its mV response is frequently expressed as % Nernst, meaning

$$\frac{\text{mV response measured}}{\text{theoretical mV response}} \times 100$$

per pH unit. The technical nomenclature used for this expression is electromotive efficiency with designation

$$\beta_e = \frac{E_x - E_s}{E_x' - E_s'}$$

where $E_x$ and $E_s$ are the observed values of emf and $E_x'$ and $E_s'$ represent emf of the same system if the glass electrode were replaced by a hydrogen cell.[8] The electromotive efficiencies of most useful glass electrodes lie between 0.95 and 1.0 (95% Nernst or better). For accurate work it is now recommended that pH meters should provide a corrective adjustment so that the glass electrode response can be corrected to the theoretical or 100% Nernst response.[64] This will be further discussed under Meters.

Occasionally an electrode will appear to give a mV/pH unit response greater than theoretical (more than 100% Nernst). One of two causes is usually responsible:[44] either the temperature compensation is incorrect or some electrode drift has occurred since standardization. From our experiences with buffers, we would be inclined to suspect an incorrect buffer even *before* the two causes listed above.

We now routinely check the zero potential for each new glass electrode and also make a notation of the span available around the isoelectric point of the meter on which the electrode is to be used. While the latter is relative and subject to other differences in the circuit (*e.g.,* reference electrode), the information is helpful in pinpointing troubles later. Incidentally, the zero potential for different reference electrodes appears to fall in a much more narrow range than for glass electrodes.

## Response Time

Some workers have classified response time curves and have correlated these somewhat to glass compositions and also different pH ranges.[11] However, they chose the initial response as correct and regarded slow creeps as changes in asymmetry potential. We have not yet found it necessary to try to distinguish some cutoff point in a reading that creeps. Any very slow responses we have seen have been attributed to a defective electrode. Our usual ranges of pH, however, do not include high values where one would expect exceptionally slow responses. With many people making readings, we would be reluctant to try to standardize end-point readings if our instrument functioned in this manner.

Response pattern and the time required to make a stable pH reading vary somewhat with the glass composition of the electrode. Once established as "normal" for a particular electrode system, however, both pattern and time should remain approximately the same. If a recorder were attached to the pH meter so that the electrode response were shown with time as the ordinate and either pH or mV as the abscissa, the response pattern would be useful. The ideal pattern would be shaped as in Figure 6-6A, indicating a steady, fast response with little creep

209

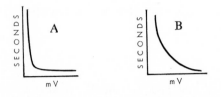

**Figure 6-6.** *Response patterns. A. Ideal. B. Slow response.*

toward the final reading. On the other hand, a curve shaped as in Figure 6-6B indicates a slow response. An alert operator learns to notice the response time and can picture this function without using a recorder. The operator must also be familiar with the normal response time pattern of the electrode being used. Some lithia glasses respond slowly, and the shapes of these curves would have to be considered in terms of lithia's own normal response. Also strongly acid or strongly alkaline solutions on transfer from weak ionic to strong or vice versa show a slow response.[44] This could be the result of a dirty electrode or even air bubbles somewhere in the system (liquid junction, reference element column, standard solution in inner reference electrode, or a capillary glass electrode if one is being used). Recently it has been suggested that letting the electrode stand in distilled water may cause a slow response time.[33] No glass electrode yet constructed has the theoretical response in all types of test solutions and over the entire practical pH range.[3] The three steps required for pH measurement are the same, however, for all glass electrodes:[1]

1. The membrane of pH sensitive glass, consisting of a three-dimensional lattice of silicon and oxygen, holds within its interstices cations of alkali metals.

2. Hydrogen ions from the solution being measured enter the lattice and displace some of the metallic cations outwards into the test solution.

3. The ionic transfer sets up an emf across the glass membrane.

The operator's first problem then is to understand what factors contribute to each step so that he may choose the proper electrode for the intended use. The first two steps are intimately associated with the composition and atomic structure of the glass membrane and are thus fixed by the choice of electrode. The third step, while also determined by the specific glass characteristics, is more specifically limited by the care with which the operator maintains the electrode and the restrictions he puts on its use within the known limitations of the glass and the rest of the system. The successful use of this indicating electrode (and indeed this entire pH meter system) can be judged by only one criterion—how consistently the electrode's sensitive surface can produce a mV response in accord with the Nernst equation. Although this discussion is related to pH response, the same considerations apply in general to other cations measured not only with glass electrodes but with other types of membranes.[56] In all cases the potentials measured are those generated through controlled ion-exchange transactions, and the response must be reproducible to within a tolerance of no more than a few tenths of a mV.

## pH Sensitive Membrane

The glass electrode's pH sensitive membrane behaves in general like a cation exchanger having uniform chemical properties. The particular values of its measured response originate as a result of ion-exchange processes, and the observed potential is the sum of diffusion and phase-boundary potentials.[24] The composition and structure of the glass determine both these parameters. The first stage of the reaction is always the diffusion of the ions into the silica lattice,[36] and hydration of the glass increases this ionic mobility.[23, 24]

As soon as the equilibrium between the solution and the glass surface is established, the diffusion potential is fixed and does not ordinarily change with time.[21] Changes that can occur in the structure of the glass will cause changes in the mobility ratio and thus in the diffusion potential. These include progressive hydration of the glass in contact with water, internal variations in the glass structure, and stress changes in the glass. Ion-exchange equilibrium constants are characteristic of the particular glass membrane.

The potential of the glass electrode, whenever it is responding with a Nernst slope to a particular ion, is the result of changes in the values of the phase-boundary potentials.[24] The cations entering and leaving the glass cause either an excessive or a deficient total charge to the glass, and an electrical potential difference builds up between the membrane-solution interfaces.[21]

The charge transfer (*i.e.,* current) has recently been stated to be "carried entirely by the cationic species of lowest charge available in any given glass. No single sodium ion (for sodium silicate glass) moves through the entire thickness of the dry glass membrane, but, rather, the charge is transported by an interstitial mechanism where such charge carrier needs to move only a few atomic diameters before passing on its energy to another carrier."[56]

## Atomic Structure of the Glass

Selectivity of the cation exchange is predetermined by its atomic structure.[36] The structure of the glass is determined by its composition during melting at high temperatures; once it is cooled below the glass transition temperature, its structure remains the same, even if its cations are exchanged with others.[21] This basic structure is formed as a lattice of silicon and oxygen atoms whose three-dimensional random structure is tetrahydral (*i.e.,* four oxygens are attached to each silicon.) Melting the silicate in the presence of alkali metal or alkaline earth metal ions "breaks" the lattice, and the size of the spatial configuration follows the atomic radius of the alkali metal ion. The structure shown in Figure 6-7 (a), known as the $(SiO)^-$ site, indicates the $Na^+$ ion held in position by a field strength typical of the structure—*i.e.,* charge of the nonbridging oxygen which can be thought of as how close the cation ($Na^+$) can approach the charge center of the anionic group.[21] Thus, the smaller the cation, the more it will be attracted in the glass structure and the less likely it is to move into the solution.

211

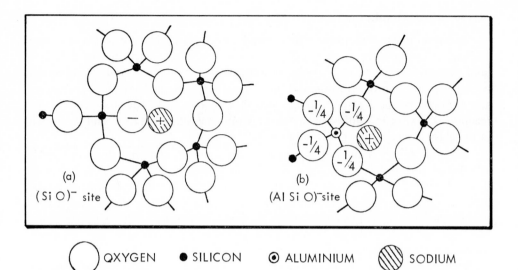

OXYGEN    SILICON    ALUMINIUM    SODIUM

**Figure 6-7.** *Schematic for exchange sites.  A. (SiO⁻) sodium silica glass.  B. (A1SiO⁻) aluminosilica glass.  (Redrawn with permission from Isard, J. O.: The dependence of glass electrode properties on composition. In* Glass Electrode for Hydrogen and Other Cations. *G. Eisenman, Ed. New York, Marcel Dekker, Inc., 1967, p. 54.)*

$H^+$, having a smaller radius, would be much preferred by this glass. Furthermore, the similar structure formed when lithium oxide is melted with the silicate contains $(SiO)^-$ sites which hold the $Li^+$ more strongly than the $Na^+$ was held ($Li^+$ coordination number being 4 and $Na^+$ being 6 or 8). The $Li^+$ ions then show little tendency to exchange with other larger cations in the solution;[3] therefore, the sodium ion errors are much less in electrodes made of lithia glasses. The selectivity for the silicate site is $H^+ > Li^+ > Na^+ > K^+ > Rb^+ > Cs^+$ and may be said to be preferentially selective to $H^+$ ions.[36]

If a trivalent or tetravalent ion such as aluminum is added into the glass structure, as shown in Figure 6-7(b), the cations are no longer associated with the negatively charged nonbridging oxygen ions but with the whole of the tetrahedral units.[36] This site has considerably lower field strength and is designated $(AlSiO)^-$ type. Very early it was recognized that the less $Al_2O_3$ glass contained, the better it was for measuring $H^+$.[23] The Corning 015 formula contains no $Al_2O_3$. The mV/pH response for this glass is shown in the upper portion of Figure 6-8.

As shown in the lower portion of Figure 6-8, if a small amount of $Al_2O_3$ is added to the glass, the alkaline error is increased to the point that the electrode becomes strongly dependent upon $Na^+$ as well as upon $H^+$. The field strength at the $(AlSiO)^-$ site defines selectivity functions that have been delineated for a family of $Al_2O_3$ glass compositions. [22, 23, 36] In general, the calculated order of ion selectivity for the alumino-silicate site is the exact reverse of that for the silicate site.[36] The alumino-silicate site is thus expected to be preferentially selective to

212

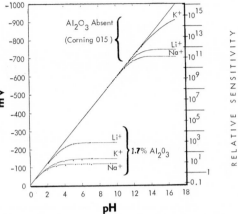

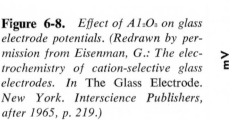

**Figure 6-8.** *Effect of Al₂O₃ on glass electrode potentials. (Redrawn by permission from Eisenman, G.: The electrochemistry of cation-selective glass electrodes. In* The Glass Electrode. *New York. Interscience Publishers, after 1965, p. 219.)*

cations other than $H^+$. It was this alumino-silicate selectivity that provided the basis for the further development of other materials for ion-selective electrodes.[56]

## Composition of the Glass

To achieve the desired pH response and at the same time to maintain reasonable electrical resistance and adequate durability of the glass electrode, the composition of the glass is of utmost importance.[4] While other oxides can form glasses, the silicates alone have sufficient chemical durability to be serviceable under ordinary conditions of use, and all but a few commercial glass compositions contain at least 50% $SiO_2$.[36]

Electrode glasses usually have at least three constituents: $SiO_2$, $R_2O$, and MO (or $M_2O_3$). R is an alkali metal and M is a bivalent or trivalent metal, the latter preferably one of the rare earth group.[3] The customary expression for composition of each constituent is in moles% of the oxides. A glass whose composition is 11 moles% $Na_2O$, 18 moles% $Al_2O_3$, and 71 moles% $SiO_2$ has the formula $(Na_2O)_{11}$ $(Al_2O_3)_{18}$ $(SiO_2)_{71}$ and is designated NAS 11-18. This is the recommended electrode for $Na^+$.[22] Electrodes currently being made for ion selectivity are commonly labeled by this formula designation, and in all probability pH electrodes will also be so labeled when we, as users, become more discriminating in our choice of electrodes.

For years the best electrode glass for measuring pH was the Corning 015 formula, which contained 22% $Na_2O$, 6% CaO, and 72% $SiO_2$[36]. Response of this glass was so well known that, while the formula is scarcely used now,[8] other glasses are described by comparison to it. The response time for this glass is about 30 seconds for buffers, and about 99% of the response occurs in 150 milliseconds.[44] It is accurate for pHs only between 2 and 8.

In the pH range below 2.0, the observed pH is too high, and the amount of error depends upon the anions present.[36] Above pH 9, relatively large departures occur, depending on the type and concentration in solution.[36] Figure 6-9 indicates

213

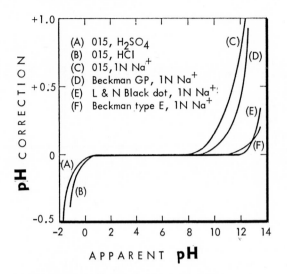

**Figure 6-9.** *Approximate acid and alkaline range of pH corrections necessary for various glass compositions at 25°C. (Redrawn with permission from Bates, R. G.:* Determination of pH: Theory and Practice. *New York, John Wiley & Sons, Inc., 1964, p. 316.)*

the approximate corrections necessary for the acid and alkaline ranges using the Corning 015 glass and several other compositions. The Beckman general purpose electrode contains $Li_2O$, BaO, and $SiO_2$; the Leeds & Northrup black dot is $Li_2O$, $La_2O_3$, and $SiO_2$; and the Beckman type E is $Li_2O$, BaO, and $SiO_2$.[3]

Substitution of $Li_2O$ for $Na_2O$ in glass greatly reduces the alkaline errors for all but the $Li^+$ ion. These glasses became available about 1940, and since that time $Li_2O$, or combinations of multiple constituents, has been used almost exclusively for glass electrodes intended for pH measurement.[36] The lithia electrodes require about 1 minute to approach within 0.01 pH unit of the final reading. These electrodes are particularly subject to slow decay in mV response if there is any tendency for the electrode to be only slightly polarized in this circuit.[44] For this reason progressively more sluggish response of the electrode is expected if the trend begins. Bates notes that some instruments are less prone to cause polarization than others and that the lithia glass electrode *can* respond rapidly.[3] He also states that the response is linear up to pH 12.5. This electrode is more durable than the Corning 015 glass[36] and also requires less water for satisfactory function;[44] it is, therefore, preferable for media which are not very aqueous. The inclusion of a divalent oxide (such as BaO) in an alkali silicate improved the electrode's durability and also its response; less of the silica skeleton is removed during the exchange of $H^+$ for the $Na^+$ ions within the structure, and reversible potentials are more likely to be obtained.[36]

An electrode made of a modified Corning 015 glass in which 5 to 6% of the $SiO_2$ was replaced by uranium oxide is reported to have 10 times the conductivity of the 015 glass at 25° and to respond linearly from pH 1 up to pH 12.[3] Useful high temperature electrodes can be made by substituting titanium dioxide for part of the $SiO_2$ in the 015 formula.

The majority of modern pH electrodes are four-component glasses: a $Li_2O$–$Cs_2O$–$La_2O_3$–$SiO_2$ system.[54] The $Cs^+$ tends to shift the upper limit of the $H^+$

function toward the alkaline region but loosens the glass structure, thus causing significant acid errors.[54] The $La^{+++}$ does not affect the upper limit of the $H^+$ function but tends to eliminate the acid errors. When both of these ions are present in the glass, their effects are summed and one obtains a glass with a wide range of $H^+$ function.

## Asymmetry

The pH-sensitive membrane of the glass electrode shows a slightly different potential even if the same solution is placed inside and outside the bulb. This is thought to result from differences in the ability of the two surfaces to absorb ions.[3] When the bulb is new, such differences arise from shape of the membrane, membrane thickness, internal glass condition as a result of annealing temperature, pH of solutions on either side of the membrane, and surface state differences.[44] Unequal stress at the two surfaces is given as the main cause of the potential difference, according to Doremus: the distortion in the holes of the silicon-oxygen network would be slightly different as the result of the difference in shape of the bulb.[21] He infers that the asymmetry effect is one of a diffusion potential alteration which, once equilibrated, will remain constant. In this case, adjustment of the zero mV response would always remove the asymmetry effects from the measurement.

Changes in the outer surface of the membrane may or may not be totally compensated in the standardization. A marked difference in the pH of the buffer and test solutions or in viscosity of the two would not be balanced.[3] Transitions between low and high pH solutions (or between low and high cation concentrations with cation electrodes) and variations of more than 20° in temperature are not compensated in the standardization.

With use, the alkali ions are gradually removed from the surface layer, leaving the silicate skeleton, and the asymmetry potential increases. If this surface is allowed to dry, a marked shift in asymmetry results and may render the electrode no longer useful, depending on how much internal membrane is left.[4] At any rate, such an electrode must be rehydrated as though it were new, may require etching away the outer surface, and may or may not be salvaged.

From a practical standpoint, the asymmetry potential becomes a concern of the user in terms of a maintenance procedure:

1. The membrane must be kept moist once it has been hydrated and put into use.[44]

2. If not to be used for extended periods, the electrode should be dried and rehydrated when again put into service.[3]

3. A regular program of controlled etching away of the outer layer of the membrane is beneficial.[36]

4. The asymmetry potential must be kept low if good reproducibility and reasonable accuracy are to be achieved in pH measurement.[48] The asymmetry potential may drift slightly from day to day but is not ordinarily subject to large or sudden fluctuations.[3] If large changes occur, suspect an adsorptive process on the surface of the glass such as grease, protein, or surface-active agents.

215

## Hydration, Deterioration and Rejuvenation of Membrane

Before the $H^+$ response can be developed, the glass membrane must be conditioned by soaking in an "activating" solution preferably for about 24 hours.[44] (Both pH- and cation-sensitive glass electrodes require the establishment of a hydrated layer on the surface of the glass). The hydrated exchange layer produced on the membrane surface is very thin;[36] while those who have studied glass membranes agree that some water is required to produce this layer, there appears to be no general agreement concerning the best aqueous solution to use. Tap water or phosphate buffer with pH 7.0 has been recommended for electrodes to be used below pH 9, and borax for those above pH 9.[3] Others suggest that the electrode be hydrated with 0.1 M HCl[8, 44] or with 0.05 M $H_2SO_4$.[8] Rechnitz's discussion of cation electrodes suggests that another possibility for the activating solution for pH electrodes would be a fairly strong buffer containing the ion of the alkali metal of the glass:*

> "Depending on the composition (solubility) of the glass, the establishment of a mature hydrated layer may require from a few hours to several days for an initially dry electrode. Preferably, a new electrode should be soaked in a moderately concentrated solution of a strong electrolyte containing the primary cation for at least 24 hours prior to use. During this time the surface layers of the glass lattice undergo hydration (accompanied by swelling) and, if the cation to be measured is different from the univalent cation or cations in the glass, ion exchange between the solution and the hydrated layer will take place to satisfy the necessary (steady state) distribution across the interface. Outer portions of the hydrated layer are constantly (if slowly) dissolving into the solution, and this hydrated layer is replenished by hydration of additional segments of the dry glass membrane."

In our institution we do not know what is the best solution for hydrating glass electrodes; we are following the manufacturer's instructions for specific electrodes. In the past, water was recommended, and the most common solution now appears to be 0.1 N HCl or buffer of about pH 7.0. In no instance have these pH electrodes been identified with exact glass compositions. This whole correlation of glass composition, reasonable expectations for exact electrode properties, and hydration procedures for best stability and durability is a badly needed study—or probably more fairly stated, badly needed information from the manufacturers.

Once hydrated, the glass electrode should be stored in an aqueous solution similar to the media being measured. Deterioration due to leaching is less than when the electrode is subjected to repeated drying and reconditioning.[4] Tap water and buffer of about pH 7 have been suggested.[44] Our glass electrodes used for aqueous solutions are left connected to the meter and kept in tap water.

Deterioration of the glass electrode is a gradual process to be expected in about 6 months to a year, whether or not it has been in constant use during that time.[3] The ion-exchange process causes changes in the silica lattice,[36] and the outer layer

---

*By permission from Rechnitz, G. A.: Ion-selective electrodes. Chem. Eng. News, *45:*156, 1967.

gradually is dissolved off while the hydration layer proceeds further into the membrane. With the deterioration of the membrane surface, the mV response of the electrode is decreased; response may be restored, within limits, by etching away the outer silica skeleton as discussed later.

Mattock has separated the causes of deterioration into three types:[44]

1. *At Intermediate pH Values.* Deterioration is caused by $H^+$ ions replacing the alkali metal ions in the surface layer. Response tends to be sluggish because of slow diffusion rate. Etching away the outer layer with HCl or even hydrofluoric acid may be necessary.

2. *At High pH.* Lattice destruction takes place. Response is very sluggish and stable pH is hard to obtain. Try rejuvenation in 0.1 N HCl for several days. After this type of destruction, rejuvenation may not be possible.

3. *At low pH.* Deterioration is probably twofold: (a) dehydration of glass surface occurs and there is local lattice "crinkling"; (b) the specific anion of the acid may rupture the Si-O bond and form Si-X bond.

Deterioration of the membrane surface can be measured by changes in the resistance of the electrode. The initial resistance of the electrode is extremely variable and is dependent primarily upon the composition of the glass and the thickness, size, and shape of the membrane.[3] Table 6-3 indicates a few general ranges to be expected for electrodes. The input impedance of meters several years ago was not as high as is currently available; therefore the resistance of the electrode received more concern because large changes in the resistance value could easily produce current in the input circuit. The impedance of $10^{13}$ to $10^{15}$ ohms now used is not affected by such resistance changes in the electrode.

Measurement of the electrode's resistance is useful as the definitive test to declare an electrode defective.[44] Measurement of resistance at this stage in the electrode's life, however, will have questionable meaning unless the value was also obtained when the electrode was new. Mattock has explained this increase in resistance with the deterioration of the membrane as related to the leaching out of the conducting alkali ion.[45] As the electrode is used, replacement of the conducting alkali ion by the strongly binding hydrogen ion reduces the conductivity (increases the resistance). A measurement of the resistance then becomes a way to determine the extent to which the leaching attack has taken place. Bates adds that as the extraction process proceeds the leached silicon-oxygen skeleton becomes thicker, with a consequent increase in the resistance.[4] We have never gone to this extent to prove whether an electrode is defective. If the electrode's zero potential cannot be made to coincide with the meter with which it is to be used and if etching the membrane with 6 N HCl does not render it usable, we have discarded the electrode. We do, however, keep two methods for measuring resistance, with the thought that sometime we may have to try to salvage an old electrode because no other is available. These methods are given under Section VI, A, 3 of the Check System for the Corning, Model 12, pH Meter (page 267).

Deterioration of the membrane surface is most easily detected by the fact that the slope must gradually be corrected more and more while the response time

217

**Table 6-3. Composition and Resistance of Various Glass Electrodes***

| Designation of Glass or Electrode | Composition of Glass | Resistance (megohms) |
|---|---|---|
| Beckman E2 | $Li_2O$, $BaO$, $SiO_2$ | 375 |
| Beckman General Purpose | $Li_2O$, $BaO$, $SiO_2$ | 150 |
| Beckman Amber | $Li_2O$, $BaO$, $SiO_2$ | 550 |
| Cambridge Standard | $Na_2O$, $CaO$, $SiO_2$ | 87 |
| Cambridge Alki | $Li_2O$, $BaO$, $SiO_2$ | 560 |
| Corning 015 | $Na_2O$, $CaO$, $SiO_2$ | 90 |
| Doran Alkacid | $Li_2O$, $BaO$, $SiO_2$ | 200 |
| Electronic Intruments GHS | $Li_2O$, $Cs_2O$, $SiO_2$ | 200 |
| Ingold U | — | 250 |
| Ingold T | — | 140 |
| Ingold UN | $Li_2O$, $SiO_2$† | 30 |
| Jena H | — | 105 |
| Jena U | — | 30 |
| Jena HT | — | 800 |
| Jena HA | — | 290 |
| L & N "Black Dot" | $Li_2O$, $La_2O_3$, $SiO_2$ | 70 |
| Lengyel 115 | $Li_2O$, $BaO$, $UO_2$, $SiO_2$‡ | 15 |
| Metrohm H | $Li_2O$, $BaO$, $SiO_2$ | 1400 |
| Metrohm X | $Li_2O$, $CaO$, $SiO_2$ | 100 |
| Metrohm U | $Li_2O$, $BaO$, $SiO_2$ | 500 |

* By permission from Bates, R. G.: *Determination of pH: Theory and Practice.* New York, John Wiley & Sons, Inc., 1964, p. 333.

† Glass described by K. Schwabe: Chem. Ing. Tech., *29:*656, 1957.

‡ Glass described by B. Lengyel and F. Till: Egypt J. Chem., *1:*99, 1958.

progressively becomes more sluggish. Both these symptoms will immediately be recognized as those that would be present if the electrode surface were "dirty." Actually our "cleaning" process for weekly maintenance is soaking the glass electrode in 0.1 N HCl; this treatment not only cleans the surface but also is a mild rejuvenation process.

For removal of a film on the electrode, Bates suggests 6 N HCl; the same treatment should be given the electrode after prolonged use in alkaline solutions of high sodium content.[3] He also states that electrodes "dead" enough to give only 22 mV/pH unit have been promptly returned to normal function by dipping them in a 1:1 hydrofluoric acid for a few seconds. (Incidentally, a waxed cup is a convenient container to use for hydrofluoric acid solutions.) Some industrial flow-meter pH installations provide for their glass electrode to be cleaned in an ultra-sonic chamber, a procedure reported not to affect the life of the electrode or the measured pH.[5]

Eventually, in normal use the membrane will either become thin enough that the slope control can no longer adjust for the change in resistance or will crack from mechanical strain.[1] In the latter case, the electrode will not respond to pH changes. Usually the meter needle can be adjusted with the electrode in the first buffer, but nothing happens when this buffer is exchanged for the next one at a different pH.

## Internal Reference Cell

However responsive the outer surface of the glass membrane of the glass electrode may be, this response could not be measured without a means of completing the electrical circuit. The inner reference electrode dipping into an electrolyte in contact with the inner surface of the glass membrane serves this purpose. The potentials involved, $E_4$ and $E_5$, are indicated in Figure 6-1.

Since this portion of the electrode is sealed, the reference electrode solution chosen for the internal standard solution must be stable over extended periods of time and over a wide range of temperatures. The buffer capacity of the solution must be fairly high because the alkali metals in the membrane will be leached out of the glass and the solution must be able to neutralize them.[3]

In addition to all these restrictions, though not required, it is convenient for the whole pH measuring system if the choice of internal reference electrode and standard solution can make the glass electrode-calomel electrode assembly zero potential. It is particularly convenient when this zero potential is chosen so as to occur at midscale, i.e., pH 7.0.

Jackson created a term, isopotential, to mean the potential at which a temperature change has no effect on the mV response of the electrical cell.[37] When the inner components of the glass electrode are chosen so that the isopotential point occurs midscale at pH 7.0, less than ideal temperature control causes minimal errors over a fairly wide pH range on each side of 7.0. Glass electrodes can be constructed so that both the zero potential point and the isopotential point co-incide—again, usually at pH 7.0 for convenience. Specifications for glass electrodes now often list both the zero and the isopotential points. These are the manufacturer's choices originally but become the user's responsibility to buy replacement electrodes which are consistent with the circuitry of the system. This will be discussed more fully under the section entitled "Meter."

The most commonly used internal reference electrode is the silver-silver chloride because its temperature coefficient can be made negative enough with the proper standard buffer to cancel the positive temperature coefficient of the calomel external reference cell.[3] A fairly high molarity of KCl is added to the chosen buffer solution in order to furnish enough Cl⁻ ions to keep the Ag–AgCl electrode stable.

219

### Alkaline Error

All glasses show some departure from the Nernst response at high pH values, and sometimes with high alkali-metal-ion concentration in only weakly alkaline solutions the measured pH is lower than the true pH[44]. These errors are not constant or easily reproducible, even for the same electrode in the same solution. The 015 glass electrode response shows the largest alkaline errors with the sodium ion, less with lithium, and still less with potassium, ammonium, and calcium as shown in Figure 6-10. These errrors are increased as the temperature rises above 25°C. For example, at 50° the Na+ error begins at pH 8; at 60° it begins between pH 5 and 6.[3]

The response in high pH solutions varies with time but inconsistently in terms of the shape of a response curve;[11, 44] it appears that slow exchange diffusion to steady state is being counteracted by a destructive effect of the alkali.[44] This is the reason for not exposing the glass electrode to high alkaline solutions for longer than absolutely necessary. The response of alkali metal errors can be reproducible, as evidenced by electrodes selective for these ions.

Separation of the so-called alkaline errors into those related to increased concentrations of OH⁻ ions and those related to the presence of Na+ and K+ brings several questions to mind. How many times have we followed a prescribed method to make up reagents and/or buffers to a specific pH above 10 (to the first decimal place[3]) and then adjusted the pH on a meter which was set with a high buffer at 9 or 10 pH? We probably made no effort to determine whether Na+ was also present and correct for it.

When comparing tables and nomograms for correction to be made in the pH value, one can't honestly tell whether, for example, the OH⁻ effect is not present

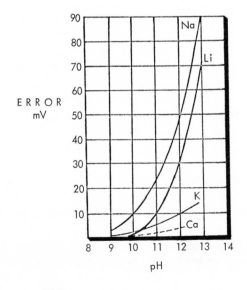

**Figure 6-10.** *Alkaline errors for Corning 015 glass. (Redrawn with permission from Isard, J. O.: The dependence of glass-electrode properties on composition. In Glass Electrode for Hydrogen and Other Cations, New York, Marcel Dekker, Inc., 1967, p. 79.)*

**Table 6-4. Alkaline Error Data for Some Commercial Glasses at 25° C\***

| Manufacturer | Glass designation | pH error | |
|---|---|---|---|
| | | 0.1N NaOH (pH = 12.9) | N NaOH (pH = 13.8) |
| Beckman Instruments, Inc. | E2 | 0.02 | 0.2–0.3 |
| (Fullerton, California) | | 0.04 | 0.18 |
| | General purpose | 0.25 | 0.70 |
| | | 0.44 | 1.43 |
| | Amber (high temperature) | 0.03 | 0.21 |
| | | 0.02 | 0.17 |
| Corning Glass Co., | Corning 015 | | |
| (Corning, N.Y.) | (≡MacInnes-Dole) | 0.98 | 2.52 |
| Electronic Instruments Ltd. | GHS | ~0.02 | 0.20 |
| (Richmond, Surrey, | (all purpose) | 0.04 | 0.19 |
| England) | BH 15 (high temperature, high pH) | — | ~0.05 |
| Metrohm A. G. | U | — | 0.10–0.20 |
| (Herisau, Switzerland) | (Universal) | 0.08 | 0.26 |
| | H | — | 0.05 |
| | (high temperature) | 0.08 | 0.15 |
| Radiometer | B | 0.03 (20°C.) | 0.18 (20°C.) |
| (Copenhagen NV, Denmark) | | | |

\* By permission from Mattock, G.: Laboratory pH measurements. In *The Glass Electrode.* New York, Interscience Publishers, p. 78.

and the correction is to be made for the $Na^+$ alone or whether the correction covers both. See Table 6-4 and Figure 6-11. Once this dilemma is faced, what can be done about it from a practical standpoint?

Measurement of high pH values (where $OH^-$ ions participate significantly) has been stated to be difficult even with low alkaline error glasses because the desorption and absorption processes change with time even with constant temperature.[44] Further, the glass electrode has a larger deviation than the hydrogen electrode at pH greater than 10, and pretreatment and storage affect the amount of alkaline error.[8] Finally, condition of the electrode surface causes variation in the alkaline error so that corrections given in tables or nomograms can only be considered approximate.[3, 8] When the error of the electrode exceeds 0.5 unit, an accurate pH value cannot be obtained through application of corrections.[3]

221

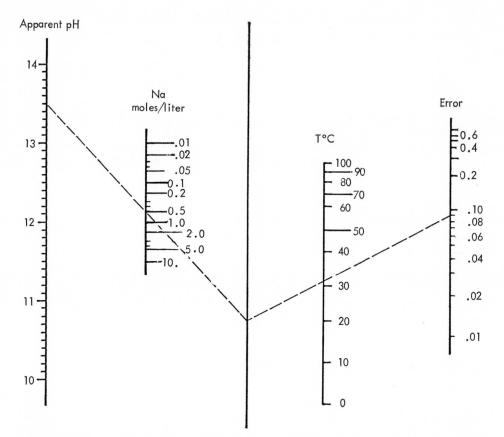

**Figure 6-11.** *Nomograph for calculation of approximate pH corrections for sodium ion error. (Reproduced with permission from Corning #476022 information sheet. Corning Glass Works, Corning, N. Y.)*

The ASTM* pH measurement method imposes three requirements on measurements above pH 10:[2]

1. The electrode used shall be of high alkalinity type and the manufacturer's instructions shall be observed.

2. The difference in potential between the glass electrode and the hydrogen electrode in the same buffer solutions in the cell being used (standardized to 25° ± 0.1) shall be no more than ± 5 mV at pH 12.8.

3. Borax buffer (pH 9.18) shall be used to standardize the system, and an alkaline phosphate buffer (pH 11.72) shall agree within ± 0.1 unit.

The inclusion in the ASTM method of the comparison of glass electrode performance to the hydrogen electrode is not limited to measurements in the high pH range; specifications are within ± 2 mV in the pH 1.10 to 9.18 range. Use of the

---

* American Society for Testing Materials, 1916 Race Street, Philadelphia, Pa.

hydrogen cell has been described for checking glass electrodes, reference electrodes, and buffers.[58] Beckman Instruments makes an inexpensive unit (hydrogen electrode cell assembly 75299).[16]

## Acid Errors

The problems encountered in acid error must also be considered in checking the response of the glass electrode. In the past acid errors had been considered of no real concern in the clinical laboratory, since routine work rarely involved pH values in that range.[44] However, acid errors can no longer be ignored if we choose to measure gastric juice acidity by electrometric pH as has been recently strongly advocated.[51, 52, 53] Moore originally stated that $H^+$ concentration (previously called "free acid") could not be equated to a titration value at any given pH but could be determined readily from a single pH measurement in unaltered gastric juice.[52] Somewhat later his data showed essentially identical values for $H^+$ concentration by pH meter and titration to pH 7.0.[55] Let's consider several additional items together with the previous two statements:

1. Moore stated that (a) $H^+$ concentration measurement of gastric juice requires that the pH meter be standardized with NBS 0.05 M potassium tetroxalate buffer (pH 1.679 at 25°C) and that (b) other buffers commercially obtained were not satisfactory although correct from pH 2 to 7.[51]

2. In the critique for the American Society of Clinical Pathologists' Continuing Education Check Sample #ST-43, Picoff and Trainer reported that their pH meter standardized at pH 4.0 fails to give a linear relationship for titrated versus electrometric gastric pH.[55] The ST-43 "gastric specimen" was stated to be pH 1.16 if read against the NBS 1.68 buffer.

3. Our evaluation of specimen ST-43 at the South Bend Medical Foundation was:
   (a) pH 1.18 when read versus our routine pH 4 and 7 buffers* (specifications of manufacturer ± 0.01);
   (b) pH 1.185 when read versus the National Bureau of Standards tetroxalate set at 1.679 at 25°C.

   The meter we used was Corning 12 with an Arthur H. Thomas combination electrode #4858-L15. The NBS textroxalate read 1.675 versus our routine pH 4 and 7 sloped calibration.

This is extremely confusing data to an individual institution trying to find ways of standardizing its own pH measurements. It is given here to point out that pH meters and electrodes vary in response. All one can do at this point is keep definitive notes and compare one's own calibration points from time to time with those of the National Bureau of Standards standard buffers.

Another point of concern in thinking of gastric pH in terms of electrometric measurements is the statement by Moore that rounding off a pH measurement of 0.98 to 1.0 creates a rounding-off error of 4.7 mEq/1 of $H^+$ which is greater than

---

\* Harleco: pH 4, m/20 Potassium hydrogen phthalate, #2106; pH 7, m/15 Potassium sodium phosphate #7531.

the difference in H[+] ion activity from pH 2.4 to 14.[52] While some meters are calibrated in terms of precision to within ± 0.003 pH unit or better, the uncertainty of the accuracy is still probably ± 0.02 pH unit—the quantity involved in the rounding-off error cited.[22, 48] For this reason we judge at the present time that we are not prepared for switching to the electrometric pH measurement of gastric acidity.

Mattock described the acid error, in general, as related to the acid's anion and its concentration.[44] In very low or negative pH solutions, some electrode glasses tend to give values that are higher than those indicated by the hydrogen electrode. Specific anion participation in surface exchange is variable as is the destructive effect produced. Some drifting occurs as a time-dependent function, causing lack of reproducibility which is much worse in concentrated acids. This behavior regularly occurs at the following molarities for the specific acid's anion: 1 M for hydrochloric; 5 M for hydrobromic; 7 M for sulfuric; and 10 M for phosphoric, acetic, and perchloric.[11] The pH error in acid solutions changes little with temperature changes.[3]

The electrodes made from improved multicomponent glasses show less acid error than the older 015 glass. Therefore, the user must check the reaction of his own electrode system for the magnitude of this error.

### Noise

In our experience noise has been traced invariably to the electrodes, but it could conceivably arise from poor grounding or other electronic malfunctioning. The causes of drift we have been able to pinpoint include the following:

1. Moisture at connections between electrode contacts in a head or cable.
2. Glass electrode with some problem within itself—never determined exactly.
3. Cables beginning to show small breaks in the wire or contacts.

Bates has pointed out that leads from high resistance electrodes must be carefully guarded from electrical leaks, as must the stem itself.[3] The stems of electrodes can be made water-repellent by treatment with silicone preparations such as GE Drifilm or Beckman Desicote and thus be protected from moisture adsorption. Bates further points out that high humidities may cause erratic behavior not observed with systems of low resistance.

### Drift

Drift seems to be related to many different causes and sometimes may not be eliminated entirely. The trick seems to be to avoid as many of the causes as possible and know when to expect the unavoidable occasions. Some electrodes will always show drift at high and low pH ranges, but even in these cases the drift can be decreased considerably by etching away the outer coat of the hydrated layer.[3, 8, 33, 44]

Drift, in general, is caused by an imperfect steady state in the hydrated layer of the glass—*i.e.,* the diffusion potential is not constant.[56] The seriousness of this instability appears to be related to the condition of the hydrated layer. It is reasonable then to expect drift from any one of the following conditions:

1. A new electrode that has not been allowed to hydrate long enough before use.
2. An electrode that has been used for some time without etching off the skeleton lattice.
3. An electrode that has been allowed to dry out and then has been put back into use without etching off the outer layer.
4. Immediately after changing from a strong ionic solution to a weak one and vice versa, or after use in high or low pH solution.
5. Use of the electrical cell soon after an obvious ambient temperature change.
6. Use of the electrical cell soon after cleaning and refilling the reference electrode.

Drift is said to be least when the electrode is left standing in a solution whose pH value is close to the value the electrode is expected to read—a compromise for general purpose would be a buffer about pH 7.[1] The direction of the drift has been noted to depend upon the pH of the solution in which the electrode was stored:[59]

1. Borate buffer (pH 9.09)—drifts toward the alkaline side.
2. Acid (0.1 N HCl)—drifts toward the acid side.
3. Phosphate (M/15)—slight drift toward alkaline side.

## METERS

Any stable high impedance potential measuring device is considered satisfactory for use with hydrogen and other cation selective electrodes.[23] Wright points out that, while meters have now reached the level of discrimination of $\pm 0.002$ pH units, their performance is still subject to six limitations.[64] He labels three of these obvious: zero stability, sensitivity, and the accuracy of the dial calibration. The input impedance must be at least a thousand times that of the highest resistance electrode used. He adds that since the pH scale proportionality is altered by the temperature control and the zero of the scale is altered by the asymmetry control,* it is vital that these controls match or exceed the main dial in fineness and accuracy of calibration.

Manufacturers have scaled the specifications for the limitations named above to provide meters which give the user an almost unlimited choice for his appropriate use. However, the general design of all these meters is based upon the same criteria:[18]

1. Measurements should not be affected by the magnitude of, or changes in the magnitude of, resistance of the pH cell (primarily this resistance is that of the glass electrode).
2. For most purposes, it is desirable that the pH meter be operative on AC current, and normal fluctuations in line voltage should not affect the meter's operation.

---

* See the list of synonyms for meter adjustment controls on page 246.

3. The meter should have provision for temperature compensation, preferably automatic. Wright *pleads* for the calibration of this control to be made directly in potential/pH ratio instead of in degrees centigrade.[64]

4. Changing vacuum tubes should not require adjustment of circuit constants. More recent counterparts could be handled by changing circuit boards.

5. Provision should be made for adding a recorder to the system without affecting the precision of measurement.

In the past, much emphasis was given to the distinction between types of meters: null-balance versus direct reading. The expected precision, accuracy and cost were directly related to the meter type differences. This is no longer true. The specifications of the electronic components themselves now are responsible for the major differences in the expected performance of the meters. The difference in measurement arrangement between null-balance and direct reading pH meters can be visualized by referring to the simple circuit in Figure 6-12. In the null-balance system the variable resistor (potentiometer), R, is adjusted until the meter balances at zero and R is calibrated in pH units or millivolts. In the direct reading systems, R is merely used to bring the ammeter reading on scale by compensating for the potentials in the reference electrode arm of the circuit. The pH or mV response is then read from the meter scale. The amplifier shown here is a triode, but this is just one of the possible choices to be discussed later. The concept that high precision required the choice of null-balance over direct reading systems has been practically phased out by the improvements in electronic components. In fact, current brochures of available circuitry continually mention components whose function description is hard for the average user to assess or for which he has difficulty in finding explanations. The conscientious user does persist until he finds these explanations, however, because he knows he must understand his meter in order to know what performance to expect.

The method used for amplification controls the pH meter's optimal capabilities for stability, linearity, and sensitivity. The user must decide first what sensitivity is required for his purposes. He may then choose the most economical instrument to provide the stability and linearity allowable within the sensitivity specifications. For example, if pH values can be accepted which have a relative accuracy of $\pm 0.1$ unit (about 6 mV), a single stage electrometer tube amplification could be chosen

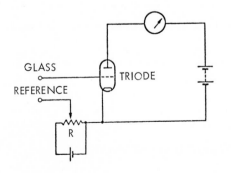

**Figure 6-12.** *Simple circuit measuring pH. (Redrawn with permission from Mattock, G.: Laboratory pH measurements. In* The Glass Electrode. *New York, Interscience Publishers, after 1965.)*

as either direct readout or null-balance. At the accuracy range of $\pm$ 0.002 pH unit (about 0.15 mV) a feedback system combined with a sophisticated modulator of some type is necessary. The new DC field effect transistor (FET) amplifiers are anticipated to provide this sensitivity also.

Adequate amplification of the low signal from the electrodes requires the pH meter circuit be designed to overcome three basic problems:

1. Provide extremely high impedance input.
2. Eliminate zero drifts from power supply or from changes in the tube grid or other circuit components.
4. Maintain proportionality accuracy while amplifying the low signal.

For many years the low-grid-current electrometer tube was used to provide the high impedance input. When directly coupled for DC amplification, this circuit has the following shortcomings:[62]

1. There is no definite zero point, and the circuit is arranged so that the meter reads zero at some finite anode current. This current varies from tube to tube and increases as the tube ages.
2. The relationship between the grid potential and consequent changes in anode current is not constant even within relatively short periods.
3. Changes in the power supply or other components are also amplified in any direct coupled amplifier.

Use of an AC amplifier produces no output voltage signal for slow drifts from changes in the power supply or circuit components, so the zero stability is excellent.[43] Use of negative feedback permits great improvement in proportionality accuracy but does not help zero stability.[62] In order to obtain the best overall performance, the trend until recently was to use a combination of electrometer tube, AC amplifier and negative feedback. In this circuit the electrometer tube and the converter from DC to AC are often separated into a portion called the preamplifier. For a concise explanation of the basic operation of the high impedance input devices and feedback stabilization, see Part I of Lewin's article on pH meters.[40]

The impedance of transistors was previously too low for these devices to serve as the first stage of amplification; the electrometer tube was therefore the only choice for this stage. Field effect transistors (FET) recently produced have a higher impedance than the majority of vacuum tubes.[26] Limited discussions of FET circuits can be found in Ewing,[26] Malmstadt, Enke, and Toren,[43] and Stott.[61]

There are now three basic types of components available for the input to the pH meter: (1) electrometer tubes, (2) vibrating capacitors (and other similar devices), and (3) field effect transistors (FET). Beyond this point the amplifier can be handled in many ways. Any of the three can be used with an AC amplifier, but the FET has also been used singly or multiply in cascade as a DC amplifier. In general, solid state electronic amplifiers have been considered preferable because of immediate warmup, relative freedom from drift, and compact size. However, a solid state amplifier is sometimes listed for an instrument even though the preamplifier contains a tube; the user may well believe that his instrument is entirely solid state. The specification sheet and often even the schematic do not give the user any definite way to tell what high input impedance device has been used. It is advisable, therefore, to ask the company specifically for this information.

From the first direct coupled single stage amplifier using the electrometer tube to the present entirely solid state systems, the numerous variations of circuitry are all aimed toward correction of the two basic problems of the electrometer tube; zero drift and lack of proportionality (or range shift). The usual operator of the pH meter cannot be expected to understand the entire circuitry of his meter; but he must know a few basic facts about the instrument:

1. Is the instrument circuit one in which zero drift or nonlinear response is expected? If so, the zero must be frequently checked, and the measurements of unknowns must be bracketed by buffers close to the unknown values.

2. Is the instrument direct reading or null-balance? This is more important in simple direct-coupled amplifiers than in the more sophisticated modifications. For the simple null-balance instrument frequent zero setting is the most necessary monitoring procedure.

3. Does the instrument use a feedback circuit? Negative feedback is the best means of reducing proportionality errors.

4. What arrangement is provided for temperature compensation in the specific meter being used? Temperature compensation is often made through a rheostat in the feedback circuit.

5. Is the amplifier AC or DC? An AC amplifier usually is able to eliminate a drift in the zero point.

6. What is the reasonable expectation for relative accuracy and reproducibility of the meter? What is the relative accuracy and reproducibility to be expected for the whole system as limited by the user's own electrodes?

## Types of Amplifiers

Some of the commonly used types of amplifiers are given below in order to point out various sources of error. More complete discussions of these and other types may be found in Bates,[3] Clark and Perley,[18] and Taylor.[62]

THE DIRECT-COUPLED, DC AMPLIFIER USING ELECTROMETER TUBE. This circuit (Figure 6-12, for example) when used for a null-balance readout is capable of relative accuracies in pH measurements to the second decimal place but requires extra precautions in technique.[62] The performance is limited by the quality of the tube and changes in the power supply. Since the input is directly connected to the grid of the tube, any variation in the power supply will also be amplified. Frequent resetting of zero and rechecking of buffers are necessary. By using several tubes to increase the gain sufficiently, feedback could be combined with this amplifier so that proportionality can be improved.[61] Negative feedback alone, however, does not compensate for grid current variations, for shifts in zero, or for supply voltage variations.[44] Examples include Beckman G, Radiometer 4, Coleman Compax 20, and Coleman 18A.[3]

228

Direct-reading instruments using feedback also provide improved linearity but likewise do not necessarily have a stable zero. The Beckman Zeromatic originally used additional circuits to read and correct zero every second. (The current Beckman Zeromatic SS-3 has been changed to FET for amplification.) Two identical amplifiers coupled in opposition can cancel out most of the internal noise or drift, but Mattock has pointed out that matched tubes age differently and cannot be relied upon to retain similar characteristics.[44]

THE AC AMPLIFIER WITH FEEDBACK. The improvements gained with use of the AC amplifier are a high degree of zero stability (drift is usually limited to *micro*volts[62]) and increased gain which extends the possible sensitivity to about 0.1 mV.[63]

The AC amplifier when used for pH measurements requires three distinct operations (*i.e.,* groups of components): input chopper (also called modulator or converter from DC to AC), AC amplifier, and the detector (also called demodulator or converter from AC to DC). These three portions of the amplifier circuit are shown by block diagram in Figure 6-13.

The converter may be either of two types based on its function. The first type receives the signal from an electrometer tube and changes it from DC to AC via a mechanical chopper. The second type, which was devised later, can serve both to receive the signal from the electrodes and also to change DC to AC. The following devices have been used for the latter type converter: vibrating capacitor (condenser), photoconductive cell, and vibrating reed. Examples of these are shown

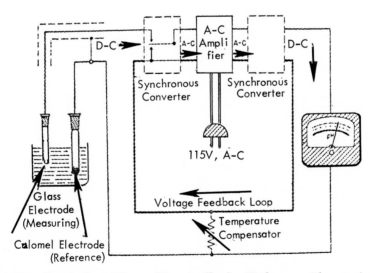

**Figure 6-13.** *Circuit for AC amplifier feedback. (Redrawn with permission from Clark, W. R., and Perley, G. A.: Modern developments in pH instrumentation. In* Symposium on pH Measurement. *ASTM Special Technical Publication #190. Philadelphia, 1956, p. 43.)*

as A, B and C in Figure 6-14. Recognition of them could possibly be made from the schematic of meters the user already has.

Electronic components are improved continually, and circuits vary so much in the details chosen to increase particular advantages or decrease disadvantages

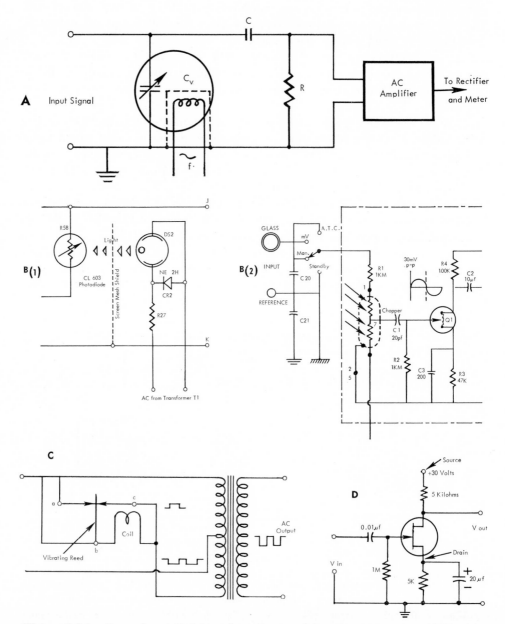

**Figure 6-14.** *Examples of high impedance input solid state components. A. Vibrating capacitor. B. (1) Photoconductor; (2) photochopper. C. Vibrating reed. D. FET.*

230

that no exact comparisons can be drawn up for component characteristics. There-fore, the following generalizations are only meant as guides.

The photochopper (photodiode) uses a neon light source operated at power-line frequency from a half-wave rectified AC line. The noise level is relatively high, sensitivity is low, and the system is temperature sensitive. When the neon gets old and begins to flicker, the signal becomes lost in the noise. The mechanical chopper is said to surpass others in its high inherent null stability,[43] but some noise is inherent from contact potentials.[44] As the contacts age and their surface conditions change, the noise increases.

The vibrating capacitor overcomes  the contact potential problems,[44] and expanded scales may set 1 or even 0.5 pH unit full scale and allow readings to be made to 0.001 pH unit.[63] A variation of the vibrating condenser, the vibrating reed, is considered by some as the only satisfactory form of amplifier for high precision pH meters.[61] The zero stability of a meter using this capacitor is greater by a factor of about 10 than zero stability in an instrument using tubes.[65] The main sources of drift are related to temperature changes and their effects on contact potentials. For highest accuracy, the instrument is best designed as null-balance, either for manual or self-balancing bridge circuit. Capabilities of accuracy of 0.01 mV and freedom from zero drift have been claimed.[3]

FET AMPLIFIERS.    The high impedance of the unipolar field effect transistor makes this device capable of being used as the input circuit for direct coupled DC amplifiers.[26, 43] (See Figure 6-14, D.) Solid state characteristics such as low noise levels and small drift are expected for pH meters using a FET cascade to obtain the necessary high gain. However, while there are several manufacturers offering these models, they are new enough that rigorous evaluations have not appeared yet.

Completely transistorized amplifiers using the FET as high impedance choppers ($10^{15}$ ohms) have been designed, and their performance is said to be considerably better than can be achieved with tubes.[61] The Beckman Century SS™ is described as having a FET direct coupled DC amplifier paralleled by a chopper stabilized AC amplifier.[15] In this combination the DC amplifier is said to provide fast response while the AC amplifier stabilizes the DC amplifier against zero drift. The reader must keep in mind that manufacturers are continually modifying meter models and should check the specifications with the company at any specific time.

## Meter Scale

Most meters capable of sensitivity to the third decimal place have an expanded scale in addition to the normal 0 to 14 pH. The expanded scale is usually full scale coverage by 1, 1.4, or 2 pH units. Recently a logarithmic scale has been added to accommodate readings for ion concentrations measured with other electrodes. The mV scale usually is indicated as $\times$ 100 and is read from the normal 0 to 14 scale; in this case the polarity of the potential is set by a switch marked $-$ mV and $+$ mV. Some meters also have an expanded mV scale for which 100 mV represents full scale deflection. Other meters, such as the Beckman Zeromatic,

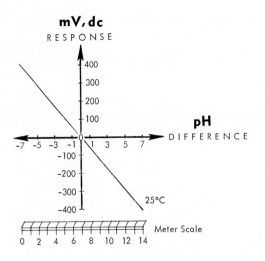

**Figure 6-15.** *Isopotential point and assignment of positions of meter scale. (Redrawn with permission from Brems, N.: Measurements of pH. Electrodes and pertinent apparatus. Acta Anaesth. Scand., Suppl., 11:199, 1962.)*

have a scale with 0 positioned above 7 on the normal pH scale and 7 increments on each side of zero indicating $\pm$ 700 mV.

For the meter design, the zero mV point may be set at any place to make the entire system (including reference and glass electrode) most practical. Note in Figure 6-15 that the line representing the mV response of the glass electrode goes through a zero mV position. This line has the theoretical Nernst response, *i.e.,* slope of 59.16 mV per pH unit change. As discussed previously, the choice of inner reference electrode and internal standard solution in the glass electrode determines the zero mV of the electrical cell; this choice now usually is made to give zero mV (zero potential point) at pH 7. The meter scale can be positioned so that the pH 7.0 point also is the zero mV of the meter circuit. The pH 7.0 point for this system then represents the zero mV point for the entire pH measuring system. When the glass electrode has its zero potential and isopotential at the same point, then one can refer to the above zero mV point as the isopotential point of the whole measuring system.

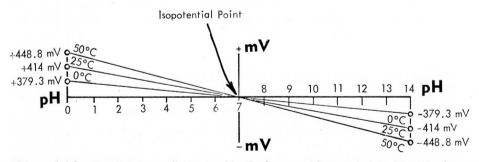

**Figure 6-16.** *Temperature effect on pH. (Redrawn with permission from Beckman Instructions for Zeromatic pH Meter: Bulletin 1382-B. Beckman Instruments, Inc., Fullerton, Calif., August, 1945, p. 4.)*

The mV change in the slope value (*i.e.*, $\frac{2.3026\ RT}{F}$) as listed in Table 6-2 can also be shown graphically as the slope rotates through the isopotential point. See Figure 6-16. In this form it is easy to see that a given temperature change makes a progressively greater difference in pH error as the measured pH is removed in either direction from the isopotential point.

Table 6-5 lists the measurement error that will result if temperature changes are not compensated.[12] For example, a 5°C difference between sample and standardizing buffer would cause no error at pH 7, a 0.02 pH unit error at a pH of 6 or 8, but would cause more than 0.1 pH unit error at a pH of 0 or 14.

## Temperature Compensation

The object of temperature compensation in a pH meter is to nullify changes in the electromotive force (emf) from any source other than a change in the true pH of the unknown solution being measured. A change in temperature has two effects:[3]

1. The slope is changed.
2. The scale position is altered—*i.e.*, zero shifts because $E_o$ and $E_J$ of the electrical cell are changed.

Adjustment of the slope to that which is correct for the temperature at which the measurement is being made can be done on some instruments with a slope-adjust potentiometer. Such an adjustment corrects not only for the temperature effect but also for any deviation the glass electrode has from the theoretical 100% Nernst response. The second means of correcting the slope is the temperature control,[6, 20] which is actually a fine adjustment of the slope control.[29] For instruments whose slope control is not accessible to the user, the temperature control is the only means of correcting the slope. If the room temperature is noted carefully and if both standard buffers and unknowns are equilibrated to room temperature, the labeled temperature on the temperature control can be ignored and the control

Table 6-5. **Measurement Error for Uncompensated Temperature Changes***

| Temperature Change (Degrees C) | pH of Solution | | | | | | | |
|---|---|---|---|---|---|---|---|---|
| | 7 | 6 or 8 | 5 or 9 | 4 or 10 | 3 or 11 | 2 or 12 | 1 or 13 | 0 or 14 |
| 1 | 0 | 0.0037 | 0.0074 | 0.0111 | 0.0148 | 0.0185 | 0.0222 | 0.0259 |
| 2 | 0 | 0.0074 | 0.0148 | 0.0222 | 0.0296 | 0.0370 | 0.0544 | 0.0618 |
| 5 | 0 | 0.0183 | 0.0366 | 0.0549 | 0.0732 | 0.0915 | 0.1098 | 0.1281 |
| 10 | 0 | 0.0366 | 0.0732 | 0.1098 | 0.1464 | 0.1830 | 0.2196 | 0.2562 |

\* By permission from Beckman Instruments, Inc.: *Instructions for Research pH Meter.* Bulletin 1226-B, April, 1964.

can be used as slope control. This will be further discussed under Measurement of pH.

The manual temperature compensator in the circuit for a direct reading meter is a variable resistor in the feedback circuit, as shown in A of Figure 6-17. The resistor must have a linear response with temperature change,[62] and the increase in amplification is set for 0.34% per 1°C.[17] Setting the temperature-adjust

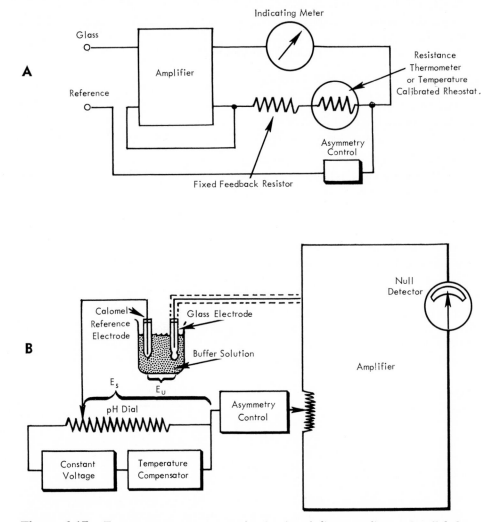

**Figure 6-17.** *Temperature compensator in circuits of direct reading and null balance meters. A. Direct reading meter circuit. (Redrawn with permission from Taylor, G. R.: pH measuring instruments. In pH Measurement and Titration. G. Mattock, Ed. London, Heywood & Company, Ltd., 1961.) B. Null balance meter circuit. (Redrawn with permission from Malmstadt, H. V., Enke, C. G., and Toren, E. C., Jr.: Electronics for Scientists. New York, W. A. Benjamin, Inc., 1963.)*

234

to the ambient temperature therefore corresponds to assigning the proper theoretical slope (*i.e.,* mV response per pH unit for that temperature). Automatic temperature compensation is made by having a resistance thermometer immersed in the solution or buffer being measured.[62] As the temperature of the solution changes, the resistance of the circuit is altered accordingly.

The temperature-adjust in the circuit of a null-balance meter (B of Figure 6-17) is also a variable resistor but is placed in the balancing circuit of the potentiometer carrying the pH dial.[43] The temperature effect on the meter zero via the $E_0$ of the electrical cell can be compensated by circuitry and is discussed by Taylor.[62] However, almost all pH meters used in the clinical laboratory bypass this adjustment by requiring that the standard buffer and unknown solutions be at the same (ambient) temperature. In this situation $E_0$ cancels out when the instrument is adjusted to the isopotential point with the zero offset (also known as asymmetry, standardization, balance, buffer-adjust, zero-adjust, and calibration control). This control, shown as Asymmetry Control in Figure 6-17, is in series with the reference electrode and is therefore a direct mV correction to the zero point. Thus, in the standardization of the direct reading meter, this zero point should be properly set first before the slope correction is made. Simple null-balance meters, such as the one shown in Figure 6-17B, are set for the proper temperature before balancing the zero point.

When the meter is used in mV readout position, the temperature and slope controls are cut out of the circuit. The zero point control is usually also cut out of the circuit, but a few meters have an additional zero mV control. The meter is then a voltmeter whose sensitivity is governed by the gain of the amplifier. The sensitivity and readability of the scale become serious concerns when considering the use of the meter for ion specific electrodes. For example, the entire normal range of 130 to 150 mEq serum sodium is covered by a 3.5 mV change.[57]

The expanded meter scale, used for more precise measurements, must obviously coincide with the normal scale. We have seen these scales lose this correlation and therefore this function must be checked.

## Grounding

In addition to the usual precautions for avoiding ground loops[60] (pages 4 to 5), pH measurements require attention to other details. Careful attention to shielding and to prevention of electrical leakage is necessary to avoid spurious effects.[11] A high impedance circuit is prone to the pickup of stray electrical signals.[60] The meter should be used in a location that is free from sources of AC radiation, such as motors or unshielded electronic instruments. The pickup problem tends to be greater with line-operated instruments than with those using batteries.[40]

The insulation of the measuring electrode circuit must be kept clean and dry throughout. The screening of the glass electrode itself obviates AC pickup and local charge effects from body movement.[44] The cable from the glass electrode (Fig. 6-4) is likewise screened for the same reasons; fingerprints on the connector or input lead surface can cause small current leakage paths. A pH meter operates at ordinary temperatures most satisfactorily at relative humidities between 20% and 60%; at 90% or higher many meters are completely useless.[3]

Antistatic spray on the meter face reduces the static charges present at low humidities. At high humidities, adsorption of moisture seriously increases electrical leakage. Meters using tubes are particularly susceptible in the leakage path from control grid to ground. Moisture can also condense in the region where the screened cable enters the cap.

Particular attention must be given to the choice of whether to ground the sample solution. An accurate measurement cannot be obtained if a direct current connection between the instrument and the sample solution occurs by any means other than through the electrodes. This situation would exist, for example, if the instrument were grounded through its power cord and the sample were in a metallic container not isolated from ground or a wet sample container sitting on a metallic stirrer. The manual for the specific pH meter should be consulted for instructions related to solution grounding. In general, the meter may be grounded only once, and if the solution is grounded, then the power plug usually is not. As shown in Figure 6-18, this principle also applies to a recorder if used with the meter. Note that the recorder lead connected to the meter is also shielded.

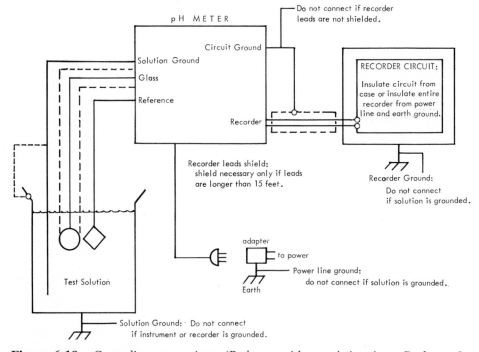

**Figure 6-18.** *Grounding connections. (Redrawn with permission from Beckman Instructions for Zeromatic pH Meter: Bulletin 1382-B. Beckman Instruments, Inc., Fullerton, Calif., August, 1965, p. 7.)*

236

Some electrodes (*e.g.,* Beckman Futura[13]) use detachable cables. The connection points of cable and electrode must be kept dry and clean in order to maintain the high impedance between the center and the outer connector pins. Any contaminant in the area should be wiped away with a tissue saturated with alcohol.

## STANDARD BUFFERS

The National Bureau of Standards has standard buffers available under the listing of Standard Reference Materials. Each lot of each buffer is provided a certificate of analysis, and lots vary by only a few thousandths of a pH unit. In 1962 Bates reassigned values for the NBS standard buffers to a third decimal place.[7] The current values for these buffers are listed in Table 6-6.

The uncertainty of the assigned $pH_s$ is given as $\pm$ 0.005 unit from 0° to 60°C and $\pm$ 0.01 unit from 60° to 95°C. For standardization of glass electrode assemblies with liquid junction, the five standards of pH 3.5 to 9.5 are considered *primary* standards. When the same pH assembly, standardized in the intermediate pH range, is used to read the tetroxalate standard, the measured pH is about 0.03 lower than the assigned value. Similarly, the calcium hydroxide standard will read about 0.03 lower than its assigned value. For this reason the assigned values of the tetroxalate and the calcium hydroxide are designated *secondary* standards. Bates further points out that, while the assigned values of these secondary standards are just as accurate as the other standards, comparable certainty cannot be placed in the standardization at pH 1.7 or 12.5 because differences in liquid junction potentials cannot regularly be calibrated out. In fact, differences are expected for all assigned buffer values when the buffers are read in a system containing a liquid junction.[45] The magnitude of these differences is evident in Table 6-7. The value listed as $pH_s$ was measured with a cell without liquid junction according to NBS standards at 25°C. The effect of the liquid junction can be assigned to the $\triangle$ pH, or the pH observed minus the $pH_s$. Beck has reported 0.003 to 0.005 error in the pH for the equimolal disodium hydrogen phosphate-potassium dihydrogen phosphate buffer measured by glass electrodes as compared to the value by hydrogen electrodes.[10] He contends that the 0.025 molal concentration is too dilute for this buffer to function as a primary standard for glass electrodes.

While these standards were chosen for their reproducibility, stability, buffer capacity, and ease of preparation,[3] no one buffer is ideal in all its properties. The NBS standard buffers are compromises of the concentration for buffer capacity versus reliability of single ion activity.[10] Mattock's description of buffer characteristics will help in the evaluation and appreciation of these NBS buffer properties.

Mattock identifies five characteristics of buffer solutions:[45]

1. *Buffer capacity* of a solution is unity when one liter of it increases one pH unit on the addition of one gram equivalent of hydroxyl ions, or decreases by one pH unit on the addition of one gram equivalent of hydrogen ions.
2. *Dilution value* is the change in pH caused by the dilution of the buffer solution with an equal volume of water.

237

**Table 6-6. Assigned Values for NBS Standard Buffers***

| Temp °C | 0.05 m Potassium tetroxalate[†] | Satd. (25°C) Potassium hydrogen tartrate | 0.05 m Potassium hydrogen phthalate[‡] | 0.025 m Potassium dihydrogen phosphate 0.025 m Disodium hydrogen phosphate§ | 0.008695 m Potassium dihydrogen phosphate 0.03043 m Disodium hydrogen phosphate§ | 0.01 m Borax | Satd. (25°C) Calcium hydroxide[†] |
|---|---|---|---|---|---|---|---|
| 0 | 1.666 | — | 4.012 | 6.981 | 7.531 | 9.464 | 13.423 |
| 5 | 1.668 | — | 4.005 | 6.948 | 7.497 | 9.395 | 13.207 |
| 10 | 1.670 | — | 4.002 | 6.920 | 7.469 | 9.332 | 13.003 |
| 15 | 1.672 | — | 4.001 | 6.897 | 7.445 | 9.276 | 12.810 |
| 20 | 1.675 | — | 4.003 | 6.878 | 7.426 | 9.225 | 12.627 |
| 25 | 1.679 | 3.557 | 4.008 | 6.862 | 7.410 | 9.180 | 12.454 |
| 30 | 1.683 | 3.552 | 4.014 | 6.850 | 7.397 | 9.139 | 12.289 |
| 35 | 1.688 | 3.549 | 4.023 | 6.841 | 7.386 | 9.102 | 12.133 |
| 38 | 1.691 | 3.548 | | 6.837 | 7.381 | 9.081 | 12.043 |
| 40 | 1.694 | 3.547 | 4.033 | 6.835 | 7.377 | 9.068 | 11.984 |
| 45 | 1.700 | 3.547 | 4.045 | 6.831 | 7.370 | 9.038 | 11.841 |
| 50 | 1.707 | 3.549 | 4.058 | 6.830 | 7.364 | 9.011 | 11.705 |
| 55 | 1.715 | 3.554 | 4.073 | 6.832 | | 8.985 | 11.574 |
| 60 | 1.723 | 3.560 | 4.089 | 6.836 | | 8.962 | 11.449 |
| 70 | 1.743 | 3.580 | 4.12 | 6.845 | | 8.921 | — |
| 80 | 1.766 | 3.609 | 4.16 | 6.859 | | 8.885 | — |
| 90 | 1.792 | 3.650 | 4.20 | 6.877 | | 8.850 | — |
| 95 | 1.806 | 3.674 | 4.22 | 6.886 | | 8.833 | — |

* From Bates, R. G.: Revised standard values for pH measurements from 0 to 95°C. J. Res. NBS *66A*:179-184, 1962.

[†]*Secondary* Standards. The other five are *primary* Standards.

[‡] Values for Reference Material 185d, July 21, 1966.

§ Values from Reference Material 186-I-c and 186-II-b, July 29, 1966.

238

Table 6-7.  The Effect of Liquid Junction on pH Values of Various Buffers*

| Solution | $\Delta pH$<br>(pH observed—pHs) | pHs |
|---|---|---|
| 0.1M hydrochloric acid | +0.012 | 1.09 |
| 0.01M hydrochloric acid<br>0.09M potassium chloride | −0.021 | 2.10 |
| 0.1M potassium tetroxalate | −0.016 | 1.51 |
| 0.05M potassium tetroxalate | −0.023 | 1.68 |
| 0.025M potassium tetroxalate | −0.009 | 1.87 |
| 0.01M potassium tetroxalate | +0.006 | 2.15 |
| 0.05M citric acid | −0.019 | 2.24 |
| 0.01M citric acid | −0.018 | 2.62 |
| 0.1M potassium dihydrogen citrate | +0.012 | 3.72 |
| 0.02M potassium dihydrogen citrate | +0.005 | 3.84 |
| 0.05M potassium hydrogen phthalate | +0.001 | 4.01 |
| 0.05M acetic acid<br>0.05M sodium acetate | −0.006 | 4.68 |
| 0.01M acetic acid<br>0.01M sodium acetate | −0.003 | 4.72 |
| 0.025M sodium bicarbonate<br>0.025M sodium carbonate | −0.006 | 10.02 |
| 0.01M sodium carbonate | −0.026 | 11.01 |
| 0.025M sodium carbonate | −0.012 | 11.16 |
| 0.01M trisodium phosphate | −0.018 | 11.72 |
| 0.05M trisodium phosphate | +0.009 | 12.04 |
| 0.01M sodium hydroxide | −0.040 | 11.94 |
| 0.05M sodium hydroxide | −0.046 | 12.62 |

* By permission from Mattock, G.: *pH Measurement and Titration.* London, Heywood & Co., Ltd., 1961, p. 172.

3. *Salt effect* is the change in pH caused by the different ionic strength produced with the addition of a salt to a buffer solution. The activity coefficients of the ions originally present change, and in dilute buffer solutions the variations may be quite significant.

4. *Temperature effects* are primarily caused by the changes in values for the equilibrium constants and activity coefficients. Generally the basic solutions have larger pH temperature coefficients than the acid solutions because of the large temperature coefficient of $pK_w$.

5. *Pressure effects* cause only slight changes in activity coefficients or dissociation constants. For practical purposes, these effects may usually be ignored.

Some of the properties of the NBS standard buffers are given in Table 6-8. The variation in the NBS buffers with temperature is shown quantitatively in Table

Table 6-8.   Properties of Seven Standard Buffer Solutions at 25°*

| Solution | $m$ | Density g./ml. | Molarity | Dilution Value $\Delta pH_{1/2}$ | Buffer value $\beta$ equiv./$pa_H$ | Temperature Coefficient $\delta pa_H/\delta t$ units/°C. |
|---|---|---|---|---|---|---|
| Textroxalate | 0.05 | 1.0032 | 0.04962 | +0.186 | 0.070 | +0.001 |
| Tartrate | 0.0341 | 1.0036 | 0.034 | +0.049 | 0.027 | −0.0014 |
| Phthalate | 0.05 | 1.0017 | 0.04958 | +0.052 | 0.016 | +0.0012 |
| Phosphate 1:1 | 0.025[a] | 1.0028 | 0.02490[a] | +0.080 | 0.029 | −0.0028 |
| Phosphate 1:3.5 | 0.008695[b] 0.03043[c] | 1.0020 | 0.008665[b] 0.03032[c] | +0.07 | 0.016 | −0.0028 |
| Borax | 0.01 | 0.9996 | 0.009971 | +0.01 | 0.020 | −0.0082 |
| Calcium hydroxide | 0.0203 | 0.9991 | 0.02025 | −0.28 | 0.09 | −0.033 |

[a] Concentration of each phosphate salt.

[b] $KH_2PO_4$.

[c] $Na_2HPO_4$.

* By permission from Bates, R. G.: *Determination of pH: Theory and Practice.* New York, John Wiley & Sons, Inc., 1964, p. 128.

6-6 and in Table 6-8 as the temperature coefficient, but the differences are more striking when viewed in graph form as shown in Figure 6-19.

The fact is self-evident, therefore, that standardization of the pH cell can be no better than the care with which the proper buffer $pH_s$ value is chosen for the prevailing temperature. In Table 6-8 note the dilution values. These figures are enough to discourage the less careful worker from dropping a prepackaged tablet into an unmeasured quantity of water and calling the product a working standard. "Buffer tablets" contain such substances as polyethylene glycol, dextrose, or glucose to aid the tabletting process.[45] While these substances may not significantly affect the pH for general work, precise work necessitates the preparation of buffer solutions by exact prescriptions.

The additional notes for the National Bureau of Standards buffers given below are taken primarily from Bates.[3] The concentrations of these standards are given as molality (m), but the difference between this and molarity (M) is negligible as shown in Table 6-8.

In the preparation of the buffer solution it is essential to use materials of high purity (NBS certified Standard Reference Material preferably) and to use freshly prepared water with specific resistance of 500,000 ohms or more (specific conductivity less than 2 micro-mhos). The buffer solutions should be stored in bottles

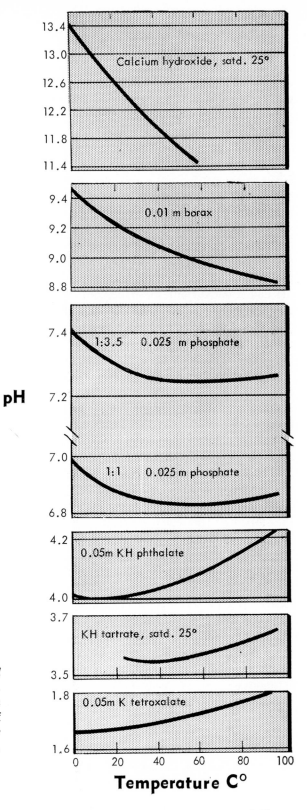

**Figure 6-19.** *NBS standard buffers at various temperatures. (Redrawn with permission from Bates, R. G.:* Determination of pH: Theory and Practice. *New York, John Wiley & Sons, Inc., 1964.)*

of resistant glass or polyethylene; the bottles need not be sterilized. Except for the tartrate solution, it is recommended that the buffers be replaced about four weeks after preparation. Refrigeration tends to retard the mold growth that appears in some of these buffers.

0.05 m POTASSIUM TETROXALATE. Weigh out 12.61 g $KH_3(C_2O_4) \cdot 2 H_2O$ and dissolve in water to one liter of solution at 25°C. The solution has excellent buffer properties but has a relatively high dilution value. The $pa_H$ of this solution is 1.679 at 25°C, but the pH on the operational scale fixed by the primary standards is usually about 1.65.

SATURATED (25°C) POTASSIUM HYDROGEN TARTRATE. An excess of the salt is shaken with water, and it can be stored in this way. Before use it should be filtered or decanted at a temperature between 22° and 28°C. This solution is particularly subject to mold growth accompanied by an increase of 0.01 to 0.10 pH unit. Consequently the buffer must be replaced every few days unless a preservative is added. A thymol crystal, about 8 mm in diameter, is sufficient for 200 ml and preserves it about 2 months. The preservative alters the pH about 0.01 unit. Because of the limited stability of the tartrate buffer, it is recommended that the phthalate solution be used instead of the tartrate solution whenever possible.

0.05 m POTASSIUM HYDROGEN PHTHALATE. Although drying is not usually essential, the crystals may be dried at 110°C for an hour and cooled in a desiccator. 10.12 g $C_6H_4 (CO_2H) (CO_2K)$ are dissolved in water and the solution is made up to one liter at 25°C. Because of the rather low buffer value, this solution should be guarded carefully against accidental contamination with strong acid or alkali. If used in a platinized hydrogen electrode, special precautions are necessary (see Bates' discussion[3]). The density of this solution changes from 1.0017 g/ml at 25° to 1.0030 at 20°.

0.025 m DISODIUM HYDROGEN PHOSPHATE, 0.025 m POTASSIUM DIHYDROGEN PHOSPHATE. The anhydrous salts are best, and each should be dried for two hours at 120°C, and cooled in a desiccator, since they are slightly deliquescent. Higher drying temperatures should be avoided to obviate formation of condensed phosphates. Dissolve 3.53 g $Na_2HPO_4$ and 3.39 g $KH_2PO_4$ in water to give one liter of solution at 25°C. The water used should not contain dissolved carbon dioxide. Boil the water 10 minutes and guard it with a soda-lime tube while cooling. The primary use for this buffer and the next one listed is in measuring blood pH at 37°C. In addition to the combined proportions of $Na_2 HPO_4$ and $KH_2PO_4$ given below, a combination may be used to provide a convenient pH 7.0 working buffer (see Table 6-9).

0.008695 m POTASSIUM DIHYDROGEN PHOSPHATE, 0.03043 m DISODIUM HYDROGEN PHOSPHATE. Prepare as in preceding directions and dissolve 1.179 g $KH_2PO_4$ and 4.30 g $Na_2HPO_4$ in water to give one liter of solution at 25°C. This buffer solution is more sensitive to contamination with carbon dioxide than is the 0.025 molal solution.

0.01 m SODIUM TETRABORATE DECAHYDRATE. This salt must *not* be dried in an oven before use. Dissolve 3.80 g $Na_2B_4O_7 \cdot 10 H_2O$ in water to give a liter

242

of solution. This borax solution is particularly susceptible to pH change from carbon dioxide absorption and should be protected.

SATURATED (25°C) CALCIUM HYDROXIDE. Pure calcium hydroxide can be shaken with water, or $CaCO_3$ can be ignited at 1000°C for an hour to give CaO, which is then carefully slaked, and the suspension is boiled, cooled, filtered, dried in an oven, and crushed. The solution should be decanted at 25°C before use. The solubility of calcium hydroxide decreases with increased temperature, and the change in solubility is sufficiently large to require correction if the temperature of saturation cannot be done at 25°C. If the temperature of saturation is between 20° and 30°C, the $pa_H$ is given by:

$$pa_H = (pa_H \text{ from Table 6-6 for } t_s) - 0.003 \ (t_s - 25),$$

where $t_s$ is the saturation temperature.

## Working Standard Buffers (secondary standards)

The cost of the National Bureau of Standards reference material has increased so much recently that it is not practical to use these buffers to calibrate the pH

Table 6-9. Potassium Dihydrogen Phosphate-Disodium Hydrogen Phosphate Working Standard*

| pH | $I = 0.05$ 25° | | | $I = 0.1$ 25° | | | $I = 0.2$ 25° | | |
|---|---|---|---|---|---|---|---|---|---|
| | A | B | β | A | B | β | A | B | β |
| 5.6 | — | — | — | — | — | — | 333 | 22.4 | 4.9 |
| 5.8 | — | — | — | 159 | 13.8 | 3.0 | 303 | 32.4 | 6.9 |
| 6.0 | 74.2 | 8.58 | 1.8 | 142 | 19.5 | 4.0 | 265 | 44.8 | 8.9 |
| 6.2 | 64.6 | 11.8 | 2.3 | 121 | 26.4 | 5.0 | 222 | 59.4 | 10.8 |
| 6.4 | 53.4 | 15.5 | 2.8 | 98.2 | 34.0 | 5.8 | 176 | 74.6 | 12.1 |
| 6.6 | 42.0 | 19.3 | 3.0 | 75.6 | 41.4 | 6.1 | 133 | 89.2 | 12.2 |
| 6.8 | 31.4 | 22.8 | 3.0 | 55.4 | 48.2 | 5.9 | 95.2 | 102 | 11.3 |
| 7.0 | 22.4 | 25.8 | 2.7 | 39.0 | 53.6 | 5.2 | 65.8 | 111 | 9.5 |
| 7.2 | 15.4 | 28.2 | 2.3 | 26.4 | 57.8 | 4.2 | 44.2 | 119 | 7.4 |
| 7.4 | 10.3 | 30.0 | 1.8 | 17.6 | 60.8 | 3.1 | 29.2 | 124 | 5.4 |
| 7.6 | 6.74 | 31.0 | 1.3 | 11.5 | 62.8 | 2.2 | 18.9 | 127 | 3.8 |
| 7.8 | 4.36 | 31.8 | 0.90 | 7.38 | 64.2 | 1.5 | 12.1 | 129 | 2.6 |
| 8.0 | 2.80 | 32.4 | 0.61 | — | — | — | — | — | — |

* By permission from *Biochemists' Handbook.* C. Long, Ed. Princeton, N. J., D. Van Nostrand, 1968, p. 32. Copyright 1968 by Van Nostrand Reinhold Company.

A ml. $0.5M$-$KH_2PO_4$ + B ml. $0.5M$-$Na_2HPO_4$ diluted to 1 l., or $A + B$ ml. $0.5M$-$KH_2PO_4$ + B ml. $0.5M$-NaOH. ( β= buffer value).

meter for routine use. A reasonable compromise is the daily use of working buffers that are checked weekly against the reference standard buffers.[1]

We find it convenient to stock commercial buffers at 4, 7, and 10 pH (stated to second decimal place) for routine use. These are bottled in 16 oz. size and initially are checked by lot number against standard reference material. Since we set at pH 7.0 and slope with either 4 or 10, these bottles of buffer are depleted at different times. As long as all three buffers can be fit on the same slope setting, we do not routinely recheck with reference buffers. At any time the three cannot be read properly (provided the glass electrode has been cleaned with dilute HCl) we check with standard reference buffers.

The additional working buffers given in Tables 6-9, 6-10, and 6-11 are useful in various ways. The combinations of $Na_2HPO_4$ and $KH_2PO_4$ listed in Table 6-9 provide a means of obtaining a pH 7.0 buffer to use for standardization of systems whose isopotential point is at that point. Another way to adjust the 0.025 m phosphate reference buffer to pH 7.0 is to add an appropriate amount of 0.1M sodium hydroxide.[6] About 40 ml of the alkali per liter of buffer solution should be required. The assignment of the pH value to the secondary buffer thus prepared must be made with a pH meter standardized to read correctly at pH 6.86, the pH of the phosphate buffer before any alkali was added to it.

The hydrochloric acid listed in Table 6-11 can be used with the tetroxalate buffer for closer monitoring of low pH values.[45, 51] Errors due to residual junction potential in dilute HCl solutions and in solutions of potassium tetroxalate are of the same sign and of about the same magnitude.[3] The sodium hydroxide with the borax and calcium hydroxide buffers serves the same purpose in the alkaline range.[3, 45]

**Table 6-10. Hydrochloric Acid-Potassium Chloride Working Standard\***

| pH | A | C | β | pH | A | C | β |
|------|-----|-----|-----|------|----|-----|-----|
| 1.10† | 512 | 0 | 48 | 1.90 | 81 | 419 | 7.4 |
| 1.20 | 407 | 93 | 38 | 2.00 | 65 | 435 | 6.0 |
| 1.30 | 323 | 177 | 30 | 2.10 | 52 | 448 | 4.8 |
| 1.40 | 257 | 243 | 24 | 2.20 | 42 | 458 | 3.8 |
| 1.50 | 201 | 299 | 19 | 2.41 | 25 | 475 | 2.4 |
| 1.60 | 160 | 340 | 15 | 2.80 | 10 | 490 | 0.8 |
| 1.70 | 128 | 372 | 12 | 3.11 | 5 | 495 | 0.4 |
| 1.80 | 102 | 398 | 9.4 | | | | |

\* By permission from *Biochemists' Handbook.* C. Long, Ed. Princeton, N. J., D. Van Nostrand, 1968, p. 30. Copyright 1968 by Van Nostrand Reinhold Company.

25°, $I = 0.1$. $A$ ml. 0.2M-HCl $+$ $C$ ml. 0.2M-KCl, diluted to 1 1. ($\beta$ = buffer value).

† $I = 0.102$.

**Table 6-11.** Hydrochloric Acid and Sodium Hydroxide Working Standards at Various Temperatures*

| $t$ (°C) | pH 0.1M-HCl | pH 0.1M-NaOH |
|---|---|---|
| 0 | 1.10 | 13.83 |
| 5 | 1.10 | 13.62 |
| 10 | 1.10 | 13.43 |
| 15 | 1.10 | 13.24 |
| 20 | 1.10 | 13.06 |
| 25 | 1.10 | 12.88 |
| 30 | 1.10 | 12.72 |
| 35 | 1.10 | 12.57 |
| 37† | 1.10 | 12.50 |
| 40 | 1.10 | 12.42 |
| 45 | 1.10 | 12.28 |
| 50 | 1.10 | 12.15 |
| 55 | 1.11 | 12.02 |
| 60 | 1.11 | 11.90 |
| 70 | 1.11 | — |
| 80 | 1.11 | — |
| 90 | 1.12 | — |
| 95 | 1.12 | — |

* By permission from *Biochemists' Handbook*. C. Long, Ed. Princeton, N. J., D. Van Nostrand, 1968, p. 21. Copyright 1968 by Van Nostrand Reinhold Company.

† Values at 37° by interpolation.

## MEASUREMENT OF pH

Before starting the actual standardization process, the operator must be sure the instrument is in a stable condition so that measurement may be done in an efficient manner—*i.e.,* accurately but also with a minimum of time involved. The instrument should have been turned on long enough for its components to equilibrate. Even some entirely solid state meters specify a 30 minute warmup period. We prefer to leave the instrument on continually and set it to standby position when not in use. Observe the reference electrode to be sure that there are a few crystals of KCl present (but no hard cake); open the air vent so that the KCl can flow through the liquid junction. In some meters this process involves the loosening and then retightening of the reference electrode into the headpiece; an electrode of this type requires this "making of a fresh junction" before each measurement.[2] Rinse the electrodes well with demineralized water and wipe once with clean tissue. (Some prefer to shake off the excess water and flush with the solution to be used next.[3])

245

The standardization process involves three steps: setting the meter to read the correct value of a standard buffer, checking the slope by reading a second buffer (correcting the slope if necessary), and rechecking the standardization. The exact standardization process for each meter must be consistent with the specific

Table 6-12. Synonyms for the Function Control Knobs of pH Meters

| Mechanical Zero Control | Balance Electrodes |
|---|---|
| Meter Adj. Control<br>  Beckman Research | Standardize Control<br>  Beckman Research |
| Mechanical Zero<br>  IL 265 | Buffer Adj.<br>  Radiometer |
| Meter Adj. Control<br>  Beckman Zeromatic | Standardizing Control<br>  Coleman Metrion 28 |
| Meter Zero Adj. Screw<br>  L&N #7401 | Balance Control<br>  IL 205 |
| Meter Mechanical Zero*<br>  Corning 12 | Standardize Control<br>  Beckman Zeromatic |
| | Standardization Control<br>  Sargent DR 30000 |
| | Standardization Control<br>  L&N #7401 |
| | Calibration Control*<br>  Corning 12 |
| | Calibration Control<br>  Orion 801 |

| Slope Control | Zero Offset Control for mV |
|---|---|
| Temperature Compensator<br>  Beckman Research | Standardizing Range Control<br>  Coleman Metrion 28 |
| Calibration Control<br>  Coleman Metrion 28 | mV Zero*<br>  IL 205 |
| Slope Control*<br>  IL 205 | Standardize Control (for mV Zero)<br>  Zeromatic<br>  (for 0-1400 range only) |
| Buffer Adjust<br>  Sargent DR 30000 | Standardization Control<br>  Sargent DR 30000<br>  (zero for mV or reference pt) |
| Temperature Compensator<br>  Corning 12 | Standardization Control (adjust to mV zero)<br>  L&N #7401 |
| Temperature Compensator<br>  Orion 801<br>  (% Nernst indicated) | Zero Adjust<br>  Orion 801<br>  (In Rel mV position calibrate can adjust<br>  over 90 mV range) |

* Term used in this chapter.

directions from the manufacturer. There seems to be no consistency in the terminology used to label the control knobs of the meters made by different manufacturers. Synonyms for these function controls are listed in Table 6-12.

The terms used throughout this chapter are designated in the following manner:

1. *Slope Control.* The mV response is adjusted to be theoretically correct (*i.e.,* 59.16 per pH unit at 25°C).

2. *Calibration Control.* The mV response range is shifted so that the correct pH value on the scale coincides with that of the standard buffer. By this manipulation the amplifier is balanced at the standard buffer response.

3. *Standardization.* The instrument is correct in its slope and the pH scale of its meter. The instrument is ready to read an unknown.

---

### General Guide for the Measurement of pH

1. Read and record the room temperature (assuming the electrode chain is at room temperature). Determine the exact value of the buffers at that temperature: for example, 4.01, 7.00, and 10.00 pH.

2. Using the 7.00 buffer, with the calibration control adjust the meter to read properly. It is quicker and more satisfactory if the value of this buffer coincides with the isopotential point of the system.[1] The pH 7 buffer satisfies this condition for most current meters.

3. Rinse the electrodes, dry them, and read the 4.01 buffer. If the value is not correct within ± 0.02 (or whatever specification is chosen), the slope is not correct. Adjust the slope (as described below) and check with 10.00 buffer.

4. Recheck the standardization before the unknowns are read. Frequently some drift occurs following the first readings, even when the electrodes have been stored in a solution whose composition is similar to that of the buffer.[44] The buffers should again be rechecked after a series of unknowns have been read. Exactly how frequently this rechecking is necessary depends entirely upon the meter and how much drift one detects with it.

---

As long as the glass electrode is clean and other factors involved remain consistent, once the slope has been adjusted properly, it should remain correct for a relatively long period of time. In order to correct the slope, the dotted line in Figure 6-20 must be pivoted around the isopotential point until the indicated pH is identical with the true pH value. In this graph the indicated 3.4 pH must be corrected to 4.0. For meters with a control designated "slope" this is a simple adjustment; many meters do not have such a control easily accessible to the user. Provided both samples and buffers are at the same temperature and provided the buffer values are being used at their correct values for the ambient temperature, the temperature compensator can be used to adjust the slope. We routinely use our meters in this fashion and keep a daily record of the position on the tempera-

247

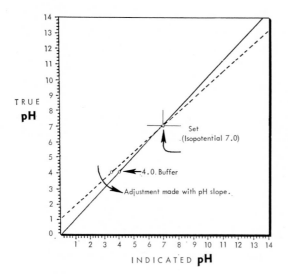

**Figure 6-20.** *Correction of the response slope. Solid line: correct slope—indicated pH coincides with true pH. Broken line: an incorrect slope in which indicated values above pH 7.0 are low and values below pH 7.0 are high.*

ture dial necessary to correct the slope. If the reading is as much as 2° different from what it was previously, the glass electrode is cleaned.

The pH 10.00 buffer should now be read to check the slope. This buffer should read correctly if the slope adjustment made with the 4.01 buffer was proper. If the correct reading cannot be obtained for both the pH 4 and 10 buffers, this is usually an indication that the glass electrode needs cleaning. Eventually, however, the deterioration of the pH response will not be corrected by simply cleaning the glass electrode, and the electrode will have to be replaced.[5] A check of the electrode resistance can prove this point.[44] Under ordinary circumstances, the pH 4 and 10 buffers can be sloped correctly, and unknowns may be read with confidence as long as their values fall between those of the buffers.

The amount of time required as "adequate" for the glass electrode to come to equilibrium varies in several ways. If the type of electrode used is a capillary for micro samples, about 10 seconds is usual for the response; dipping bulb electrodes usually require 1 to 3 minutes for pH values in the intermediate range of pH 3 to 9. Outside this range, the response usually is slower. At pH values above 10 the electrode may be very sluggish even when the electrode is one labeled "low alkaline error type."[45] If the same electrode is then immediately used to read a pH value in the intermediate range, the operator is prone to cause inaccuracies by not allowing the electrode enough time to stabilize. The sluggishness caused by using the electrode in alkali can be eliminated by soaking in dilute HCl, but that caused by using the electrode in strong acids is best overcome by soaking in water.[45]

Time for equilibration is variable in other circumstances also. It may take 15 minutes for an automatic temperature compensator to reach temperature equilibrium in a sample solution if the solution temperature is other than ambient.[39] If the temperature range of the sample overlaps the operating temperature ranges of two types of electrodes, the better choice is the one designed for the lower temperature range. A reading that drifts slowly to its end point is said to be a normal response when a dilute solution is read immediately after the standard buffer.[47] Presumably this is caused by slow desorption of buffer from the glass surface.

The use of the temperature-adjust for slope control as given above assumed availability of a buffer that coincided with the isopotential point. Dicker has shown that a buffer that does not coincide with the isopotential point may be used in a similar manner by correcting the slope first and then adjusting the zero offset.[20] We find it much easier to provide the buffer at the isopotential point than to explain to several different operators how to use some other buffer for this purpose.

Sample volume should be the same for the standard buffer and the unknown solution for two reasons. First, the flow of KCl through the liquid junction will be the same only when the proportion of head-to-sample is the same for buffer and unknown. A very small sample could show a pH change from the salt effect of added KCl. Secondly, if the volume of test solution is too small, relative to the surface area of the bulb of the glass electrode, changes in pH through adsorption or solution of the glass become serious.[3]

With good technique and reasonable maintenance of the instrument, routine operation of pH meters for measuring aqueous solutions should provide reliable values to $\pm$ 0.02 pH units or better. Bates lists the difficulties encountered as traceable to one or more of the following:[3]

1. Scratched or cracked bulb of glass electrode.
2. Cracked or broken internal assembly of the glass or calomel electrode.
3. Electrodes not properly cleaned.
4. Contamination of the potassium chloride solution of the calomel electrode or salt bridge.
5. Interruption of the flow of potassium chloride solution from the calomel electrode by clogged aperture or fiber.
6. Inaccurate buffer solution.
7. Instability of sample being tested or unusually high resistance of the solution.
8. Worn-out battery, imperfect, or incorrect battery connections.
9. Defective or worn-out tubes.
10. Humidity effects.

A compilation of common symptoms and possible causes of improper function of pH meters is given in Table 6-13.

By using Table 6-13 in conjunction with the check system which follows, we have been able to identify most of the malfunctions we have encountered with pH meters.

Almost all pH meters available currently can provide values to $\pm$ 0.02 pH units using the general points of measurement given above. If values are to be measured to $\pm$ 0.005 pH unit or better ($\pm$ 0.1 mV or less), several extra considerations are necessary.[45]

1. The pH meter must be capable of adequate discrimination. A meter using a vibratory capacitor has been recommended, but several current meters using other input devices can now meet such specifications.

**Table 6-13. Various Symptoms and Possible Causes of Improper Function of pH Meter**

| Symptom | Possible Cause |
|---|---|
| A. Instrument completely inoperative; calibration control does not move meter needle | 1. Instrument not plugged into the wall outlet or instrument improperly grounded<br>2. Fuse<br>3. Electrode improperly plugged in<br>4. Loose cable contacts if cables are separate; defective cable<br>5. Insufficient KCl in reference electrode; junction plugged; cracked glass electrode<br>6. Open circuit |
| B. Instrument cannot be standardized | |
|    1. Amplifier cannot be balanced with meter shorted | 1. Batteries<br>2. Tubes (refer to specific manual)<br>3. Current leakage: poor insulation, grounds, or contacts |
|    2. Meter needle responds to calibration control but can't be set at isopotential point with standard buffer solution (offset beyond adjusting ability of meter) | 1. Glass electrode: cracked, coated, or dehydrated; if new, wrong zero potential<br>2. Short circuit in electrode plug or cable<br>3. Reference electrode: clogged or defective internal element; unsaturated or contaminated KCl |
|    3. Incorrect slope: buffers of pH 4, 7, and 10 (having been proved all right) do not read properly | 1. Dirty glass electrode<br>2. Defective glass electrode<br>3. Defective slope control (or temperature compensator) |
|    4. Normal scale and expanded scale do not correspond | 1. Electronic adjustment |
| C. Instrument can be standardized but response is unsatisfactory | |
|    1. Erratic kicks of meter needle (especially with movement in vicinity of electrode) | 1. Poor connection in cable, cap of electrode, or contact point<br>2. Inadequate grounding<br>3. Poor liquid junction: clogged; unsaturation or bubbles in reference internal element |
|    2. Erratic movement of meter needle when standardization control is adjusted | 1. Dirty contact surfaces |
|    3. Drift | 1. Reference electrode: insufficient flow of KCl; unstable response from recent cleaning or change in temperature |

**Table 6-13 (Continued)**

| Symptom | Possible Cause |
|---------|----------------|
| | 2. Current leakage: zero drift from power supply or bad tube |
| | 3. Improper grounding |
| | 4. Glass electrode: not properly hydrated; dirty |
| | 5. Change in pH of solution |
| 4. Sluggish response | 1. Normal for some glass electrodes |
| | 2. Deteriorated or dirty glass electrode; improperly hydrated glass electrode |
| | 3. Bad tubes in some meters |
| 5. Poor reproducibility | 1. Plugging of reference electrode junction; air bubble in internal element; unstable from recent change of temperature or KCl |
| | 2. Zero drift (especially in meters using tubes) |
| | 3. Change in temperature of buffers or sample |
| | 4. Dirty glass electrode; air bubble at inner contact lead |

2. Erratic liquid junction potentials must be minimized. A ceramic plug seems satisfactory as the type of junction. Ionic strength must be similar for the standard buffers and unknowns to assure similar junction potentials.

3. Inadequacies of the specific glass electrode used must be compensated as much as possible. These effects include use in pH regions where response is non-theoretical, slow response, asymmetry potential drifts, and inner reference electrode instability.

4. Instability of the external electrode must be controlled. Usually instability can be traced to temperature variation, variation in the concentration of the KCl (or other electrolyte), or contamination of the KCl.

5. Insufficient temperature control can affect all the preceding considerations. Thermostating both electrodes and sample is required for this level of discrimination. It is better to introduce precontrolled temperature sample solutions to the electrodes held in a suitable chamber than to transfer the electrodes to different vessels containing the solutions.

6. Standardization before and after measurement is necessary. The buffers used must be as close as possible to the unknown's pH—certainly within one pH unit.

## CHECK SYSTEM FOR THE pH METER

The overall performance of the system (*i.e.,* electrode chain and meter) must be judged on the basis of six points: reproducibility (at low, intermediate, and high pH ranges), noise and/or drift (this is primarily zero stability), response time, sensitivity, linearity, and accuracy. Bates points out that these should be checked at least annually, including the accuracy of the standard cell, if the instrument has one.[3] However, manufacturers of instruments using the standard cell emphatically state that the user should not tamper with this circuit; following Bates' recommendation then would mean that either the instrument would have to be returned to the factory or a qualified serviceman from the factory would have to check the meter annually.

In our institution we have not been able to operate a whole year without having to go over each of the above points to isolate a malfunction. Therefore, our operation has been based on the belief that "adequate scale length (*i.e.,* slope) is the ultimate general criterion of performance of a pH measuring system."[45] Our routine use involves making the notations shown in Figure 6-21.

Every time the instrument is used:

1. Note and record ambient temperature.
2. Set the instrument to read the exact value for the pH 7 buffer at that temperature.
3. Read a second buffer whose value is close to that expected for the unknown. Record this value. If the value is outside the acceptable range (we use ± 0.02 pH unit), slope the instrument until the buffer reads its correct value for the prevailing temperature. Record the slope notation. For an instrument without a slope control we use the manual temperature compensator and record the "temperature number" that makes the slope correct.

| DATE | READING for 4.01 | READING for 10.00 | ROOM temp °C | SLOPE reading | GLASS ELECTRODE soaked 0.1 N HCl | REF. ELECTRODE | |
|---|---|---|---|---|---|---|---|
| | | | | | | junction ck | change KCl |
| | | | | | | | |
| | | | | | | | |
| | | | | | | | |
| | | | | | | | |
| | | | | | | | |
| | | | | | | | |
| | | | | | | | |
| | | | | | | | |
| | | | | | | | |
| | | | | | | | |
| | | | | | | | |
| | | | | | | | |

**Figure 6-21.** *Daily record sheet for Corning 12 pH Meter.*

At any time that the % Nernst for the electrode changes more than 2% or the temperature setting on the compensator is more than 2° away from the room temperature we check to find out why. Usually cleaning the glass electrode in 0.1 N HCl will bring the response back to normal. If the cleaning does not correct the response, we then go through the system below to isolate the problem as involving the meter or the electrodes.

Under good-performance conditions, the glass electrode is cleaned weekly. The reference electrode is checked monthly: its liquid junction portion is examined and cleaned if necessary, the internal element is examined, and the KCl is replaced. When a combination electrode is used, the weekly cleaning of the glass bulb portion makes it necessary to take care of the reference electrode portion at the same time.

## CHECK SYSTEM FOR THE CORNING MODEL 12 pH METER

The following outline is specifically made for the Corning Model 12 (direct reading, expanded scale) pH meter. The details can be altered slightly to make it apply to any meter. Each point in the outline includes directions for doing the tests and evaluating the test results. We have attempted to make the outline as complete as possible, but the experienced user will soon become accustomed to picking priority checkpoints, depending upon the symptoms. These function tests are all within the capability of the user to run, but often the follow-up of the symptoms thus detected will have to be completed by an electronics technician. Repairs, of course, must be made only by a qualified serviceman.

Before the instrument operator starts through the check system, he must have already convinced himself that the malfunction of the instrument is not some simple point of technique he has overlooked or taken for granted. The most likely symptom, in our experience, has always been that the instrument could not be sloped properly. Before starting this point-by-point check, he should have already followed the instructions pertaining to daily use—*i.e.,* (1) try fresh buffers; (2) clean the glass electrode. If there still is a problem, the systematic approach is to determine the nature of the problem, attempt to isolate the problem, correct the problem if possible, but—above all else—consult the manufacturer or a qualified service technician *before* attempting any adjustment or procedure he is not absolutely sure he is capable of handling.

## I. Preliminary Step

### I. Instrument on and Mechanically Zeroed

A. If the instrument appears completely inoperative, *i.e.,* the pilot light is not on with the function switch in standby:

1. Check to see that the electric cord is plugged into the wall socket and is properly grounded. Is the wall socket functional for something else plugged into it?

*Continued on page 254*

253

2. Check the pH meter fuse and replace it if it is blown. If the fuse blows again, have an electrician locate the problem.

B. If the instrument appears operative, check to see that the meter needle reads exactly zero. If it does not, adjust the mechanical zero while the meter is in standby position.

We have our instrument on in standby position at all times. Not only does this mean that the instrument can be used at any time, but high internal humidity is minimized.

## II. Functional Symptoms of the Problem

### II. Functional Characteristics

A. Standardize the instrument with buffers for general operation. Check first in the 0 to 14 pH range. Record all readings.

1. *Reproducibility*—Read each buffer three times:
   a. pH 4.01
   b. pH 7.00
   c. pH 10.01

2. *Noise and/or Drift*—For 10 minutes observe the readings of the buffers:
   a. pH 7.00
   b. pH 4.01

3. *Response Time*—Determine with a stopwatch how long it takes the instrument to equilibrate when changing buffers from:
   a. pH 7.00 to 4.01
   b. pH 7.00 to 10.01

4. *Linearity*—Record the room temperature. Read the following NBS standard buffers in mV response:
   a. pH 1.679
   b. pH 4.008
   c. pH 6.862
   d. pH 9.180

B. Repeat the 4 steps of A using the expanded scale.

These function characteristics for each pH meter are fairly well known by the operator, but they change somewhat from time to time. Also, the user sometimes tends to remember vague general terms. As factual data this information is useful in looking for the causes of problems. Electrode condition has an effect on these readings, and an alert user can sometimes decide, at this point, that the glass electrode needs to be cleaned better with stronger hydrochloric acid. Or if the

254

electrode has been used for an extended period in the alkaline range or at high temperature, it may need to be replaced (or put aside for less precise use). It is useful at times to plot the mV response (checkpoint 4) versus the correct pH value for the prevailing temperature. For example, the electrode showing the results of long exposure to high alkalinity would be less linear in that range. Incidentally, if the linearity of the system is known to be correct, an incorrect buffer can best be identified by such a plot.

## III. Isolation of the Problem

The shorting lead that comes with the meter is used in the following tests. Remove the electrode leads from the meter and plug in the shorting lead between the input and the reference connections. The meter may now be checked separately to determine its functional characteristics; whether the controls can balance the amplifier; and, what the offset voltage is at the zero mV position on the scale. By including a resistor of high value in the shorting circuit, the meter can be screened for current leakage; this resistor can be added to the shorting lead if it was not provided originally.

The meter can be checked for additional items by using a pH/mV test unit (Section V). However, enough information can usually be obtained with the shorting lead (including resistor) for the manufacturer's service department to take over the problem.

---

### III. A. Amplifier Balance

1. While the Function Switch is in standby position, short the input to the reference with the alligator clip attached to position A in the diagram of the shorting lead.

2. Move the Function Switch to the pH mode, 0 to 14 scale. The meter needle should move to about midscale.

3. Move the Calibration Control fully clockwise (CW) and record pH reading; then fully counterclockwise (CCW) and record. For this meter the range covered between CW and CCW should be about pH 5 to 9.

4. Switch to 0 to 1 (expanded scale); set the Range Switch on pH 7.

5. Adjust the meter to zero with the Calibration Control; switch the Range Switch to pH 6. The meter should now read exactly 100 (full scale deflection). If it does not read properly, an adjustment is required for either the 0 to 1 step or 0 to 1 full scale deflection.

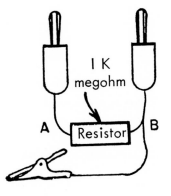

---

## III. B. Meter Zero mV Position

1. With the Range Switch at zero, switch to $+$ mV and $-$ mV in the normal output range (0 to 14).
2. Repeat using the expanded range (0 to 1).
   The meter should read zero within $\pm 1\%$ of full scale at all times.

## III. C. Current Leakage Screening Test

1. Change the alligator clip on the shorting lead from position A to position B. This adds 1000 megohms resistance into the shorting circuit.
2. Repeat steps 1 and 2 of III. B. The same response should be obtained in spite of the added resistance. If the meter shows an increased response, current leakage is present.

## III. D. Function Characteristics

1. *Reproducibility*
   a. Leave the shorting lead as in III. C, 2.
   b. In pH mode, 0 to 14 scale, adjust the meter to 7 with the calibration control. Move the function switch to standby.
   c. Move the switch from standby back to pH and note the meter reading. Repeat twice and record.
2. *Noise and/or Drift*
   Leave the pH7 settings and observe the readings for 10 minutes.
3. *Response Time*
   a. Using calibration control, set the meter to read pH 14 (*i.e.,* full scale deflection).
   b. With a stopwatch, measure the time it takes the meter needle to reach pH 14 when the function switch is moved from standby to pH. The time required should not be more than 10 seconds.
   Repeat steps 1, 2, and 3 for pH mode, expanded scale.

The calibration control will be able to obtain varied ranges in step III. A. 3 for different meters. The wider this range, the more choice is available for electrodes that can be used with the meter. Beckman meters can be adjusted almost to the scale limit in both directions from pH 7.

The function characteristics are more important here than they were with the electrodes in the circuit. Deviations from the expected response or changes with time indicate an electronic problem that must be corrected.

256

## IV. Recalibration of Meter without a Potential Bridge

Replacement of any circuit components requires that the meter be recalibrated. A potential bridge accurate to 0.1% is the proper input source to use.[2, 3, 19] While not as accurate, the following procedure can be used until the meter can be properly serviced.

---

### IV. Calibration Using Buffers

A. Short the input to reference. With the Function Switch set on standby adjust the mechanical meter zero to read zero.

    1. In pH mode, expanded scale, adjust the Calibration Control until the meter reads 7.00. Lock Calibration Control in this position.

    2. Change the Range Switch to 6 and adjust the 0 to 1 FSD so that the meter reads 100 mV (full scale deflection).

B. Remove the shorting lead and connect the reference and glass electrodes to the meter.

    1. Read the mV response for buffers of pH 7.00 and 4.01.

    2. Look up the exact buffer values for the exact room temperature. Calculate the slope (mV per pH unit) from the buffer values and the mV difference between them.

C. Adjust the 0 to 1 step control until the measured slope is exactly equal to the calculated slope. Adjusting the 0 to 1 step control CCW will increase the mV response. Repeat step A, 1 through C, to be sure the adjustment is correct.

D. Short the input to reference again. In pH mode, expanded scale, Range Switch on 7, adjust the 0 to 14 FSD control until the meter reads exactly pH 7.

E. Remove the shorting lead and put the electrodes back in place.

    1. Using the pH 4.01 buffer, with meter in pH mode, expanded scale, adjust the temperature compensator until the meter reads the correct pH for the buffer at the ambient temperature.

    2. Mechanically adjust the temperature control knob on its shaft until the exact ambient temperature coincides with that indicated on the temperature compensator.

---

## V. Use of the pH/mV Test Unit

The test unit we use is the Heath model EUA 20-12,* which costs about $35.00. This unit uses a 1.35 V mercury battery and the resistors are listed in the specifications as only 1% tolerance. Initially we were skeptical that this degree of precision would be great enough to evaluate our pH meters to the second

---

\* Available from Heath Company, Benton Harbor, Mich.

decimal place. It has proved to be an invaluable tool in this capacity, and its precision appears to be better than one would expect. The pH output is provided from 0 to 14 in steps of 1 pH unit each, with variable output resistance up to 1000 megohms. A switch provides for the pH output voltage to be made equivalent to that at temperatures of 10°, 25°, 50°, and 90°C. In the x1 or x10 mV selector switch position, the voltage output is 0 to 70 mV in fourteen steps of 5 mV each or 0 to 700 mV in steps of 50 mV each.

Our unit has been modified slightly to add the following capabilities:[25]

1. Equivalent output voltage for temperature of 37°C.

2. Increased sensitivity to provide full scale 1.4 mV, 14 mV or 1.4 pH at 25°C.

3. Polarity reversal switch. This eliminates the necessity to reverse leads physically while performing a check procedure.

The circuit, including the modifications, is shown as Figure 6-22.

Other test units are available, but we have had no experience with them. Photovolt Electronic Tester, Model 25* is a line operated unit using an RCA voltage reference tube. The schematic for this unit has been published,[41] and the accuracy of the reference voltage is stated as equivalent to approximately ± 0.02 pH unit. Radiometer Type PHN2a pH Calibrator† contains standard cells. The resistors in this unit are specified as 0.1%. The cost of both these test units is about $100. After questioning various pH meter manufacturers we get the impression that a testing unit constantly precise to 0.1% and versatile enough to check out the entire circuitry of the meter completely would cost approximately $1,000. For this reason we have used the Heath Test Unit and referred problems beyond our capabilities to the manufacturer of the specific instrument.

### Test Procedure for the Meter Section of the pH Measuring System Using the Heath Test Unit

The following test procedures can be used for all types of pH meters by including the proper adapter if the shielded test lead provided with the unit does not fit the input connector of the meter. The limitations of the "within 1%" specified by the resistors in the unit can be exceeded with some degree of assurance if the unit is checked periodically against a high precision meter such as the Orion 801.‡

Before starting any of these procedures, be sure that the pH meter is operative and that it has been plugged in long enough to have reached sufficient warm-up equilibrium. Most meters have a standby position for this purpose. Also be sure that the mechanical meter zero is reading properly; if adjustment of this setting is necessary, be careful to follow the instructions in the manual for the specific instrument. Meters vary considerably in the procedure for this simple operation.

---

* Photovolt Corporation, New York.

† Radiometer, The London Company, Westlake, Ohio.

‡ Orion Research Inc., Cambridge, Mass.

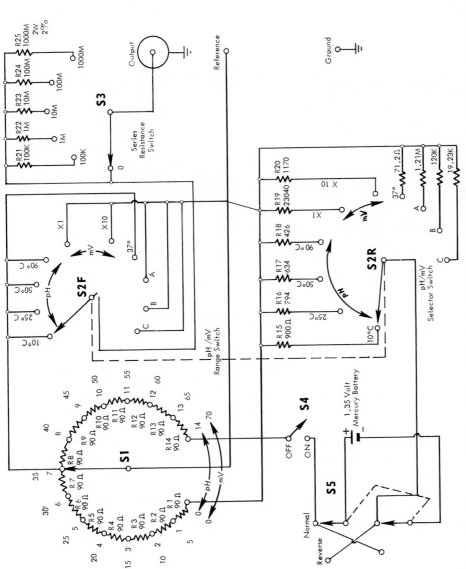

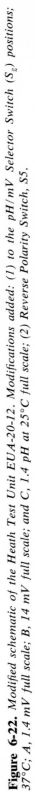

**Figure 6-22.** *Modified schematic of the Heath Test Unit EUA-20-12. Modifications added: (1) to the pH/mV Selector Switch ($S_2$) positions; 37°C; A, 1.4 mV full scale; B, 14 mV full scale; and C, 1.4 pH at 25°C full scale; (2) Reverse Polarity Switch, S5.*

259

## *V. A. General Response Characteristics*

Connect the test unit to the pH meter as shown in Figure 6-23.

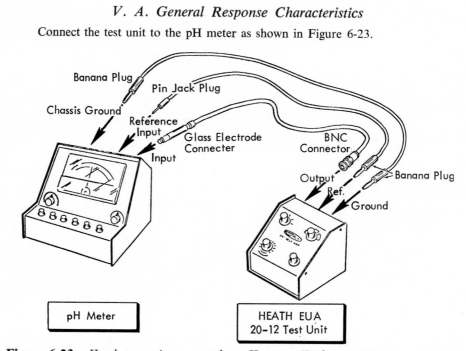

**Figure 6-23.** *Heath test unit connected to pH meter. (Redrawn with permission from Heath Operation of the pH/mV Test Unit, Model EUA-20-12. Heath Company, Benton Harbor, Mich., December, 1965.)*

1. *Response Time*
   a. Set the test unit controls:
      Series Resistance Switch to 100 M.
      pH/mV Selector Switch to 25°C.
      pH/mV Range Switch to pH 7.
      Off-On Switch to ON.
   b. Turn on the pH meter in the pH mode and set the temperature control to 25°C.
   c. Adjust the calibration control of the meter until the indicator reaches exactly pH 7.
   d. Change the meter switch from Standby to pH, and with a stopwatch measure the time required for the meter to reach its stable reading. Repeat with the test unit Range Switch changed to pH 10 (or limit of amplifier range).

   Tolerance should be less than 10 seconds; for many meters it is less than half this amount.

2. *Noise and/or Drift*
   After the meter has reached its stable reading in Step d above, observe the reading for 10 minutes. There should be no drift; if noise is present at all, it should be less than ± the smallest division on the meter scale.

260

3. *Reproducibility*

Repeat Section 1. d. three times for each range switch setting of the test unit. Record each reading.

Readings should agree within the readability of the meter—*i.e.*, less difference than the smallest scale division.

4. *Sensitivity*

a. Set the test unit controls:

Series Resistance Switch to 100 M.

pH/mV Selector Switch to 1.4 mV (position A of our modified unit); Reverse-Polarity Switch in + mV position.

pH/mV Range Switch to 0.

Off-On Switch to ON.

b. Turn on pH meter in + mV mode, expanded scale; Range Switch on 0.

c. Rotate the test unit Range Switch stepwise from 0 to 14 and record the meter response. If the sensitivity cannot be read with these settings, change the Selector Switch to 14 mV (position B) and repeat. Repeat until the response can be judged reproducible at its lowest mV level. Specifications for the specific meter will be found in its instruction manual. Meters used satisfactorily at the discrimination of 0.02 pH unit level will usually respond well between 0.2 and 0.4 mV.

---

With the exception of V. A. 4., instructions for these responses will be noted to be identical to those checked under Section II using the meter with buffers. These performance tests for the meter can be done with the test-resistor-shorting lead as given in Section III. C. We prefer to use the test unit because we think it is a more positive approach in that the input to the meter is being changed.

The electronics of the meter portion of the pH measuring system must perform precisely and without noise or drift. If defects are noted, repairs require the services of a qualified electronics technician. Most manufacturers are now using designs in which modules or electronic boards are exchanged in the field and all actual repair work is done at the factory.

The primary use of the sensitivity test given as 4, is to establish that there is no change in response from time to time.

---

## V. B. Linearity in Both pH and mV Modes

Connect the test unit to the meter as shown in Figure 6-23.

1. Check in pH mode first.

a. Set the test unit controls:

Series Resistance Switch to 100 M.

pH/mV Selector Switch to 25°C; Reverse-Polarity Switch in — mV position.

pH/mV Range Switch to pH 7.

Off-On Switch to ON.

*Continued on page 262*

    b. Turn on the pH meter in pH mode and set its temperature control to 25°C.

    c. Adjust the Calibration Control of the meter until the indicator reaches exactly pH 7.

    d. Switch the pH/mV Range Switch from pH 7 to 14 and from pH 7 to 0 in increments of 1 pH unit. Record the exact reading for each from the meter.

Tolerance suggested is ± 0.02 units. See discussion below.

2. Check in mV mode.

    a. Set the test unit controls:
      Series Resistance Switch to 100 M.
      pH/mV Selector Switch to x10 mV.
      pH/mV Range Switch to 0.
      Off-On Switch to ON.

    b. Turn on the meter in mV position, expanded scale.* The calibration and temperature controls are automatically cut out of the circuit in most meters in mV position. In some, however, a zero mV control is provided (occasionally a relative mV position is available to measure mV steps, and the calibration control may adjust the mV to zero). If there is a zero mV control, adjust it to 0; if not, record this initial mV reading.

    c. Switch the test unit's pH/mV Range Switch through each of its fourteen positions and record the mV output. The pH meter has a + mV and a − mV position. Use this in conjunction with the Reverse-Polarity Switch on the test unit for the most convenient manner of reading the entire range. Record all values.

    d. Compare the mV output from the test unit to that read from the pH meter. Original tolerance of the test unit is ± 1%, but if the unit has been compared to a precise meter, the user may set his own tolerance.

---

* Range Switch setting + expanded scale reading $\times$ 100 = mV.

The only reliable way to check or calibrate the meter output is in mV. The check in pH mode is included to detect some gross malfunction either in that response or in the temperature compensator. We have found this useful when the normal range and expanded scale pH response do not agree. With our modification of the test unit to include more sensitive full scale mV and pH response, we have been able to prove the misadjustment was in the expanded scale of the meter. Bates points out that a calibration curve should be constructed when corrective adjustments cannot be made to satisfy the entire output range, if the magnitude of the error warrants such a procedure.[3] He allows the cumulative error at the extreme ends of the range to be ± 5 mV and any 100 mV increment within 1%. The ASTM specifications are almost identical: ± 1 mV per 100 mV increment and calibration curve required for cumulative error greater than ± 6 mV.[2] We believe these tolerances to be a little wide for the instruments currently available; about half that range seems consistent with the values we get.

### V. C. Accuracy of the Temperature Compensator

Connect the test unit to the meter as shown in Figure 6-23.

1. Set the test unit controls:
   Series Resistance Switch to 100 M.
   pH/mV Selector Switch to 25°C.
   pH/mV Range Switch to pH 7.
   Off-On Switch to ON.
2. Turn on the meter in the pH mode and set the temperature control to 25°C.
3. Adjust the calibration control of the meter until the indicator reaches exactly pH 7.
4. Switch the test unit pH/mV Range Switch to pH 4, 0, 10, and then 14. Record the pH readings from the meter.
5. Change the test unit Selector Switch to 10° and repeat the readings as in 4. Record the exact readings of the meter. Repeat for Selector Switch setting of 50° or any other desired temperature.
6. The temperature control of the meter should be correct within 1° for most meters. Consult the instrument manual if it is necessary to correct the compensator. Often the difficulty is that the knob has slipped on the shaft of the temperature control.

Table 6-14. Test Unit Output Voltages—in pH Mode at Five Temperatures

| pH Reading (a) | Output Voltage in Millivolts (b) | | | | |
|---|---|---|---|---|---|
| | 10°C | 25°C | 37°C | 50°C | 90°C |
| 0 | 393 | 414 | 431 | 449 | 505 |
| 1 | 337 | 355 | 369 | 385 | 433 |
| 2 | 281 | 296 | 308 | 321 | 360 |
| 3 | 225 | 237 | 246 | 256 | 288 |
| 4 | 169 | 178 | 185 | 192 | 216 |
| 5 | 112 | 118 | 123 | 128 | 144 |
| 6 | 56.2 | 59.2 | 61.5 | 64.1 | 72.1 |
| 7 | 0 | 0 | 0 | 0 | 0 |
| 8 | −56.2 | −59.2 | −61.5 | −64.1 | −72.1 |
| 9 | −112 | −118 | −123 | −128 | −144 |
| 10 | −169 | −178 | −185 | −192 | −216 |
| 11 | −225 | −237 | −246 | −256 | −288 |
| 12 | −281 | −296 | −308 | −321 | −360 |
| 13 | −377 | −355 | −369 | −385 | −433 |
| 14 | −393 | −414 | −431 | −449 | −505 |

(a) pH as read off the pH/mV Range Switch.
(b) Millivolt output voltage between Output and Reference terminals corresponding to theoretical values at five Centigrade temperatures (selected by the pH/mV Selector Switch).

If there is an error in the mV response of the meter itself, the error will also show in this test procedure. Therefore, the linearity (or accuracy) of the meter should be verified before checking the temperature compensation. Automatic temperature compensators can be checked in the same fashion,[3] but during the test the resistance thermometer must be immersed in a bath regulated to the desired temperature. A cross check of the mV response provided by the test unit for the specific temperature may be made by using the test unit Selector Switch at that temperature and the Range Switch in pH while reading the response in mV on the pH meter. Comparison can be made with the output voltages listed in Table 6-14. Since we routinely use the temperature compensator as a slope control for the pH meter, specific values for the compensator do not concern us. We do think this test procedure has a valid use in locating the source of difficulty when an instrument cannot be sloped properly.

---

### V. D. Check for and Measurement of Current Leakage in the Input Circuit of the pH Meter

Connect the test unit to the pH meter as shown in Figure 6-23.

1. Set the test unit controls:
   Series Resistance Switch to 10 M.
   pH/mV Selector Switch to 25°C.
   pH/mV Range Switch to pH 7.
   Off-On Switch to ON.
2. Turn on the pH meter in the pH mode and set the temperature control to 25°C.
3. Adjust the calibration control of the meter until the indicator reaches exactly pH 7.
4. Switch the series Resistance Switch from 10 M to 1000 M. Record any changes in the pH reading of the meter.
5. Repeat step 4 for pH meter settings of 4, 10, and any others desired.
   The leakage current can be calculated from:

$$\text{Leakage current} = \frac{(\text{pH change}) \times (\text{volts/pH})}{\text{resistance change}}$$

For example: if 10 M gave a reading of pH 4.00 and 1000 M gave 4.02, the pH change was 0.02.

$$\frac{0.02 \times 59.2 \times 10^{-3}}{(1000 - 10) \times 10^{6}} = \text{approximately } 1 \times 10^{-12} \text{ amperes}$$

Tolerance should be checked from the specific instrument manual, but almost all meters currently have no more than $10^{-12}$ amperes specified.

If leakage current does develop in a pH meter, it is a problem for the experienced electronics technician—not for the user. However, seemingly insignificant factors such as fingerprints on the input plugs or other sensitive components may produce some change. A sufficiently high leakage current can cause an apparent decrease in the mV response of the instrument, and the decrease can become great enough that the amplifier cannot be balanced. We have never experienced a problem traceable to leakage current. After discussing current leakage with service representatives, we have concluded that as long as the response on the "screening test" (III. C) does not exceed tolerance there is no need to measure the current leakage.

## VI. Check of Glass and Reference Electrodes

If the defects originally present when the function characteristics were recorded in Section II were not present when the meter was checked separately in Section III, there is no alternative to blaming the electrode chain for the problem.

The usual directions for checking the electrodes of a pH measuring system are to substitute the suspect electrodes with some known to be good. This is frustrating to the operator for two reasons primarily: first, even electrodes bought as spares, and carefully kept as such, deteriorate to varying degrees with time. So who knows whether a substituted electrode is "known to be good"? Second, if substitution did render the instrument satisfactorily operative, what was wrong with the electrode removed? Can the electrode be cleaned, rejuvenated, or altered some other way to salvage the piece of equipment? Electrodes are expendable items, but we have found that the cost can be lowered considerably by salvaging some electrodes which *"just don't work right" on a given day*.

VI. A. GLASS ELECTRODES. The glass electrode, in our experience, has caused more problems than the reference electrode. A regular weekly cleaning with 0.1 N HCl has greatly extended the period of satisfactory use of this electrode. When the electrode doesn't respond properly after its weekly cleaning, we try 6 N HCl. The recommended hydrofluoric acid for "last resort" cleaning has not seemed practical to us in our general laboratories, and we have not used it. We have cleaned some electrodes with dilute solutions of HCl and NaOH in a cycling process and found it helpful a few times. In general, if the glass electrodes have not worked satisfactorily after the 6 N HCl, we have discarded them.

If we can assume that, at this point, the user has cleaned the glass electrode through the full treatment including 6 N HCl and that the electrode does not respond properly, there are three checks to prove the electrode defective: physical examination with a magnifying lens, measurement of zero potential, and measurement of the electrode's resistance. The technologist must keep in mind that the pH measurement takes a good glass electrode, a good reference electrode, and a good electrolyte bridge between them. Neither electrode should be assumed defective until proven so.

265

## VI. A. 1. Broken or Cracked Membrane

With a good lens:

a. Examine the pH sensitive bulb for cracks or scratches.

b. Look for cracks in the glass stem or the seal of the cap to the stem.

c. Is the wire from the cap continuous to the inner electrode? If the electrode has a shield inside the stem, the wire may not be visible. Often a platinum lead comes through the cap and is joined to silver wire on which the silver chloride is deposited; if there is a break in the wire, it is usually at the junction.

d. Is there a bubble lodged around the silver/silver chloride terminal portion of the inner electrode?

e. If the cable is removable, check for continuity. If the cable is not removable gently try to turn the center pin contact of the cap; it should not be loose.

The separate chamber for the bulb portion of the electrode which contains the inner electrode may have different shapes and varied amounts of internal standard solution. If the space is such that a bubble is present, the bubble can lodge around the electrode and decrease the mV response of the electrode. It is possible in some electrodes to manipulate the electrode to dislodge the bubble and correct the problem.

Much attention was originally given to the color of the silver–silver chloride electrode,[38] but the varied processes used in manufacturing these elements cause somewhat different shades of gray-black (brownish-black for some). The color should not noticeably change, but any change is almost impossible to detect. If the inner reference standard gets cloudy, it may or may not be defective. Usually there is some silver chloride present in this solution, and it can cause clouding without damaging the electrode. All these physical observations really only satisfy the questioning viewer. If the electrode is defective, it will test unsatisfactory in one or both the following tests.

## VI. A. 2. Measurement of Zero Potential of Glass Electrode

Short the meter input to reference with the shorting lead. Set temperature control to 25°.

a. With the meter in pH mode, adjust the meter to read 7.00 (or whatever the zero potential of the electrode is supposed to be). Lock the calibration knob in place.

b. Remove the shorting lead; plug in the electrodes.

c. Using a pH 7.00 buffer, read the mV response. Tolerance is specific for each electrode but usually is less than $\pm$ 15 mV.

We have found it is a good practice to check the zero potential of new electrodes to establish a base line for this test. As long as the amplifier can be balanced with a given electrode pair, the pH meter can usually operate satisfactorily. As mentioned when doing test Section III. A. 3. considerable range is allowed in most meters so that different electrodes can be used. The significance of this zero potential as a test procedure is in determining the changes that may occur with time. Many of these changes occur within the inner reference electrode, and eventually the amplifier can no longer be balanced with the aged electrode. However, a dirty electrode will have an increased zero potential, and this possibility must be eliminated before this test is performed.

### VI. A. 3. Resistance of the Glass Electrode

An increase of about 3- to 5-fold in the resistance of the glass electrode generally means the electrode has become defective. There are two points worthy of note:

a. To recognize a 3- to 5-fold increase in resistance one must have measured the resistance of the electrode when it was new.

b. The resistance values being considered are large differences and related to general "ballpark figures," examples of which were listed in Table 6-3, page 218.

The hydration state of the electrode will greatly affect the measured resistance, so before measuring the electrode be sure it is in its normal "in-use" state of hydration. A dry electrode may have a resistance which is several hundred times as much as that obtained when the same electrode is hydrated. The usual electrode will also increase manyfold when the temperature is markedly lowered; therefore, note the ambient temperature, and if possible, see that it is about 25°C.

Measurement of resistance can be made by either of the two following methods. The first method is quoted directly from Mattock,[44] and the circuit is given in Figure 6-24:

The cell should be set up with an external reference system identical to the inner reference system of the glass electrode. Thus for the inner reference of

Ag; AgCl 0.1$M$ HCl

the cell should consist of

glass electrode $\parallel$ 0.1$M$ HCl $\parallel$ AgCl;Ag

The open-circuit e.m.f. ($E_G + E_S$) is first measured, and then the glass electrode cell + series cell (which may be a Weston cell or other stable e.m.f. source) is shunted by the resistor R to give an e.m.f. $E_R$. If the glass electrode cell has a resistance $R_G$, $R_G = R(E_G + E_S - E_R)/E_R$. Best results are obtained when $R_G \approx R$(i.e., $E_G$

267

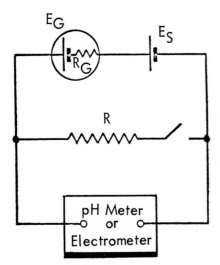

**Figure 6-24.** *Circuit for the measurement of resistance of a glass electrode. (Redrawn with permission from Mattock, G.: Laboratory pH measurements. In The Glass Electrode. New York, Interscience Publishers, after 1965, p. 81.)*

$+ E_S \approx 2E_R$). If drift is observed from dielectric absorption current decay in the glass, it is advisable to wait for stabilization of the voltage before noting the reading.*

The second method uses components of the electrode itself.[32] This circuit is shown in Figure 6-25. The electrode being measured is shown as A; B is the inner reference silver/silver chloride electrode and cap from a broken glass electrode identical to A. The bridge solution should consist of a buffer of approximately the same pH as the internal standard solution (usually pH 7.0) to which a small amount of silver chloride has been added. The voltage source is a 1.35 mercury battery. The meter shown is a sensitive ohm meter, but if this meter is not available, the meter scale of a pH meter can be calibrated by using a series of resistors in place of the electrical cell in the same circuit. We were cautioned about two points in this procedure:[32]

---

* By permission from Mattock, G.: Laboratory pH measurements. In *The Glass Electrode.* New York, Interscience Publishers, after 1965.

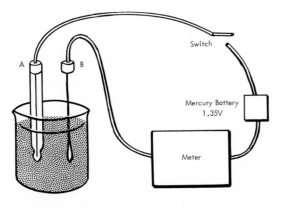

**Figure 6-25.** *Circuit for measuring resistance of glass electrode.*

1. Never leave the switch closed for more than 3 to 5 seconds at a time and repeat no more than necessary. This precaution avoids polarizing the electrode.
2. The differences in resistance must be large to be significant. If, for example, the electrode being checked ordinarily has a resistance of about 100 megohms, when it becomes defective, it will measure 300 megohms or more. A cracked glass membrane, on the other hand, will produce a very low resistance.

VI. B. REFERENCE ELECTRODES.    The appearance of the calomel reference electrode was described on page 199.  The points to be noted will be repeated here.

---

### VI. B. 1. Appearance of the Calomel Reference Electrode

a.  KCl solution: sufficient to cover most of the inner element; few crystals present; not caked over bottom.
b.  Inner column: Mercury at the top intact; no air bubbles in the calomel; color of the calomel, silver gray.
c.  Air vent (filling hole): not plugged but open only when electrode is in use.
d.  Liquid junction opening: appears clean and not clogged.

---

The liquid junction opening may be such that observation alone will not be sufficient. Direct observation of electrolyte flow through a paladium annulus, fiber, or fritted junction is not possible.[14] Development of a wet spot when a filter paper is held to one of these junctions does not tell more than that *some* electrolyte is being absorbed; sufficient flow can be proved by the response of the electrode in the test VI.B.2.b.

In order to distinguish the malfunction caused by a plugged liquid junction from that of a faulty calomel column, it is necessary to run two tests: (a) check of electrode resistance, and (b) response of the electrode to KCl versus that of a buffer.

---

### VI. B. 2, a. Check of Electrode Resistance

(1)  Immerse the electrode to a depth of about one inch in a beaker of saturated KCl solution.
(2)  Using an ohm meter connect one lead to the reference electrode cable jack and place the other lead tip into the beaker of KCl solution.
(3)  Measure the resistance of the electrode. A resistance greater than about 10 K ohms indicates either a clogged junction or a faulty internal column.

---

269

Usually the good electrode will have about 2 to 3 K ohms resistance, and the 10 K ohms thus represent a threefold increase. One must be sure of the specifications for the electrode before calling it defective. For example, the Beckman ceramic junction reference electrode is normally expected to have about 10 K ohms resistance; the quartz junction about 20 K ohms.[13] Therefore, the resistance value for a defective electrode of these types would have to increase to about 30 or 60 K respectively.

---

### VI. B. 2, b. Response to KCl Versus Buffer[14]

(1) Plug the test electrode and known-to-be-good reference electrode into the reference and glass electrode inlets to the meter (an adapter may be necessary for the glass electrode input position). Connect the good electrode to the glass electrode inlet.

(2) Set the meter to read in mV and record the response when both electrodes are immersed in buffer solution.

(3) Immerse both electrodes in saturated KCl solutions and record the mV response. Identical electrodes, both good, should read $0 \pm 5$ mV in the KCl solution. If the reading is not zero ($\pm 5$ mV) in the buffer solution, the liquid junction is plugged.

If the mV response of both electrodes is the same in both buffer and KCl but the reading is not zero ($\pm 5$ mV), the internal element of the electrode being tested is defective.

---

Several ways are available to try to unplug a clogged junction:

1. Plug the air vent and hold the electrode under hot water for about one minute. Then place the electrode in cool water. If the outlet has opened, a small stream of KCl will flow. Pressing the sleeve over the air vent may exert enough pressure to release the plug.

2. Boil electrode tip gently in a solution of KCl and let the tip remain immersed while the solution cools.

3. Dilute nitric acid can be substituted for the solution in which the tip is boiled as in #2 above). If this does not unplug the electrode, discard it.

4. A *fiber junction* can be slightly ground in an effort to free it when clogged. Caution: a grinding process should never be used on any other type junction.[14]

If the internal element is judged defective, there is one possibility for correcting it: clean the outer jacket and refill with fresh KCl. If this procedure does not help, the electrode must be discarded.

The crude measurement of the mV potential of the reference electrode, as described below, bears little resemblance to the determination of the standard potential of the calomel half-cell. In the routine use of the pH meter, when the calibration control cannot balance the amplifier, there may be at least three possibilities: the meter circuit itself, the glass electrode, or the reference electrode.

270

We use this test procedure to eliminate the reference electrode as the causative agent in the same way that we eliminate the glass electrode by the value of its zero potential. Reference electrodes of the same catalogue number from the same manufacturer are expected to check with each other more closely than are glass electrodes.

### VI. B. 3. Potential of the Reference Electrode

Connect the test unit (Fig. 6-23) and reference electrode as shown in Figure 6-26.

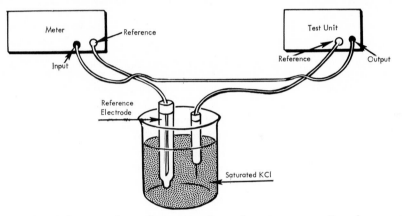

**Figure 6-26.** *Reference electrode, test unit, and meter connection for measuring electrode potential.*

    a.  Set test unit controls:
        Series Resistance Switch to 100 M.
        pH/mV Selector Switch to x10 mV.
        pH/mV Range Switch to 0; polarity switch to − mV.
        Off-On Switch to ON.

    b.  Set the pH meter to read mV response; we prefer the expanded scale, but either can be used.

    c.  Increase the Range Switch of the test unit from 0 to 15, 20, 25, 30, and 35 settings. Record the meter reading and the polarity of the mV response. Calculate the potential of the electrode from the difference between input and meter reading. See example in Table 6-15.

Tolerance between electrodes is expected to be about ± 5 mV, but with this procedure ours have been about ± 15.

As can be seen from Figure 6-26, no refined equipment is used for this test. The lead from the reference post of the test unit into the KCl bridge is a common test lead with one terminal jack simply placed in the beaker of KCl. The information gained from the procedure is enough to indicate a defective reference elec-

271

Table 6-15.  Example of Calculated Reference Electrode Potential

| Input from Test Unit | Meter Reading (expanded scale) | Calculated mV Response |
|---|---|---|
| −150 | −126 | −276 |
| −200 | − 76.5 | −276.5 |
| −250 | − 26.5 | −276.5 |
| −300 | + 23.5 | −276.5 |
| −350 | + 74.5 | −275.5 |

trode insofar as its suitably for use as part of the particular meter-electrode combination.

## VI. B. 4. KCl Used for the Salt Bridge

The salt bridge is expected to contain a saturated solution of analytical grade potassium chloride whose pH is neutral. The saturation is judged by the presence of KCl crystals in the bottom of the container. We have received some solutions marked "saturated" which contained no crystals. We do not think this is a satisfactory solution, and the manufacturer has replaced the material. The neutrality can be roughly checked by measuring the pH of a diluted sample of the KCl; we have never found this to be a problem.

If the purity of the KCl is not high enough, one contaminating material that will affect the pH measurement is the presence of even trace amounts of bromide.[45] Mattock suggests the following test to determine the presence of bromine.[45]

    a. Drop a small quantity of chromic acid into a sample of the saturated solution of KCl.

    b. Into the vapor, quickly insert a filter strip which has previously been dipped into a solution of the sodium salt of fluorescein. The presence of bromine will turn the color of the strip from yellow to brown.

We have never obtained a KCl solution whose purity we felt was questionable and so have not used this test. The original reference includes a method for purifying the material if desired.

## REFERENCES

1. Adams, A. P., Morgan-Hughes, J. O., and Sykes, M. K.: pH and blood gas analysis, Part I. Anaesthesia, 22:575, 1967.

2. ASTM: E 70-52T; pH of aqueous solutions with the glass electrode. 1967 Book of ASTM Standards, Part 30. Philadelphia, American Society for Testing Materials.

3. Bates, R. G.: Determination of pH: Theory and Practice. New York, John Wiley & Sons, Inc., 1964.

4. ———: Electrodes for pH measurement. J. Electroanal. Chem., 2:93, 1961.

5. ———: Electrometric pH determination. Chimia, 14:111, 1960.

6. ———: Meaning and standardization of pH measurements. In Symposium on pH Measurement. ASTM Special Technical Publication #190, Philadelphia, 1956.

7. ——: Revised standard values for pH measurements from 0 to 95°C. J. Res. NBS., *66A:* 179, 1962.

8. ——, and Covington, A. K.: Behavior of the glass electrode and other pH-responsive electrodes in biological media. Ann. N. Y. Acad. Sci., *148:*67, 1968.

9. ——, and Guggenheim, E. A.: Report on the standardization of pH and related terminology. Pure Appl. Chem., *1:*163, 1960.

10. Beck, W. H., Bottom, A. E., and Covington, A. K.: Errors of glass electrodes in certain standard buffer solutions at high discrimination. Anal. Chem. *40:*501, 1968.

11. Beck, W. H., Caudle, J., Covington, A. K., and Wynne-Jones, W.F.K.: Precise measurements with the glass electrode: the time variation of EMF. Proc. Chem. Soc., 110, 1963.

12. Beckman Instructions for Research pH Meter: Bulletin 1226-B. Beckman Instruments, Inc., Fullerton, Calif., April, 1964.

13. Beckman Instructions, 81618: The Use and Care of Futura Electrodes. Beckman Instruments, Inc., Fullerton, Calif., April, 1969.

14. Beckman Instructions for Zeromatic pH Meter: Bulletin 1382-B. Beckman Instruments, Inc., Fullerton, Calif., August, 1965.

15. Beckman Bulletin 7147-A: Beckman pH Meters. Beckman Instruments, Inc., Fullerton, Calif., May, 1969.

16. Beckman Bulletin 86-T: Supplies for pH Meters. Beckman Instruments, Inc., Fullerton, Calif., 1968.

17. Brems, N.: Measurements of pH. Electrodes and pertinent apparatus. Acta Anaesth. Scand., Suppl. *11:*199, 1962.

18. Clark, W. R., and Perley, G. A.: Modern developments in pH instrumentation. In *Symposium on pH Measurement.* ASTM Special Technical Publication #190. Philadelphia, 1956.

19. Corning Service Manual for Model 12 pH Meter. Corning Glass Works, Corning, N. Y., September, 1967.

20. Dicker, D. H.: The laboratory pH meter. Amer. Lab. 73, February, 1969.

21. Doremus, R. H.: Diffusion potentials in glass. In *Glass Electrodes for Hydrogen and Other Cations.* G. Eisenman, Ed. New York, Marcel Dekker, Inc., 1967.

22. Eisenman, G.: Particular properties of cation-selective glass electrodes containing $Al_2O_3$. In *Glass Electrodes for Hydrogen and Other Cations.* New York, Marcel Dekker, Inc., 1967.

23. ——: The electrochemistry of cation-selective glass electrodes. In *The Glass Electrode.* New York, Interscience Publishers, (no date—after 1965).

24. ——: The origin of the glass electrode potential. In *Glass Electrodes for Hydrogen and Other Cations.* New York, Marcel Dekker, Inc., 1967.

25. Ensman, R., and Yount, R.: Personal communication. Indiana University, Bloomington.

26. Ewing, G. W.: *Instrumental Methods of Chemical Analysis.* New York, McGraw-Hill Book Co., 1969.

27. Feldman, I.: Use and abuse of pH measurements. Anal. Chem. *28:*1859, 1956.

28. Fischer, R. B., and Peters, D. G.: *Basic Theory and Practice of Quantitative Chemical Analysis.* Philadelphia, W. B. Saunders Co., 1968.

29. Gleason, D. F.: pH measurements. Arch. Intern. Med. *116:*649, 1965.

30. Gold, V.: *pH Measurements: Their Theory and Practice.* New York, John Wiley & Sons, Inc., 1956.

31. Guggenheim, E. A.: A study of cells with liquid-liquid junctions. J. Amer. Chem. Soc. *52:*1315, 1930.

32. Haadad, I.: Personal communication. Instrumentation Laboratory, Inc. Lexington, Mass.

33. Hanlon, T.: Personal communication. Corning Glass Co., Corning, N. Y.

34. Heath: Operation of the pH/MV Test Unit, Model EUA-20-12. Heath Company, Benton Harbor, Mich., December, 1965.

35. Hills, G. J., and Ives, D. J. G.: The calomel electrode and other mercury-mercurous salt electrodes. In *Reference Electrodes: Theory and Practice.* D. J. G. Ives and G. J. Janz, Eds. New York, Academic Press, 1961.

36. Isard, J. O.: The dependence of glass-electrode properties on composition. In *Glass Electrodes for Hydrogen and Other Cations.* G. Eisenman, Ed. New York, Marcel Dekker, Inc., 1967.

37. Jackson, J.: The glass electrode, temperature-potential relationships. Chem. & Ind. 7, January 3, 1948.

38. Janz, G. J., and Taniguchi, H.: The silver-silver halide electrodes. Chem. Rev. *53:*397, 1953.

39. Leeds & Northrup: Instruction Manual for #7401 pH Meter. Bulletin 177166, 1965.

40. Lewin, S. Z.: Chemical instrumentation, #5. pH meters, Part I. J. Chem. Educ. *36:*A477, 1959.

41. ———: Chemical instrumentation, #5. pH meters, Part II. J. Chem. Educ. *36:*A595, 1959.

42. Long, C., Ed.: *Biochemists Handbook.* Princeton, N. J., D. VanNostrand, 1968.

43. Malmstadt, H. V., Enke, C. G., and Toren, E. C., Jr.: *Electronics for Scientists.* New York, W. A. Benjamin, Inc., 1963.

44. Mattock, G.: Laboratory pH measurements. In *The Glass Electrode.* New York, Interscience Publishers, (no date—after 1965).

45. ———: *pH Measurement and Titration.* London, Heywood & Co., Ltd., 1961.

46. ———: The accurate measurement of pH. Part II, Sources of experimental error in pH measurement. Lab. Pract. *6:*521, 1957.

47. ———: The accurate measurement of pH. Part III, Discussion of examples. Lab. Pract. *6:*577, 1957.

48. ———, and Band, D. M.: Interpretation of pH and cation measurements. In *Glass Electrodes for Hydrogen and Other Cations.* G. Eisenman, Ed. New York, Marcel Dekker, Inc., 1967.

49. Meloan, C. E.: Electrodes. In *Instrumental Analysis Using Physical Properties.* Philadelphia, Lea & Febiger, 1968.

50. Milazzo, G. M., and Bombara, G.: Reference electrodes and tensions. J. Electroanal. Chem. *1:*265, 1960.

51. Moore, E. W.: Determination of pH by the glass electrode: pH meter calibration for gastric analysis. Gastroenterology, *54:*501, 1968.

52. ———: Hydrogen and cation analysis in biological fluids in vitro. In *Glass Electrodes for Hydrogen and Other Cations.* G. Eisenman, Ed. New York, Marcel Dekker, Inc., 1967.

53. ———, and Scarlata, R. W.: The determination of gastric acidity by the glass electrode. Gastroenterology, *49:*178, 1965.

54. Nicolsky, B. P., Schultz, M. M., Belijustin, A. A., and Lev, A. A.: Recent developments in the ion-exchange theory of the glass electrode and its application in the chemistry of glass. In *Glass Electrodes for Hydrogen and Other Cations*. G. Eisenman, Ed. New York, Marcel Dekker, Inc., 1967.

55. Picoff, R. C., and Trainer, T. D.: Physiology of gastric juice. ASCP Commission on Cont. Educ. ST-43, January, 1969.

56. Rechnitz, G. A.: Ion-selective electrodes. Chem. and Eng. News, *45:*146, 1967.

57. Sekelj, P., and Goldbloom, R. B.: Clinical application of cation-sensitive glass electrodes. In *Glass Electrodes for Hydrogen and Other Cations*. G. Eisenman, Ed. New York, Marcel Dekker, Inc., 1967.

58. Sibbald, P. G., and Matsuyama, G.: Hydrogen cell assembly for standard electromotive force measurement. Anal. Chem., *35:*1718, 1963.

59. Siggaard-Andersen, O.: Factors affecting the liquid junction potential in electrometric blood pH measurement. Scand. J. Clin. Lab. Invest., *13:*205, 1961.

60. Stacy, R. W.: *Biological and Medical Electronics*. New York, McGraw-Hill Book Co., Inc., 1960.

61. Stott, F. D.: *Instruments in Clinical Medicine*. Philadelphia, F. A. Davis Co., 1967.

62. Taylor, G. R.: pH measuring instruments. In *pH Measurement and Titration*. G. Mattock, Ed. London, Heywood and Company, Ltd., 1961.

63. Willard, H. H., Merritt, L. L., Jr., and Dean, J. A.: *Instrumental Methods of Analysis*. Princeton, D. VanNostrand Co., Inc., 1965.

64. Wright, M. P.: pH measurement with the glass electrode. In *A Symposium on pH and Blood Gas Measurement*. London, J. and A. Churchill, Ltd., 1959.

65. Wynn, V. and Ludbrook, J.: A method of measuring the pH of body fluids. Lancet, *1:*1068, 1957.

# 7

# Coulter Counters

Electronic cell counters have become increasingly more popular, not only for counting the red and white blood cells but also, with the additional modules, for simultaneously determining the hemoglobin and then calculating other related values. Coulter models A, B, or F, in our opinion, can be calibrated and relied upon to count accurately all cells whose volume exceeds that indicated by the Threshold setting. While Haemocytometer counts have been used by some operators to reassure themselves that the Coulter was counting properly, we think this procedure is useless in that the precision and accuracy of the Coulter far exceeds that of the technologists' manual counts. We recognize, however, that for these Coulter counts to be accurate, the instrument must be functioning properly in every respect, the specimen must fairly represent what it purports to represent, and the operator must be able to assess the validity of the results.[25]

With the appearance of the Coulter Model S, a whole new set of considerations has become necessary. Since all the actual numbers which print out for different tests of the blood sample can be varied by adjusting voltage settings, some sample must be declared a standard to which all settings can be adjusted. Several modified blood preparations are currently being sold as standards. To date we have found no such material entirely satisfactory for use as the primary standard. The only alternative is to standardize the Coulter S settings from bloods run on one of our other Coulter Counters (either Model A or F), which we closely monitor and consider the master instrument. The proper calibration of any of the Coulter Counters is complicated by the differences in the size of white blood cells in different diluent-lysing agent combinations. These considerations will be discussed fully later. We are convinced that it is absolutely mandatory to calibrate the master

276

Coulter for its equivalent cubic micron value per threshold unit and to monitor closely the counting process with a specific quality control system. Such a system must include basic counting technique (including sample and diluents), check procedures to ascertain that the instrument is functioning properly, instrument calibration, outline for adequate routine instrument maintenance, and some means of evaluating daily the test results obtained on the instrument.

## BASIC COUNTING TECHNIQUE

The basic counting technique must take into consideration:

1. The collected sample. What anticoagulant has been used and how much?
2. The dilution of the sample. What diluent is satisfactory for the RBC, the WBC; what lysing agent can best be used for the WBC; what automatic dilutors can be used, and what is their accuracy and precision?
3. The physical mechanics of presenting the diluted sample to the instrument for counting.

A recent report by Brittin et al.[4] showed not only that blood collected in sodium or potassium salts of EDTA* was the sample of choice but also that, stored at refrigerator temperatures, these bloods gave stable values for at least 24 hours for RBC, WBC, hemoglobin, hematocrit, MCV, MCH, and MCHC. If left at room temperature, the same bloods gave white blood counts which were essentially the

* Vacutainers, containing $Na_2EDTA$ or containing $K_3EDTA$, Becton Dickinson, Rutherford, N. J.

277

same. The RBC, however, though virtually unchanged numerically, had swollen about 1 to 3%. Such a sample would then be unsatisfactory for the hematocrit, MCV, or MCHC. The effect is the same whether these test values are produced by calculations from centrifuged hematocrits or by the measured MCV on an instrument such as the Coulter S.

The amount of EDTA per cubic centimeter of blood should not exceed 2 mgm/cc.[17] A safe rule is to insist that the BD Vacutainers containing enough anti-coagulant for 7 ml blood be filled to at least half their capacity. While the cyanmethemoglobin value is not affected by excess EDTA, the centrifuged hematocrit value is reduced, and manually calculated MCV and MCHC are inaccurate.[14] On the other hand, excess EDTA is said to have no effect on the MCV of the red cells suspended in Isoton and measured on the Coulter $S^2$ or the Coulter F with a computer module attached.[14] These varied effects of excess EDTA can cause apparent discrepancies when a particular sample is checked with different instruments unless the user is aware of the possibilities.

Inadequate mixing of the sample has been pointed out as the most common cause of error in the instruments that perform and/or calculate all seven parameters simultaneously.[24] A rocking or rotating automatic mixing device is highly recommended; from 5 to 15 minutes is usually required, depending upon the efficiency of the device. It is virtually impossible to detect from the test values printed out or the scan of the differential that the sample has not been mixed adequately. For this reason some users spot-check hematocrits or hemoglobins as part of a quality control system. Such a spot-check may or may not catch the poorly mixed stat sample someone hurried to put on the instrument. As a means of catching such errors, large institutions such as the National Institutes of Health have sometimes programmed their instrument system to display the most recent previous report on the same patient while the current work is being done.[10] Those of us in even the smallest institution can control this source of error ourselves by insisting upon a specific manner and time for mixing the sample.

## DILUENTS

The primary requirements for diluents used in blood cell enumeration are:

1. That the diluent be an electrolyte of suitable conductivity to satisfy the theoretical and practical considerations of electronic counting;
2. That the diluent maintain the morphologic integrity and the volume of the cell being enumerated during the period of exposure; and
3. That the diluent contribute few particles to the count.

When the Coulter instrument is restricted to counting a red or a white cell suspension, it is relatively easy to calibrate the instrument and to choose settings that will count all the cells. It is an entirely different matter to choose a diluent capable of precisely maintaining the red cell volume so that one can measure the mean cell volume and calculate the resulting hematocrit. And it is yet a further challenge to find a single diluent that can maintain the red cell volume and also satisfactorily be used with a lysing agent to count accurately the smallest of the white blood cells present.

278

## Diluents for Erythrocytes

Normal saline used alone cannot maintain the precise red cell volume. The most important single consideration in obtaining constant volume is said to be the pH of the diluent.[5] With a lowering of the pH of the diluent, the normal red blood cell swells until it reaches its maximum size at pH 5.4; its minimum size occurs at approximately pH 8.1 in phosphate buffers. Although normal red cells begin to hemolyze at a pH of 5.13 $\pm$ 0.08, the abnormal cells found in hemolytic anemia, pernicious anemia, or leukemia can begin to hemolyze at a pH of 7.1.[28] For these reasons many buffered solutions have been suggested whose pH values range between 7 and 8. Saline buffered with TRIS and adjusted to pH 7.4 gives a mean red cell volume of 92 $\pm$ 0.9 $\mu^3$.[6] Oulie solution[16, 21] is saline with phosphate buffer at pH 7.55. Williamson solution is another saline and phosphate buffer combination with a pH of 7.3.[8] While all of the above solutions appear to be able to maintain the red cell volume, the most commonly used solution is some modification of Eagle's solution.[5, 14, 25] This solution has a pH of about 7.5, and the osmolality is approximately 280 to 325 mOsm/liter, depending upon the exact composition.

The composition of one of these modified Eagle's solutions is as follows:

---

### Eagle's Solution

| | |
|---|---|
| $NaH_2PO_4 \cdot H_2O$ | 0.14 gm |
| NaCl | 6.8 |
| Glucose | 0.9 |
| $NaHCO_3$ | 2.2 |
| $MgCl_2 \cdot 6 H_2O$ | 0.19 |
| $CaCl_2$ | 0.2 |
| KCl | 0.4 |

Dissolve the salts in water and make up to a volume of one liter. Filter through a 0.8$\mu$ Millipore filter and store in the refrigerator.

---

Isoton* is one such solution commercially available; the producer holds the tolerance from batch to batch so that no more than 1% difference should occur in the measured MCV of red blood cells. This solution is currently widely used, and because it is used with the Coulter Counter S, appears to be the solution of choice for the master Coulter to which the Coulter S is standardized.

If a Coulter Counter is used only to count cells and not to measure MCV, saline is a satisfactory diluent. The 0.9 gm % NaCL should have 1 cc of neutral formalin added per liter. Since sodium chloride is a neutral salt, the water used to make the diluent will affect its pH; the water should have a pH between 6 and 7.[29] While saline can be used for routine counting, this Coulter Counter, however, must be calibrated with Eagle's solution or Isoton, as discussed later.

---

* Coulter Diagnostics, Inc. Hialeah, Fla.

279

### Diluents and Lysing Agents for Leukocytes

Even though Coulter Counters have been used for more than 10 years to count blood cells, there appears to be no consensus on the choice of diluent and lysing agent for leukocytes. Brittin, in his recent evaluation of the Coulter S, used Isoton to count the RBC on his Coulter A and Cetrimide-citrate-saline for the WBC.[3] Originally this latter solution was cited as preferable because the stromatolyzing takes place almost instantaneously and base line noise on the oscilloscope is practically absent.[9] A combination of saponin-citrate-saline was said to provide valid white counts but a 10 to 15 minute period was required for proper stromatolysis. D'Angelo and Lacombe also considered Cetrimide-saline combination as rapidly toxic to white blood cells; they found saponin-saline alone unreliable in that the count increased and then decreased rapidly.[9] Our experience with saline and saponin has been generally satisfactory as long as the saline included neutralized formalin and was made from water of good quality. Occasionally a bad lot of saponin was encountered several years ago; recently we have had no problem with the saponin from Coulter.

Allen reported a WBC reagent with which he could produce white cell distribution curves even for the abnormal cells of leukemia.[1] This diluent contains EDTA, sucrose, ethanolic formalin, picric acid, and saponin. His average CV was 0.8% for counts between 2,500 and 187,000 compared to haemocytometer counts. The chief advantage of this diluting fluid is that it can preserve WBC for more than 24 hours without shrinking them. The diluent, however, cannot be used to count RBC, and one must again use two different diluents for routine counting of blood cells.

A sodium chloride-sodium acetate-formalin diluent adjusted to pH 6 has been recommended for use with saponin for white counts.[20] Red blood cells swell in this diluent, however, so it cannot be used if the MCV is being measured.

Popular commercially available lysing agents for leukocytes include saline and saponin* or Zaponin-saline,* Isoton and Zap-Isoton,* or Isoton and Lyse S.* Each of these lysing agents produces a different peak height (*i.e.,* cell size) for the same white cell suspension. One must be very careful, therefore, that the threshold chosen for counting the suspension is low enough to accommodate the maximum "shrinkage" of the smallest white cell, the small lymphocyte. It has been our experience that this cell can be as small as $40\mu^3$ in the Isoton-Zap-Isoton solution; it is about 85 $\mu^3$ in a saline-saponin solution.

Therefore, one cannot change at will from one diluent-lysing agent combination to another. One must choose the "stromatolyzing solution based on consideration of all types of abnormal cells. . . . A simple check on a few normal bloods, or replicates on the same blood, affords little proof of the quality of a stromatolyzing solution for use in counting WBC electronically."[13] If the cells remain intact, one can then proceed to determine the smallest cell volume that must be included in the threshold setting. This procedure is discussed under Calibration.

---

* Coulter Diagnostics, Inc., Hialeah, Fla.

Whatever lysing agent is chosen, its reaction must be checked. Saponin we make weekly and check when made. Other ready-to-use materials should certainly be checked for each change in lot number or preferably at weekly intervals.

---

### Lysing Time

1. Prepare 50 cc of a 1:500 suspension of WBC in the diluent usually used.
2. To this suspension add the appropriate amount of the lysing agent usually used and start a stopwatch.
3. At *one minute* intervals for *20 minutes* repeat white blood counts, suspending the cells by gentle swirling every *5 minutes*.
4. Post the acceptable time range for the lysing agent. The lysing time that is acceptable falls within the range that gives counts that do not vary by more than ± 2%. For our saponin, this period is usually 2 to 20 minutes.

---

## DILUTING EQUIPMENT

While it is desirable to check the calibration of all volumetric glassware, pipettes, and dilutors, we find it a physical impossibility. Spot-checking of pipettes can most easily be done by comparing dilutions of dye to those made with National Bureau of Standards certified pipettes as described by Ellerbrook.[12] We have found that Accupettes* generally check well with their specified tolerance. These are TC pipettes available with ½ or 1% error limits.

Dilutors are more likely to be suspect than good pipettes and flasks. Of the many on the market, we have not been able to find one which is unequivocally trustworthy. We use several different ones and believe the delivery of each should be checked daily. Since most of these are set to deliver 10 cc, it is convenient to check their output against previously checked Kimax† volumetric flasks. Output should be checked each morning before beginning to use the dilutor.

The first delivery should be discarded and the next three should be measured. Dilutors that both aspirate the sample and dispense it diluted must be checked by manual dilutions. Leaky connections can allow the total dispensed quantity to remain correct, but the amount of aspirated sample can be incorrect.

It is difficult to assign a separate precision for the diluting process and the counting procedures. Through the years we have found Richar and Breakell's[26] original acceptance limits easy to maintain. For counting the same dilution, repeats should check within 2%; for different dilutions, counts of aliquot should be within 7%. These are overall laboratory performance limits and one single individual might be able to establish a narrower range. Brittin recently has reported his Coefficient of Variation for RBC by hand dilution in Isoton as 1.4%.[4]

---

\* Available from Scientific Products, McGraw Park, Ill.

† Corning Glass Works, Corning, N. Y.

## THE ESSENTIALS OF GOOD TECHNIQUE

Good technique must be applied with *every* count with the Coulter Counter. With care the dividends are accuracy and freedom from uncertainty. Without care, results at best are dubious and at worst are merely approximate guesses.

Counting a control suspension does not serve as a control of the process unless uniform technique is invariably applied. The control count may be a valid indicator of instrument and operator performance for a specific count; however, carelessness with the next sample or instrument failure could cause the next count to be totally unacceptable. Control suspensions are useful but cannot be relied on as the sole means of monitoring the counting procedure. Good technique and consistency from count to count are essential, and *care* must become a habit.

Before starting the counting for the day, the background count of the diluent must be determined at both RBC and WBC instrument settings. In the following directions saline and saponin are mentioned; the same procedure should be applicable to whatever diluent and lysing agent are used. Minor changes such as the period of time the WBC should stand after adding the lysing agent will be necessary for specific materials. With Isoton, RBC dilutions appear stable somewhat longer than three minutes, but it is well to count these suspensions immediately, especially if the MCV is being measured. The nomenclature in the directions is that for the Coulter Counter, Model A, but the procedure is essentially the same for other models.

---

## *Counting Technique*

1. Count the background of the diluent three times at the proper instrument settings for RBC, and average the second and third count. Hereinafter, the term count refers to three consecutive counts made and reported as the average of the second and third. Record the counts. If the count is over 200, the diluent must be refiltered before use.

2. Flush the system well with diluent from the reservoir and record the count at the same settings. If the count is over 200, this will be indicative of particle contamination of the reservoir diluent and/or the connections to it.

3. To 10 cc of diluent add 0.1 cc saponin and again count background at the settings used for the leukocyte count. The count should be less than 50; if greater, the possibility of saponin contamination should be considered. (Steps 1, 2 and 3 are not performed with each count; these are done daily and also whenever a question arises.)

4. Add 0.02 cc blood to 10 cc diluent and mix gently. This is the primary dilution. Transfer from the primary dilution, 0.1 cc to 10 cc diluent, and count for red cells *in less than three minutes after the dilution.*

5. The primary dilution is used for white cells that may be counted conveniently in groups of 10. Add 0.1 cc saponin to each of the primary dilutions, which are counted within the time limits established by the saponin check on that batch. This is usually 2 to 20 minutes.

6. The tube containing the suspension to be counted is inverted *once,* poured into a 15 cc beaker, and placed on the platform.

7. Open the control stopcock, and clear the reset switch. Close the stopcock.

8. Glance at the mercury as it traverses the loop section of the manometer and be sure it travels at the proper speed. With experience, a glance will suffice. Listen to the cadence of the count and watch the pattern on the oscilloscope.

9. The counts are to be made as described above. The second and third counts of the set must agree with one another within 2% of the recorded count; *e.g.,* 5,000,000 ± 100,000. (This is an impossibility if polarity shift occurs.)

10. White cell counts over 100,000 should be rediluted,[19] so that the suspension contains no more than 50,000 cells. We redilute white cell counts that are over 65,000. Red cell counts should be corrected when very high white cell counts are observed on the sample, since white cells are not eliminated in the red cell suspension.

11. Correct both red and white counts for coincident passage, using the tables furnished with the instrument.

---

We began repeating the background count after flushing because one counter developed a growth of fungus inside the latex tubing from the diluent reservoir. The first indication was a sporadic increase of red cell count that was about 500,000 too high. After flushing, background counts on the diluent at erythrocyte settings were found to be 5,000. This experience also taught us to change the tubing at 6 month intervals.

The first count of the three for each dilution could be higher than the other two because of bubbles in the suspension. Look at all three values and watch for polarity shift—*i.e.,* counts that are higher or lower as related to the position of the relay switch. For example, 425, 450, and 428 for consecutive counts would indicate polarity shift. Bubbles might give counts such as 460, 425, and 428. Some diluents are more prone to bubble than others.

The user of the Coulter Counter should make it a habit to watch the oscilloscope pattern, listen to the cadence, and glance at the mercury as it traverses the manometer tube. The scope pattern will show a steady image with peaks at approximately the same height when all is going well. Figure 7-1, A is an example of such a pattern for RBC. If the orifice starts to plug, the peaks will show a slight increase in height; the pattern will be interrupted with vacant spots; blurring may occur; and the pattern may flash on and off the screen. An example of this pattern is B of Figure 7-1. The cadence will be regular until the orifice begins to plug; then, it also becomes irregular. This change in cadence is easier heard in the slower leukocyte count, but it is also detectable in the RBC by the experienced operator. Any irregularity in the sound indicates that the count is invalid. The mercury travel time becomes slower with a plugging orifice, and a glance is enough for a good operator to note the difference.

283

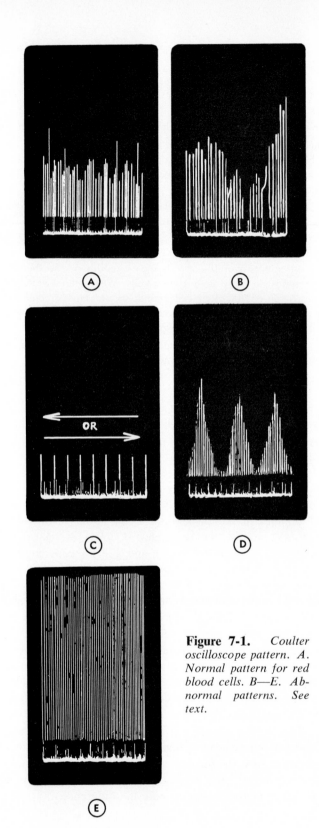

**Figure 7-1.** *Coulter oscilloscope pattern. A. Normal pattern for red blood cells. B—E. Abnormal patterns. See text.*

# BASIC INSTRUMENT FUNCTION CHECKS

Before actually calibrating the instrument, the operator must establish that his counting technique is precise (page 282) and that the instrument itself is functioning properly. The checks we use for this purpose are diluent background count, mercury travel time, polarity shift, and threshold zero. After the instrument has been calibrated, the best check we have found to ascertain that the electronics have mtaintained their linearity is the proportionality of the calibration factor at different gain and aperture current settings. This check will be discussed after the calibration procedure.

## Diluent Background Count

Directions for counting the diluent background are included in the count procedure on page 282.

## Mercury Travel Time

Two electrodes within the manometer loop mark the precise volume of 0.5 cc. When the mercury travels around the manometer loop and contacts the first electrode ("start" electrode), the instrument starts to record the count. It continues to count until the mercury contacts the second electrode ("stop" electrode).

For the count to be valid, this mercury travel time must remain consistent.

---

### *Mercury Travel Time*

1. Present any cell suspension for counting as usual.
2. With a stopwatch, measure the period of time required for the mercury to travel between the "start" and "stop" electrodes.
3. Repeat three times to check consistency.

Tolerance: time required from start to stop points on the manometer loop should be 13 to 17 seconds.

---

Too long a travel time is usually caused by a plugged orifice. A short travel time results from leaks in the manometer system, stopcocks, or the orifice headpiece connection. An inconsistent time can result from any of the above or from dirty mercury.

A decreased speed of mercury travel causes positive errors in the counts, and conversely, an increased speed of travel causes negative counting errors. Red cell counts were regularly observed to be about 1,000,000 too low when an air leak developed around the "start" electrode in the manometer loop. The decrease in count will be apparent before the visible salt encrustation develops on the outside of the tubing.

### Polarity Shift

A white cell suspension is recommended to check for polarity because relatively high threshold settings are required for counting these suspensions. When a polarity shift is present, the higher threshold settings always show the change first.

---

### *Polarity Shift*

1. Present any white cell suspension for counting with the Aperture Current and Gain set as usually used.
2. Take two consecutive counts at each threshold setting, starting at 50. Be careful to use each side of the relay for the two counts; if the relay switch must be clicked more than once, be sure not to lose account of which side of the relay switch has been used.
3. If the two counts agree within ± 2%, there is no polarity shift. If the counts do not agree, check three or more consecutive counts to be sure the discrepancy is related to polarity—*i.e.*, the first and third counts agree, and the second and fourth are lower or higher than the other pair.
4. If a polarity shift is present, check lower threshold settings and determine where it begins.

---

Originally we naively believed there was only one cause of polarity shift, the one given in the manual in which feedback from the electrode adds to the count on one polarity and subtracts from it on the other. The average of two consecutive counts is then valid and correct. Since then, we have had many instances of polarity shift. After our electronics serviceman has corrected the polarity, we have often repeated counts to see how correct they would have been if we had averaged the original counts and continued using the instrument. Sometimes the average count would have been correct. At other times, however, either the higher or the lower count would have been more accurate. We are now convinced that the polarity must be corrected as quickly as possible, and any counts taken during periods of polarity shift should be viewed with suspicion and used with great caution.

One cause of polarity shift can be a buildup charge on the orifice tube. As soon as a polarity shift is detected, the operator should either clean the orifice tube and try it again or substitute orifice tubes while the one is being cleaned. Two other causes can be (1) dirty contacts or a defective relay switch or (2) a phase inverter circuit not tuned properly. Correction for these causes may be beyond the scope of most operators and should be undertaken only after consultation with the manufacturer or a competent electronics repairman.

### Threshold Zero Check

The base line and the threshold line should merge when the threshold dial is moved to zero. When they do not merge, the dial may be physically misaligned on the shaft, or the electronic response may not be linear and go through zero. Because the two lines appear to merge does not guarantee that the electronic setting is correct. The following test will detect incorrect adjustment of Threshold Zero at the sensitivity that will affect routine use. A more stringent modification of this test can be used as part of the electronic check of the instrument and is given on page 293.

The gain is such that by raising it two increments (*e.g.,* from 4 to 6) the pulse height is doubled. By doubling the Threshold Setting and raising the Gain two increments, one should get the same count within the reproducibility limits of the instrument. If the counts check, the electronic system (for the particular aperture current used) is linear in response and goes through zero.

---

## Threshold Zero Check

1. With the Aperture Current set in its usual position, count a cell suspension twice at Gain 4 and a Threshold setting of 10.

2. Count the same cell suspension twice at Gain 6 and Threshold 20.

3. Repeat for Gain 2 and Threshold 5.

All counts should check with $\pm 2\%$. If they do not, adjust the Threshold Zero Set Screw and repeat the test until the counts do check.

---

## CALIBRATION OF THE COULTER COUNTER

The Coulter Counter counts all particles present in the solution which are larger than the size determined by the Threshold dial setting. Calibration of the instrument is the determination of how many cubic microns each division of this threshold scale represents, *i.e.,* the value of the calibration factor for a specific Aperture Current and Gain setting. The diluent used can affect the calibration factor and therefore must also be taken into consideration. The small lymphocytes may easily be smaller than the size of cell counted if the exact size determined by the threshold setting is not known continually. This is especially true for a diluent-lysing combination that badly "shrinks" the leukocytes.

Provided that proper details of counting procedure are followed, the counting of cells involves only two considerations in the Coulter:

1. Use of an Aperture Current that will make the majority of the peaks of the cells being counted fall at slightly over one-half the height of the oscilloscope screen; and

2. Selection of a Threshold value low enough to be below *all* the peaks of the cells and high enough to miss the "noise" (or "grass") of debris or background interference.

With aging of instrument components, polarity shifts, or changes in diluent characteristics (both diluent conductivity and diluent effect upon the cells being

287

counted) the calibration factor changes. Therefore, one must have a permanent "benchmark" calibration to which the instrument can continually be compared to know exactly what size cells are being counted. Additionally, if several counters are used in the same institution, it is highly desirable to be able to set them all to count the same size cells. If the instruments count exactly the same size cells, the resulting counts should agree within $\pm 2\%$.

Comparison of the calibration factor from time to time and for different Aperture Current and Gain settings is an extremely valuable check on the electronics of the instrument; this will be discussed later.

### Determination of the Calibration Factor

Calibration is accomplished by performing several erythrocyte mean cell threshold (MCT) curves on the instrument and relating these to the volumes they represent in terms of threshold divisions on the dial. One can thus determine in cubic microns the volume that is equivalent to one division on the threshold dial. The calibration factor should be established as the average of factors obtained on at least three fresh normal blood specimens representing the total normal MCV range. Individual calibration factors for these bloods should not vary among themselves by more than $\pm 0.2$ cubic microns.

We prefer to use blood collected in Vacutainers containing $Na_2$ or $K_3$ EDTA but the samples should contain at least 5 cc of blood. Excess EDTA shrinks the red cells, and the hematocrit is too low. The microhematocrit (Strumia et al.[27]) has been shown to be 1 to 3% lower than the macro method because the packing of cells is more complete.[23] For this reason the micro method is preferable.

---

### Calibration Procedure

The following calibration procedure is somewhat modified from that suggested by Magath[19] and Grant et al.:[15]

1. The microhematocrit should be determined five times and averaged.

2. Prepare a 1:50,000 dilution of the blood in Eagle's solution or Isoton. A 1:500 dilution can be conveniently made with 0.02 cc blood in 10 cc diluent. Mix by gentle inversion. Dilute 1 cc of the suspension to 100 cc in a volumetric flask. Mix gently and transfer an aliquot into a 50 ml beaker. Count from this beaker.

3. With control stopcock open, clear the reset switch. Do not close the control stopcock. Allow the suspension to flow through the orifice and observe the pattern on the oscilloscope.
   With the ACS switch, select a setting that will allow the majority of the peaks to fall a little less than half the height of the oscilloscope screen. This is then the preferable ACS for the calibration. Gain is usually set at 4 or 5. On our instruments the ACS setting proves to be 5, with a gain of 4.

4. Count the suspension twice at selected ACS with Threshold set at 5, and record as shown in Column 2 of the Calibration Sheet, Figure 7-2. In recording, omit the last two digits and record the third figure to the nearest whole number.

*Continued on page 290*

| #1 Threshold Settings "t" | #2 Cell Counts at different "t" readings | #3 Average cell counts from Column #2 draw graph from Column #3 | #3 corr. for Coincidence | #4 Average "t" settings between successive "t" settings | #5 Subtract successive cell counts in Column #3 draw graph from Column #5 | #6 Total volume to obtain multiply Column #5 by Column #4 |
|---|---|---|---|---|---|---|
| 5 | 478 / 474 | 476 | 535 | | | |
| | | | | 7.5 | 0 | |
| 10 | 474 / 480 | 476 | 535 | | | |
| | | | | 12.5 | 33 | 412.5 |
| 15 | 448 / 450 | 449 | 502 | | | |
| | | | | 17.5 | 182 | 3185.0 |
| 20 | 299 / 295 | 297 | 320 | | | |
| | | | | 22.5 | 151 | 3397.5 |
| 25 | 161 / 163 | 162 | 169 | | | |
| | | | | 27.5 | 64 | 1760.0 |
| 30 | 102 / 102 | 102 | 105 | | | |
| | | | | 32.5 | 49 | 1592.5 |
| 35 | 57 / 55 | 56 | 56 | | | |
| | | | | 37.5 | 26 | 975.0 |
| 40 | 30 / 30 | 30 | 30 | | | |
| | | | | 42.5 | 15 | 637.5 |
| 45 | 15 / 15 | 15 | 15 | | | |
| | | | | 47.5 | 7 | 332.5 |
| 50 | 8 / 8 | 8 | 8 | | | |
| | | | | 52.5 | 3 | 157.5 |
| 55 | 5 / 5 | 5 | 5 | | | |
| | | | | 57.5 | 2 | 115.0 |
| 60 | 3 / 3 | 3 | 3 | | | |
| | | | | 62.5 | 1 | 62.5 |
| 65 | 2 / 2 | 2 | 2 | | | |
| | | | | 67.5 | 2 | 135.0 |
| 70 | | | | 72.5 | | |
| 75 | | | | 77.5 | | |
| 80 | | | | 82.5 | | |
| 85 | | | | 87.5 | | |
| 90 | | | | 92.5 | | |
| 95 | | | | 97.5 | | |
| Repeat 5 | 470 / 473 | OK | | | | |
| | | | | Total Cell Count: total Column #5 | 535 | Total volume total Column #6 12762.5 |

$$\frac{\text{Column \#6}}{\text{Column \#5}} = MCT = \frac{12762.5}{535} = 23.9$$

$$\frac{MCV}{MCT} = \frac{87.8}{23.9} = 3.67 \text{ cubic microns per threshold division}$$

Calibration Sheet: MW blood in Isoton
Average Hct. = 47

Coulter Model A #542
6/25/70    ACS = 5
Gain = 4
Gain trim = 4.4

**Figure 7-2.** *Calibration sheet for Coulter Counter.*

5. Quickly count and record the value for each 5 T increment. It is unnecessary to count past the setting which gives a value 2% of the original count. After the last T setting has been counted, return to 5 T and recount to verify that no cell loss has occurred from lysis during the counting period.

6. Correct all counts over 100 using the Coincidence Loss Tables and record the corrected count. (Fig. 7-2, Column 3).

7. Subtract the corrected count at 10T from that at 5T and record opposite 7.5T (Fig. 7-2, Column 5). Continue to do this for successive pairs of T until the data are complete.

8. Multiply each midpoint T (Fig. 7-2, Column 4) times the recorded difference (Column 5) and enter the result in the Total Volume Column (Column 6).

9. Find the total for Column 5 (Fig. 7-2). This is the total cell count and should agree within a few cells of the count recorded at 5T initially.

10. Find the total for Column 6 (Fig. 7-2). This is the total volume of the cells counted.

11. Calculate:

$$\frac{\text{Total Column 6}}{\text{Total Column 5}} = \text{Mean Cell Threshold (MCT)}$$

(Values obtained for all MCTs should check within 0.5)

$$\frac{\text{Hematocrit} \times 10}{\text{Total Column 5}} = \text{Mean Cell Volume (MCV)}$$

$$\frac{\text{MCV}}{\text{MCT}} = \text{Calibration Factor, in } \mu^3$$

12. Average the calibration factors obtained using the normal blood samples. This Calibration factor and the ACS, Gain, and Gain Trim settings should be put on a permanent record for future use.

---

### Threshold Setting for Counting Red Blood Cells

Once the calibration factor has been established, the next step is the choice of Threshold settings for WBC and RBC counts. While texts list the smallest observed RBC to be about $50\mu^3$ in size, the fact that some cells drop out at a Threshold setting of 10 indicates the presence of smaller cells. The dropout of the cells at specific sizes is easily seen from a modified Price-Jones curve, which will be discussed later.

In our original calibration work it appeared that we lost red blood cells when the Threshold setting represented about $35\mu^3$. We arbitrarily chose 17.5 $\mu^3$ as the "benchmark" for orienting the size to some figure safely below the smallest drop-out size. In order to count all cells 17.5 $\mu^3$ or larger, divide this figure by the calibration factor to obtain the Threshold setting. For example, the original calibration factor for our master instrument was 3.5 $\mu^3$. Thus,

$$\frac{17.5}{3.5} = 5$$

or the proper setting for the Threshold dial to count RBC on that instrument.

## Threshold Settings for Counting White Blood Cells

During our original calibration work on the Coulter Counters, we were able to measure small lymphocytes from a chronic lymphatic leukemia patient and found them to be about 87 $\mu^3$ when suspended in saline-formalin diluent containing saponin. To be certain we could count mature lymphocytes at the Threshold setting chosen for WBC, we arbitrarily used 52.5 $\mu^3$ as the "benchmark." This size was well below the measured volume and appeared also to be about halfway between the "grass" and the shortest peaks on the oscilloscope. The Threshold setting chosen for counting WBC then would be

$$\frac{52.5}{3.5} = 15 \text{ T.}$$

We have continued to use this "benchmark" and the above diluent-lysing combination for all our Coulter Counters.

When Isoton-Zap-Isoton is the diluent-lysis combination, the leukocytes "shrink" enough that a different "benchmark" is necessary for calibration. For these reagents we have chosen 30 $\mu^3$ and calculated the T setting for WBC accordingly. However, on some of our Model A Coulters, these pulse heights are only about one-fourth the height of the oscilloscope. In order to bring the peak height up to at least half the oscillocope we must change the ACS to 6 or 7. On these instruments we now count the RBC and WBC at different ACS settings. This procedure makes it imperative that we know the calibration factors for the additional Aperture Current Settings. However, since we also use these ACS calibration factors for electronic checks, no additional work is involved in maintaining the values.

## THE CALIBRATION FACTOR AS A CHECK FOR ELECTRONICS

The calibration factor attains one of its most important uses in evaluating the electronic system of the Coulter Counter. The electronic system of the counter is linear in respect to its function and the responding threshold value.[7] Comparison of MCT values or calibration factors can then be used to check this electronic linearity. *As long as the linearity holds, the system is functioning properly.*

---

### Calibration Checks

MCTs are performed on red cells in Eagle's or Isoton solution at ACS 5, Gain 2; ACS 5, Gain 4; and ACS 5 Gain 6. Another MCT is then per-

*Continued on page 292*

formed at ACS 4, Gain 4; and another at ACS 3, Gain 4. Calibration factors are obtained for the instrument at each combination of ACS and Gain described.

For example: Instrument #542:

| Calibration Factor | ACS 5, Gain 2 | is 7.14 |
| Calibration Factor | ACS 5, Gain 4 | is 3.50 |
| Calibration Factor | ACS 5, Gain 6 | is 1.74 |
| Calibration Factor | ACS 4, Gain 4 | is 6.7 |

**Table 7-1. Conversion Factors, Aperture Current***

| Aperture Current Setting | Aperture Current Value of Calibration | | | | | | | |
|---|---|---|---|---|---|---|---|---|
| | 1 | 2 | 3 | 4 | 5 | 6 | 7 | 8 |
| 1.... | 1.00 | 1.98 | 3.92 | 7.65 | 14.6 | 26.6 | 45.5 | 67.8 |
| 2.... | 0.505 | 1.00 | 1.98 | 3.86 | 7.38 | 13.4 | 23.0 | 34.2 |
| 3.... | 0.255 | 0.505 | 1.00 | 1.95 | 3.72 | 6.76 | 11.6 | 17.2 |
| 4.... | 0.131 | 0.259 | 0.514 | 1.00 | 1.91 | 3.48 | 5.95 | 8.84 |
| 5.... | 0.0685 | 0.135 | 0.269 | 0.524 | 1.00 | 1.82 | 3.12 | 4.64 |
| 6.... | 0.0376 | 0.0746 | 0.148 | 0.288 | 0.550 | 1.00 | 1.71 | 2.55 |
| 7.... | 0.0216 | 0.0435 | 0.0861 | 0.168 | 0.321 | 0.585 | 1.00 | 1.49 |
| 8.... | 0.0150 | 0.0292 | 0.0581 | 0.113 | 0.216 | 0.392 | 0.671 | 1.00 |

* If measurements are made at an aperture current setting different from that used to calibrate the threshold dial, the observed threshold reading must be corrected. To determine the appropriate factor, see aperture current setting used and under the appropriate value of the calibration aperture current read the factor. This factor is a multiplier.

**Table 7-2. Conversion Factors, Amplifier Gain***

| Gain Setting | Gain Value of Calibration | | | | | |
|---|---|---|---|---|---|---|
| | 1 | 2 | 3 | 4 | 5 | 6 |
| 1........ | 1.00 | 1.41 | 2.00 | 2.82 | 4.00 | 5.64 |
| 2........ | 0.707 | 1.00 | 1.41 | 2.00 | 2.82 | 4.00 |
| 3........ | 0.500 | 0.707 | 1.00 | 1.41 | 2.00 | 2.82 |
| 4........ | 0.355 | 0.500 | 0.707 | 1.00 | 1.41 | 2.00 |
| 5........ | 0.250 | 0.355 | 0.500 | 0.707 | 1.00 | 1.41 |
| 6........ | 0.177 | 0.250 | 0.355 | 0.500 | 0.707 | 1.00 |

* If measurements are made at a gain setting different from that used to calibrate the threshold dial, the observed threshold reading must be corrected. To determine the appropriate factor, see gain setting being used and under the appropriate value of the calibration gain read the factor. This factor is a multiplier.

292

With Tables 7-1 and 7-2, the calibration factors should be freely interconvertible from one ACS to another and from one Gain to another.[22] For example, for the instrument above, proportionality of the calibration factors clearly exists:

| *Calibration Factor* | | *Conversion Value* | |
|---|---|---|---|
| ACS 5, Gain 4 | | ACS 5 to ACS 4, Table 7-1 | |
| 3.49 | × | 1.91 | = 6.685 |
| ACS 4, Gain 4 | | ACS 4 to ACS 5, Table 7-1 | |
| 6.7 | × | .524 | = 3.51 |
| ACS 5, Gain 2 | | Gain 2 to Gain 6, Table 7-2 | |
| 7.14 | × | .250 | = 1.71 |
| ACS 5, Gain 6 | | Gain 6 to Gain 2, Table 7-2 | |
| 1.74 | × | 4.0 | = 6.96 |

Calculate similar conversions for Gain 4 to Gain 2, Gain 4 to Gain 6, ACS 3 to 4, etc. Since the calibration factors are all based on multiple countings of a single suspension, the control limits of ± 2% prevail. The calculated factors (from conversion) should check within 2% of the observed factors. The ACS and Gain settings should be those usually employed in counting, although any three or more may be used.

The proper electronic operation of the Coulter Counter is assured so long as the proportionality demonstrated above exists. As aging of the instrument occurs, the calibration factors may change, but the proportionality will persist, since aging of the components occurs proportionately. We recommend that this calibration check be performed at six month intervals or whenever a question arises regarding the validity of electronic function. If proportionality does not hold, the threshold zero should be carefully checked before contacting the manufacturer for assistance.

## Fine Threshold Zero Adjustment Using MCT

The Threshold Zero check already described is satisfactory for routine use of the Coulter Counters. For precise volume measurements or for checking the electronics when there is a questionable value for ACS or Gain conversion, a very fine threshold zero check and adjustment may be made.

---

### Fine Threshold Zero Adjustment Using MCT

1. Prepare a 1:50,000 suspension of a particle suspension whose concentration is about 5 million/cmm. If erythrocytes are the particles used, they should be in Eagle's or Isoton solution. Count several times at the settings ordinarily used for erythrocytes.

*Continued on page 294*

293

2. Repeat the counts at increments of 5 T settings, then in increments of 1, and then of ½ T, until a T is attained which gives half the original count. This is the approximate MCT.

3. Take several counts at the approximate MCT setting and average them.

4. Double the T setting and the Gain. (Gain is doubled by moving up two divisions.) Make several counts and average.

5. Halve the original T setting and Gain. Make several counts and average.

6. The count obtained at the new settings should be within 2% of the count obtained with the T setting of the approximate MCT. If it is not, adjust the Threshold Zero Dial Set Screw until the counts do check within 2%.

7. Again align the base line and threshold line on the oscilloscope screen. If the dial does not now indicate a setting of zero, carefully correct the adjustment of the dial face knob on its shaft.

---

## PROBLEMS IN ROUTINE USE OF THE COULTER

Some of the problems and their corrections presented here are not those that technologists can diagnose and correct themselves and will require the service of an electronics technician. Noting the symptoms, though, may be helpful. Many of the problems can be solved by medical technologists or, better still, prevented.

1. *No count.* The reset counter or one of the decade tubes may be the site affected. In our laboratory the reset counter didn't work when (a) the V13 tube was burned out, (b) the mechanical arm of the relay was bent, (c) the Thyratron tube either did not fire or did not cut off, and (d) the reset itself was defective. The decade tubes have been responsible only when a tube in that bank was defective. Any of us can replace tubes, but to replace the relay or the reset counter may require the electronics technician.

2. *Continuous counting.* On two occasions our Coulter continued to count: once when the ground from the stand to the counter was broken (disconnecting the mercury to chassis ground), and again when a bad reset counter fed noise into the decade units. Both situations required repair by our electronics man.

3. *Low counts.* Low counts have usually been traceable to the diluent. RBCs are lost when the pH falls below about pH 5.5, and this drop in pH can easily occur with saline diluent if the formalin used in the diluent is not kept neutralized. Formalin should always be stored with neutralizing marble chips in the bottom of the bottle.

   WBCs can be lost from a diluent whose pH is too high (alkaline). High pH usually happens when formalin is *not* in the diluent and when the pH of the so-called "reagent water" creeps up because of a depleted deionizer or a dirty still. We have already called attention to the problem of the diluent-lysing combination badly "shrinking" the cells to a size that they are not counted. Other causes for low counts have been a cracked orifice, a leak in the headpiece stopcock, or a shifting threshold zero. The last was corrected by replacing a V7 tube.

4. *High counts.* We have had high counts from three rather bizarre causes. First, WBCs were fragmented, and counts rose from 10,000 to about 100,000 in 5 minutes. Hyamine, used as a lytic agent instead of saponin (at that time good

saponin was not always available), caused this phenomenon; we were never able to prevent it, although others reportedly had successfully used this material. Recently a user of Cetrimide reported the same problem, but the fragmenting was less than we had seen with hyamine.

At another time, an extremely high WBC (RBC satisfactory) was corrected by changing the orifice tube. The same orifice worked fine later, and the exact cause is a mystery. Consultation suggested a charge had built up on the orifice surface, causing a feedback, but the point was never proved.

The third inordinately high count was one that intermittently speeded up during the counting procedure. It was traced to noise from the vacuum pump. A saline bottle can pick up noise and feed it back through the electrodes. Prevention of such noise pickup chiefly involves cleanliness, especially around the manometer stand. Little details of maintenance, such as wiping up spilled liquids, dust, and bits of mercury and keeping the tubing and cord free of kinks, all help.

5. *Miscellaneous items.* It is impossible to operate a Coulter Counter long without experiencing a loss of vacuum. Why is it lost? The most common cause is a leak in the connection between the hose and the pump. Or perhaps, the hose has a kink in it. Worse yet, perhaps it only kinks slightly, and the vacuum pressure has to be regulated to make the instrument function. As it is regulated, if somehow the kink is released, suddenly the mercury surges over into the orifice. After such experiences, the technologist proceeds cautiously when readjusting the vacuum regulator. Before adjusting the vacuum, he checks the stopcock and the tubing resilience, the fit of the hose on the pump, and the fit of the stopper in the vacuum bottle. The vacuum regulator itself may become corroded and stick. Repairmen no longer take a faulty regulator apart. They replace it. In our laboratory we still tear it apart and clean the surfaces, especially the little steel ball. A former problem was having saline pour through the regulator because glass bypass parts were inserted upside down. This appears to have been eliminated by slight differences in the shapes of the glass parts.

6. *Electronic interference.* At some time every Coulter operator has seen interference patterns on the oscilloscope. C, D, and E in Figure 7-1 are examples of different types of such patterns. The 60 cycle pattern seen in C is the most likely cause of problems. The instrument requires grounding in a three-prong outlet, but, as discussed in Chapter 1, grounds are not always adequate. These regular standing pulses occur when the common and ground sides of the line are not alike. Often turning on a centrifuge or a neon light may cause the pulses to increase in height. The height of the pulses will depend upon the Aperture Current Setting, but they often are high enough peaks to count. The easiest way to recognize them is to note that they appear to move horizontally. Whether they go from left to right or vice versa depends upon the position of the sweep adjust knob. It has been our experience that inserting the grounding plug in the same double outlet with the instrument will remove this interference. (See page 4.)

The pulses seen in D result when some extraneous material grounds the beaker holding the cell suspension or the platform holding the beaker. These can be produced at will by holding the beaker while attempting to count the suspension. The same type of pulse is seen when one touches the screw holding the external electrode while the instrument is counting; in this case the pulses are higher.

The pattern shown in E results from either the external electrode being outside the cell suspension or air being pulled through the orifice while the instrument is counting. Patterns D and E are accidental incidents that can be quickly detected and avoided. They should cause no problem in routine counting.

## PERIODIC CLEANING AND MAINTENANCE

Overall cleanliness of all parts of the Coulter system must be a conscientious effort if the instrument is to function without downtime. Dust and lint should be kept away from the instrument as much as possible, and dusting, preferably with a vacuum cleaner, is to be encouraged. Dust particles can be harmful in many ways—from errors in counting, if present in the cell suspension, to fouling the contacts of the polarity reversal relay.

The headpiece and electrodes must be kept especially clean. Ample flushing with water and a mild detergent after using the instrument helps a great deal; Isoterge* is recommended for this purpose. The external electrode can be wiped off with a tissue to avoid dirt or fungus which would otherwise accumulate. We have seen this electrode neglected for such a period of time that fungus growth hung from the bottom in stringlike formation; in this instance the operator had originally asked for help in finding the reason for extremely erratic counts. In addition to adding counts to the suspension, such a coating interferes with the normal function of the electrode in maintaining stable signal with reversal of the current.

A dirty orifice tube should be cleaned immediately upon removal with due respect for its high cost. Old grease should be removed before a mild detergent wash is applied. Cautious use of a long, nonabrasive tool will loosen the dirt. We use cotton-tipped applicator sticks and find that the vigorous rinsing eliminates fibers that may be dislodged from the swab. To check whether the orifice itself is clean and intact, fill the orifice tube completely with water, and with very gentle pressure on its top opening with the fleshy part of the palm of the hand, force liquid through the orifice. If the circumference of the orifice is clean and undamaged, the stream will emerge at a clearly defined right angle to the long axis of the tube. Stubborn deposits around the orifice may require slightly more drastic procedures. Soaking in Clorox solution and prodding with a short-bristled camel's hair brush will usually remove such a deposit. An orifice that is regularly rinsed will not build up this much deposit unless it is allowed to become dry and salts and dirt crystallize on its surface.

Sludge above the mercury in the upper collection bulb of the manometer does not in itself hinder operation but will eventually work down into the manometer loop section. As a result, the mercury column usually splits, and the manometer then must be taken off and cleaned. The count will also be affected if accumulated dirt in this section slows the mercury or fouls the start and stop contacts.

An erratic mercury level or squealing indicates a dirty bleed regulator. This may be remedied by disassembling and cleaning the diaphragm and diaphragm

---

* Coulter Diagnostics, Inc., Hialeah, Fla.

receiver with an acetone-soaked swab. As mentioned, these regulators are usually replaced by the servicemen who do not now attempt to clean them. This problem of the Model A Coulter has been greatly reduced on the Model F in that the glass bypass tube is placed high and the diluent does not easily drain into other parts. The regulator valve itself has been removed in the Coulter F, and the vacuum is regulated by a variable length of hose. Problems can arise with this arrangement if the tubing is not replaced before it becomes old and cracked.

Slime accumulates inside the latex tubing connections even more readily than in the glass parts. If this growth occurs in the tubing of the side arm flush system, some of this material can break loose and backflush through the orifice. These particles can significantly change a count done just after the side arm has been flushed. All latex tubing should be replaced at least every six months.

It is easy to keep the maintenance "downtime" of the Coulter Counter at half an hour by keeping on hand a clean spare orifice tube and manometer and cleaning the remainder of the parts in place on the stand. It is difficult to say how frequently maintenance will be necessary, since the interval will be governed by the degree of use and the amount of flushing that is regularly applied. Any indication of minor malfunction traceable to dirt is a signal to clean whichever part may be responsible, and the general maintenance can well be conducted at the same time. As a minimum, the following spare parts should be kept on hand: orifice tube, manometer, a set of electronic tubes, beaker electrode, control headpiece, and bypass tube.

## CHARACTERISTICS OF A GOOD CONTROL SUSPENSION

New commercial control suspensions are being offered from time to time, but none has, in our opinion, been entirely satisfactory. In general, the suspensions for red cell count and hemoglobin appear much more satisfactory than those for the other parameters. To date, the materials added to simulate a white cell suspension have not been acceptable.

For the control suspension to assure that the patient's count is valid, the control "cells" must be the same size and react like the patient's cells. When the electronic components age and the pulse heights become lower under certain conditions, the most likely cells to be missed are the very small lymphocytes. A control suspension that has "cells" much larger than these cells will not detect such a problem, nor will an inert particle, such as latex, detect changes in blood cells caused by variations in the strength or reaction time of diluent-lysing reagent.

In evaluating a control suspension we consider the size of the cells, the uniformity of size, their tendency to aggregate, their measured diameter with the ocular micrometer before and after addition of the lysing agent, and their reaction in the diluent and in the diluent plus the lysing agent. These evaluations are made from a microscopic examination of a wet mount, repeating counts on the Coulter Counter while observing the pattern on the oscilloscope, a plot of a frequency distribution curve, and a stained smear.

297

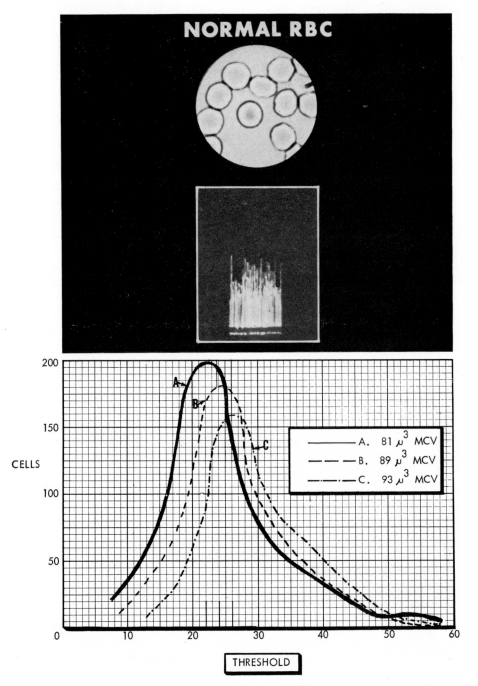

**Figure 7-3.** *Normal red blood cells suspended in Eagle's solution: microscopic view, oscilloscope pattern, frequency distribution curve. (Counted on Coulter Model A, ACS 5, Gain 4.)*

Figure 7-3 shows normal red blood cells by microscopic view, their pattern on the oscilloscope, and the frequency distribution curves that span the normal range for MCV. A good control suspension for RBC should very closely resemble these characteristics, although a cell slightly smaller would also function satisfactorily. The frequency distribution curve should approximate gaussian distribution. Such curves can be plotted from the values obtained by running an MCT curve as was done for calibration. The threshold size is used from the Column 4 figures and the number of cells from Column 5 (Fig. 7-2). This is often called a modified Price-Jones curve—modified in that this curve is a plot of relative volumes and the Price-Jones plots use diameters of cells.

Control A, Figure 7-4, is a latex suspension. The microscopic preparation shows the two distinct disadvantages of this material: the variation in size and the very large size of some particles compared to normal RBC. It is apparent from the oscilloscope pattern that the instrument gain could decrease markedly before any change would be evident in the latex count. The Price-Jones curve indicates that there is absolutely no uniformity in size of the particles. Another disadvantage of the latex is that it will not reflect the changes in blood cells caused by differences in the osmolality of the diluent or the lysing action of the stromato-lyzing reagent.

Control B in Figure 7-5 is a suspension of stabilized RBC. The cell size is smaller than normal RBC but, depending upon the threshold setting used, probably would count satisfactorily unless the cells become lysed. Actually, the cells did appear to lyse, and different lot numbers were not always the same size, as indicated in the frequency distribution curves.

Controls C and D in Figure 7-6 were made by the same manufacturer. C is the RBC control, and D is the WBC control. We have used Control C for several years and have found it satisfactory. Control D appears to be a nucleated RBC whose size is larger than we are willing to use for a WBC control. At the time we tried Control D we were using a saline-saponin reagent for counting, and the Isoton-Zap-Isoton reaction should be checked.

Other control materials suggested in the literature include *Calvatia cyanthiformis* or *C. fragilis* spores[25] (tend to aggregate unsatisfactorily), formalin killed *Candida albicans*[18] and prepare-it-yourself stabilized RBC.[30] Others recommend repeating samples from the previous day.[4, 11] Brittin *et al.* recognized the danger of a gradual change, undetectable at any single time, and recommended an overall statistical evaluation.[4] A good control suspension is very much needed. Until one appears that is satisfactory in all parameters, the conscientious operator can only choose the one with the least limitation.

## QUALITY CONTROL PROGRAM

The procedures we use for assuring accuracy in electronic counts fit into several fundamental categories: every count, daily check, weekly, and six month checks. The check sheet we use is shown in Figure 7-7.

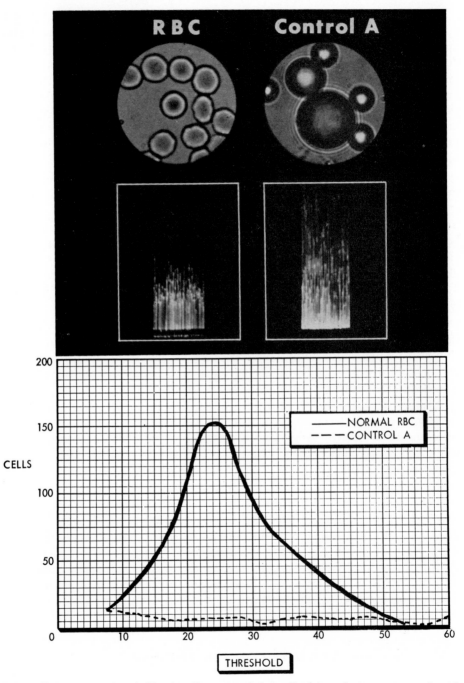

**Figure 7-4.** *Normal red blood cells suspended in Eagle's solution compared with Control A: microscopic view oscilloscope pattern, and frequency distribution curve. (Counted on Coulter Model A, ACS 5, Gain 4.)*

300

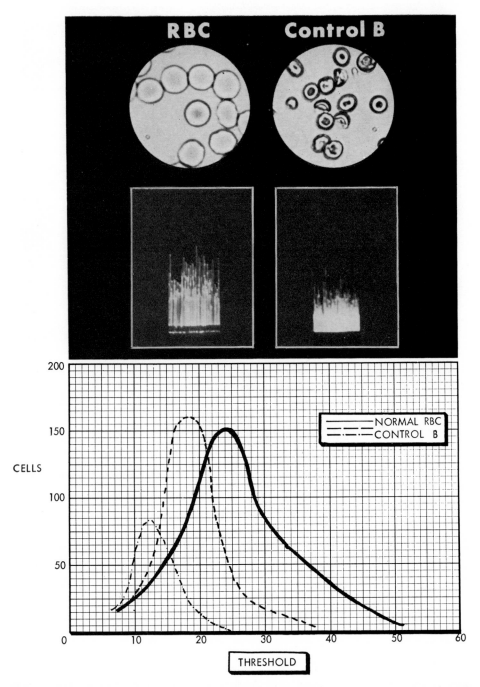

**Figure 7-5.** *Normal red blood cells suspended in Eagle's solution compared with Control B: microscopic view, oscilloscope pattern, and frequency distribution curve. (Counted on Coulter Model A, ACS 5, Gain 4.)*

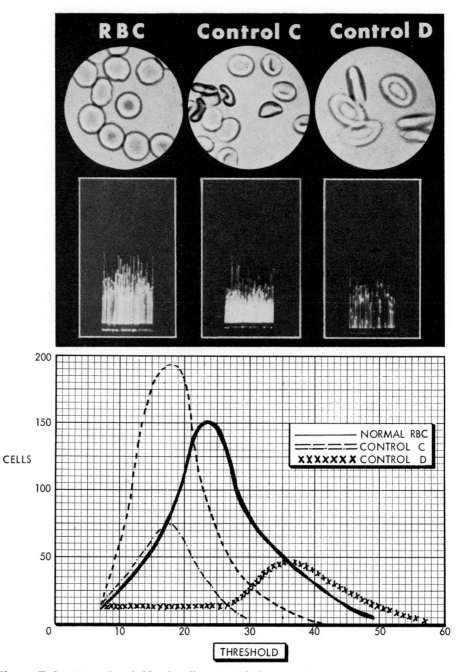

**Figure 7-6.** *Normal red blood cells suspended in Eagle's solution compared with Control C and Control D: microscopic view, oscilloscope pattern, and frequency distribution curve. (Counted on Coulter Model A, ACS 5, Gain 4.)*

# COULTER COUNTER CHECK

Hospital _____  Instrument # _____  Month _____

| Date | DAILY | | | | | | | | | WEEKLY | | | | | | 6 MONTHS | |
|---|---|---|---|---|---|---|---|---|---|---|---|---|---|---|---|---|---|
| | Dilutor Check | RBC (<200) | | | WBC (<50) | | Hg (Sec.) | Control | | Orifice | Pump | Saponin lysis | Threshold Zero | | | Change Latex Tubing | Cali-bration Check |
| | | Saline | Flush | Albumin | Saponin Without | With | | RBC | WBC | | | | 5 | 10 | 20 | | |
| 1 | | | | | | | | | | | | | | | | | |
| 2 | | | | | | | | | | | | | | | | | |
| 3 | | | | | | | | | | | | | | | | | |
| 4 | | | | | | | | | | | | | | | | | |
| 5 | | | | | | | | | | | | | | | | | |
| 6 | | | | | | | | | | | | | | | | | |
| 7 | | | | | | | | | | | | | | | | | |
| 8 | | | | | | | | | | | | | | | | | |
| 9 | | | | | | | | | | | | | | | | | |
| 10 | | | | | | | | | | | | | | | | | |
| 11 | | | | | | | | | | | | | | | | | |
| 12 | | | | | | | | | | | | | | | | | |

**Figure 7-7.** *Coulter Counter check sheet used at the South Bend Medical Foundation, Inc.*

Each "every count" step, including background count, must be accomplished exactly as outlined until it becomes a firm habit (page 282). Good habits include meticulous attention to all details in the introduction of samples plus alertness to potential problems involving cadence sounds, scope pattern, and polarity shift.

In daily operation, division of labor often makes it necessary for a number of individuals to perform parts of a complete blood count. From the slide used for the differential, the WBC should be estimated and written down for comparison with the Coulter count. This procedure will detect gross errors that might occur if samples of blood are accidentally interchanged.

The technologist should also attempt to correlate all parts of the complete blood count from the appearance of the stained blood smear. The newer systems that take up the sample and do the entire count, except the differential, leave no check and balance system for detecting errors such as inadequate mixing. This error is extremely difficult to detect unless a very gross inconsistency is evident. For this reason, mixing should become a constant concern of all those persons involved in the counting and related procedures. The schedule for other checking procedures is:

Daily Checks

1. A background count of the diluent (RBC and WBC settings) and of the diluent plus the lysing agent at the WBC setting.
2. Recording the mercury travel time.
3. Counting the control suspension at both RBC and WBC settings and recording on the graph.

Weekly Checks

1. Changing the orifice tube and cleaning the one removed.
2. Oiling the vacuum pump.
3. Checking the lysing agent and posting the acceptable lysing time near the instrument.
4. Checking the Threshold zero.

Six Month Checks

1. Checking the calibration factor for the instrument.
2. Changing the latex tubing.

After all efforts have been made to use the Coulter Counter properly for counting or sizing blood cells in the clinical laboratory, the final responsibility for evaluating the accuracy of electronic counts in terms of compatibility with the other findings still rests with the technologist doing the differential.

## REFERENCES

1. Allen, J. D., and Gudaitis, A. V.: Diluting fluid for electronic counting of leukocytes and hemoglobin determinations. Amer. J. Clin. Path. *33:*553, 1960.
2. Brittin, G. M., Brecher, G., and Johnson, C. A.: Elimination of error in hematocrit produced by excessive EDTA. Amer. J. Clin. Path., *52:*780, 1969.

3. ———:Evaluation of the Coulter Counter Model S. Amer. J. Clin. Path., *52:*679, 1969.

4. ——— and Elashoff, R. M.: Stability of blood in commonly used anticoagulants. Amer. J. Clin. Path., *52:*690, 1969.

5. Collier, H. B.: Some problems in the use of the Coulter Counter for erthrocyte total counts and volume distribution. J. Clin. Path., *21:*179, 1968.

6. Cook, J. S.: Size distribution of human erythrocytes with an electronic counter. J. Lab. Clin. Med., *70:*849, 1967.

7. Coulter, J., Jr.: Personal communication.

8. Craine, K., and Waft, A. D.: Red cell volume distribution histograms for establishing the normal range using the Coulter Plotter, Model J. J. Clin. Path., *20:*913, 1967.

9. D'Angelo, G., and Lacombe, M.: A practical diluent for electronic white cell counts. Tech. Bull. Reg. Med. Tech., *32:*196, 1962.

10. Dutcher, T. F.: Hematology—automation and quantitation. In *Advances in Automated Analysis*. Vol. 1. Technicon International Congress, 1969.

11. Dutra, F. R.: Monitoring the quality of blood cell counts with replicate determinations on routine samples. Amer. J. Clin. Path., *46:*286, 1966.

12. Ellerbrook, L. D.: A simple colorimetric method for calibration of pipets. Amer. J. Clin. Path., *24:*868,1954.

13. Feichtmeir, T. V., Nigon, K., Hannon, M. A., Bird, D. B., and Carr, L. B.: Electronic counting of erythrocytes and leukocytes. Amer. J Clin. Path., *35:*373, 1961.

14. Ferro, P. V., and Sena, T.: The effect of anticoagulant concentration on centrifuged and electronic hematocrits. Amer. J. Clin. Path., *51:*569, 1969.

15. Grant, J. L., Britton, M. C., Jr., and Kurtz, T. E.: Measurement of red blood cell volume with the electronic cell counter. Amer. J. Clin. Path., *33:*138, 1960.

16. Helleman, P. W., vZwet, J. L., and Geleijnse, M. E. M.: Electronic counting of erythrocytes, leukocytes, and platelets. In *Standardization in Haematology, III*. CH. G. de Boroviczeny, Ed. Bibl. haemat. *24:*54, 1966, Basel, Karger.

17. Lampasso, J. A.: Error in hematocrit value produced by excessive ethylenediaminetetraacetate. Amer. J. Clin. Path., *44:*109, 1965.

18. Lappin, T. R. J., and Sanderson, F. M.: An artificial leukocyte control suspension. J. Clin. Path., *23:*65, 1970.

19. Magath, T. B., and Berkson, J.: Electronic blood cell counting. Amer. J. Clin. Path., *34:*203, 1960.

20. Nevius, D. B.: Osmotic error in electronic determinations of red cell volume. Amer. J. Clin. Path., *39:*38, 1963.

21. Oulie, C.: Telling av de Röde Blodlegemer, ved deres Elektriske motstand. Nord. Med., *62:*1421, 1959.

22. Peacock, A. C., Williams, G. Z., and Mengoli, H. F.: Rapid electronic measurement of cell volume and distribution. J. Nat. Cancer Inst., *25:*63, 1960.

23. Pennock, C. A., and Jones, K. W.: Effect of ethylenediamine-tetra-acetic acid (dipotassium salt) and heparin on the estimation of packed cell volume. J. Clin. Path., *19:*196, 1966.

24. Pinkerton, P. H., Spence, I., Ogilvie, J. C., Ronald, W. A., Marchant, P., and Ray, P. K.: An assessment of the Coulter Counter Model S. J. Clin. Path., *23:*68, 1970.

25. Pruden, E. L., and Winstead, M. E.: Accuracy control of blood cell counts with the Coulter Counter. Amer. J. Med. Techn., *30:*1, 1964.

26. Richar, W. J., and Breakell, E. S.: Evaluation of an electronic particle counter for the counting of white blood cells. Amer. J. Clin. Path., *31:*384, 1959.

27. Strumia, M. M., Sample, A. B., and Hart, E. D.: An improved microhematocrit method. Amer. J. Clin. Path., *24:*1016, 1954.

28. Van Kampen, E. J., Graafland, C. A., and Hasselman, J. J. F.: The pH-resistance of erythrocytes. Clin. Chim. Acta., *2:*95, 1957.

29. Winstead, M.: *Reagent Grade Water: How, When, and Why?* Amer. Soc. Med. Technologists, Houston, Texas, 1967.

30. Zucker, S., and Brosious, E.: Preparation of quality control specimens for erythrocyte counting, hematocrit and hemoglobin determinations. Amer. J. Clin. Path., *53:*474, 1970.

**APPENDIX**

**EVALUATION OF INSTRUMENTS IN THE CLINICAL LABORATORY**

I. General

  A. Capital cost
    1. Basic unit
    2. Optional extras

  B. Tests the machine can perform and the method used
    1. Principle of each test
    2. Other methods that can be substituted for tests
    3. Possibility of isolating the channels (or module) for discrete analysis

  C. Rate of analysis
    1. Claimed by manufacturer
    2. Actual

  D. Standards recommended

  E. Space and service required by the machine
    1. Floor area
    2. Bench space
    3. Shelves
    4. Drainage
    5. Electricity
    6. Water
    7. Gas
    8. Weight of machine

  F. Training required of the staff
    1. For operation in routine use
    2. For maintenance
    3. For trouble-shooting

  G. Repair and/or maintenance service available
    1. Detailed manual including schematic
    2. Service contract from manufacturer (or other outside company)

II. Samples

  A. Type of sample
    1. Type and concentration of suitable anticoagulant
    2. Preparation of sample required (protein free filtrate, dilutions, etc.)

B. Volume of sample
   1. Method of changing volume
   2. Method of recalibrating volume

C. Mechanism for rejection of unsuitable sample (alarm for clots, haemolysis, etc.)

D. Method of function of sampler (single sample, multiple samples, turntable)

III. Reagents

A. Reagents required
   1. Supplied by manufacturer
   2. Prepared in laboratory (including details of preparation)

B. Method of dispensing reagents and regulating volumes per hour
   1. Possibility and ease of changing volumes
   2. Necessary time intervals between sampling and addition of specific reagents
   3. Method of achieving efficient mixing of sample with reagents

C. Composition of components exposed to reagents
   1. Life expectancy of tubing and other parts
   2. Reagents and solvents that are specifically prohibited

IV. Instrumentation

A. Detailed specifications for each instrument (colorimeter, fluorometer, cell counter, etc.)

B. Cuvettes
   1. Size and composition
   2. Matched
   3. Provision for rinsing
   4. Effect of bubbles in the system
   5. Interchangeability of other sizes of cuvettes

C. Mechanism for recording and displaying the signal output
   1. *If graphical display,* method of calculating final figures
   2. *If printout*, details of actual figures and number of significant figures
   3. Possibility of interfacing the system to a computer
      1. Method
      2. Difficulty
      3. Cost

308

D. Range of concentration satisfactorily handled by each channel

E. Coordination and presentation of outputs *in multichannel instruments*

F. Standardization of each channel
1. Number of set points that control the calibration curve
2. Restandardization procedures needed
3. Provision for automatically subtracting the blank from the test result
4. Provision for correction for nonlinearity of the calibration curve

## OPERATION EVALUATION

I. Accuracy of results (Compare to reference methods and determine acceptable error for each test.)

A. Check normal and abnormal bloods (or other type sample where appropriate).

B. Spread comparison evaluation over approximately 6 months and include at least 100 values.

C. Measure linearity of response over the complete concentration range.

II. Precision—(Established after accuracy has been determined.)

A. Repeat same sample twenty times (or one machine batch if turntable type sample is used) and determine the acceptable errors.

B. Determine precision for at least three different concentrations, including those most critical in clinical evaluations.

C. Check day-to-day precision with some stable control sample. Instrument drift is very difficult to detect if no such control is available.

III. Carry-over or cross contamination

A. Determine how many samples are affected by carry-over from one abnormal sample.

B. Establish the differences in concentration range that produce significant carry-over for each test.

C. Check the carry-over to the blank or error after use of a blank.

IV. Reliability

A. Assess the reliability of the instrument over a prolonged time, *e.g.,* 6 months.

B. Include in the assessment the following:
1. Test results.
2. Standards.

3. Controls.

4. Clinical correlations (*i.e.,* samples did not include interfering substances).

V. Running costs: (Determine the average cost per test.)

A. Reagents, standards, controls and water.

B. Consumables, such as sample cups, tubes, chart paper, etc.

C. Repairs and maintenance. Assess these in relation to any maintenance contract, if applicable.

D. Time spent by staff preparing samples, operating machine and in daily maintenance.

E. Depreciation over 5 years.

## REFERENCES

1. Broughton, P. M. G., Buttolph, M. A., Gowenlock, A. H., et al.: Recommended scheme for the evaluation of instruments for automatic analysis in the clinical biochemistry laboratory. J. Clin. Path., 22:278, 1969.

2. Sharp, A. A., and Ballard, B. C. D.: An evaluation of the Coulter S counter. J. Clin. Path., 23:327, 1970.

# Index

Page numbers in *italics* refer to illustrations; page numbers followed by t refer to tables.

312

313